Masters of Osteopathy

MASTERS OF Osteopathy

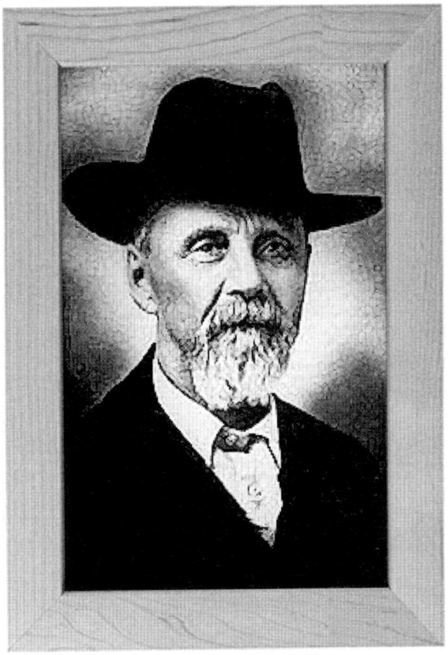

William Thomas Crow, D.O., F.A.A.O.

and

Terence C. Vardy, D.O., M.App.Sc.

Eastland Press ▸ Seattle

Published by Eastland Press, Inc.
P.O. Box 99749 Seattle, WA 98139, USA
www.eastlandpress.com

ISBN: 978-0-939616-87-9
Library of Congress Control Number: 2018957823

Printed in the United States of America

2 4 6 8 10 9 7 5 3 1

Book design by Gary Niemeier

This book may also be purchased from Eastland Press in digital format as an eBook: *www.eastlandpress.com.* Access to a website with video demonstrations of each of the 166 techniques may be purchased at: *https://www.osteomasterstechniques.com/product/video-access/*

Dedication

To John Peckham, the doctor who introduced me to the power of Osteopathy, and my wife, Janet, who has put up with me through medical school, practice, and the writing of this book.

—William Thomas Crow. D.O., F.A.A.O.

Table of Contents

INTRODUCTION, *xv*

ACKNOWLEDGEMENTS, *xvii*

SOURCE MATERIALS, *xix*

1

The Philosophy of the Osteopathic Masters in their Own Words, 1

Structure – the Basic Determinant of Body Function ··· 1

The Osteopathic Concept of Etiology ··· 5

Treatable Diagnosis of Osteopathic Lesions ··· 8

The Osteopathic Philosophy of Carl Philip McConnell and Charles Clayton Teall ··· 14

The Osteopathic Philosophy of Ernest Eckford Tucker ··· 23

The Osteopathic Philosophy and Principles of Anne Wales, D.O. ··· 30

Lippincott's Statements on Dr. Sutherland's Philosophy ··· 33

2

Techniques for the Head, 35

Tucker's Posterior OA Technique ··· 35

Tucker's Posterior OA (Anterior Atlas) Technique ··· 37

OA Release Technique (1938 Yearbook) ··· 38

Wales' Occiput Technique ··· 39

Brooks Walker and Elliott Blackman Technique for the Occiput ··· 40

Wales' Technique – the Base Spread ··· 42

3

Techniques for the Cervical Region, 45

West's Lateral Cervical Technique ··· 45

West's Scalene Technique ··· 46

West's Anterior Cervical Technique ··· 47
Hazzard's Technique for the Atlas #1 ··· 49
Hazzard's Technique for the Atlas #2 ··· 50
Hazzard's Technique for the Atlas #3 ··· 51
Ernest Eckford Tucker on Cervicals ··· 52
Tucker's Posterior Cervicals ··· 53
Tucker's Anterior Cervical Techniques ··· 55
Sutherland's Technique for the Cervicals ··· 56
Sutherland's Cervical Flexion Dysfunction Techniques ··· 57
Sutherland's Cervical Rotation Side-Bending Dysfunction Techniques ··· 58
Sutherland's Condylo-Atlantal Dysfunctions ··· 59
Wales' Cervical Vertebrae Technique ··· 60
Crow's OA Technique and Upper Cervical Technique ··· 62
Crow's Lower Cervicals Technique ··· 63

4
Techniques for the Thoracics, 65

Tucker on Thoracics ··· 65
Dorsal Region: Movements ··· 66
Tucker's Thoracic Technique ··· 69
Tucker's Prone Thoracic Technique ··· 70
Tucker's Supine Thoracic Technique ··· 71
Tucker's Upper Thoracic (T1-T3) Technique #1 ··· 72
Tucker's Upper Thoracic (T1-T7) Technique #2 (Side-Bending Technique) ··· 73
Sutherland's Thoracic Vertebrae Principles of Technique ··· 74
Sutherland's Thoracic Diagnosis – Palpation for Motion ··· 74
Sutherland's Technique for Thoracic Flexion Dysfunctions ··· 76
Sutherland's Technique for Thoracic Extension Dysfunctions ··· 76
Sutherland's Technique for Thoracic Side-Bending Rotation Dysfunctions ··· 78
Wales on the Thorax and Ribs ··· 78
Release Technique for the Erector Spinae Muscles and Longitudinal Ligaments of the Spine ··· 79

5
Techniques for the Ribs, 81

Wales' Sternal Release Technique ··· 81
West's First Rib Technique #1 ··· 82
West's First Rib Technique #2 ··· 84
West's First Rib Supine Technique ··· 85

Tucker on First and Second Ribs ··· 85
Tucker's First Rib Technique #1 ··· 86
Tucker's First Rib Technique #2 ··· 88
Sutherland's Rib Dysfunctions and Technique ··· 89
Sutherland's First Rib Technique ··· 89
Wales on Ribs ··· 90
Wales' 1st and 2nd Ribs Technique ··· 91
Sutherland's 2nd and 3rd Ribs Technique ··· 92
Sutherland's Alternate Technique for Upper Ribs ··· 94
Wales' Rib Technique ··· 94
Hazzard's Rib Technique ··· 96
West's 2nd to 6th Ribs Technique ··· 97
Hazzard's Rib Technique for Ribs 3 to 10, Seated ··· 98
Hazzard's Rib Technique for Ribs 3 to 10, Side Lying ··· 100
Tucker's 3rd through 10th Ribs Technique ··· 100
Tucker's Rib Technique #1 ··· 103
Tucker's Rib Technique #2 ··· 104
Tucker's Rib Technique #3 ··· 105
Sutherland's 4th to 10th Ribs Technique ··· 106
West's 6th to 10th Ribs Technique, Seated ··· 107
West's 6th to 10th Ribs Technique, Side Lying ··· 108
Sutherland's Two Techniques for Rib Dysfunctions Associated with Hyper Extension of the Thoracic Vertebrae ··· 109
Sutherland's Technique for the Floating Ribs 11 and 12 ··· 111
Wales' Technique for Treating the 11th and 12th Ribs ··· 111
Tucker's Floating Ribs (11th and 12th) Technique ··· 113
Tucker's Floating Ribs Technique #1 ··· 114
Tucker's Floating Ribs Technique #2 ··· 115

6

Techniques for the Lumbar Region, 117

Tucker on the Lumbar Spine ··· 117
Tucker's Lumbar Spine Technique #1 ··· 121
Tucker's Lumbar Spine Technique #2 ··· 122
Tucker's Lumbar Spine Technique #3 ··· 123
Tucker's Lumbar Spine Technique #4 "The Corkscrew" ··· 124
Sutherland's Lumbar/Sacral Region Technique ··· 126
Wales on the Thoracic Lumbar Junction ··· 127

7

Techniques for the Sacrum and Pelvis, 129

Techniques for the Sacrum and Pelvis, 129
Sutherland's Diagnosis of Respiratory Dysfunctions of the Sacrum ··· 130
Wales' Differential Technique ··· 131
Wales' Pelvic and Lower Extremity Fascial Release Technique ··· 133
Wales' Technique for the Anterior Sacroiliac ··· 134
Sutherland's Techniques for the Innominates ··· 135
Sutherland's Technique for the Posterior Rotation of the Innominate Diagnosis ··· 136
Sutherland's Technique for a Posterior Rotation of the Innominate Treatment ··· 137
Sutherland's Technique for an Anterior Rotation of the Innominate Diagnosis ··· 139
Sutherland's Technique for an Anterior Rotation of the Innominate Treatment ··· 140
Sutherland's Pubic Symphysis Technique ··· 142
Crow's Alternate Pubic Symphysis Technique ··· 143
West's Pelvis Technique ··· 144
West's Iliolumbar Technique ··· 145
Wales' Coccyx Technique ··· 146

8

Techniques for the Lower Extremities, 147

Tucker on Treating the Femur and Hip ··· 147
Tucker's Femur and Hip Technique ··· 148
Sutherland's Hip Techniques ··· 149
Sutherland's Technique for Internal Hip Rotation – Method One ··· 150
Sutherland's Technique for External Rotation of the Hip – Method One ··· 151
Sutherland's Hip Joint Diagnosis – Method Two ··· 152
Sutherland's Technique for External Rotation of the Hip – Method Two ··· 153
Sutherland's Technique for Internal Rotation of the Hip – Method Two ··· 154
West's Sartorius Technique ··· 155
Sutherland's Tibiofemoral Diagnosis ··· 156
Sutherland's Tibiofemoral/Medial Condyle Technique ··· 156
Sutherland's Tibiofemoral/Lateral Condyle Technique ··· 157
Wales' Fibula Technique ··· 158
Wales' Tibia Technique ··· 159
Wales' Subtalar Joint Technique ··· 160
Wales' Tarsal Arch Technique ··· 161
Wales' Talus, Calcaneus, Tarsal Arch Technique ··· 162
Wales' Comment on Feet ··· 163

Wales' Morton's Neuroma Technique ··· 164
Wales' Bootjack Technique ··· 165
Wales' Bunion Technique ··· 166
Crow's Ankle Sprain Technique ··· 167
Wales' Fibula and Interosseous Membrane Release Technique ··· 168
Wales' Outer Longitudinal Arch/Cuboid Release Technique ··· 169
Wales' Dropped Navicular/Cuneiform (Keystone) Technique ··· 170
Sutherland's Foot Technique per Wales ··· 171
Cochrane's Foot Exercise ··· 172
Wales on Short Leg Syndrome ··· 172
Wales on Psoas/Soleus Contraction ··· 173

9
Techniques for the Upper Extremities, 175

Tucker's Clavicle Technique ··· 176
Sutherland's Clavicle Technique ··· 177
Wales' Depressed Clavicle Technique ··· 178
Wales' Clavicle Technique #2 ··· 179
Tucker's Shoulder Joint Technique ··· 179
Sutherland's Technique for the Internal Rotation of the Humerus ··· 181
Sutherland's Technique for the External Rotation of the Humerus ··· 182
Tucker's Technique for the Bicipital Tendon ··· 183
Wales' Shoulder Diagnosis and Technique #1 ··· 184
Wales' Shoulder Technique #2 ··· 185
Wales' Scapula Technique ··· 186
Sutherland's Ulna Technique ··· 188
Sutherland's Radius Technique ··· 189
Wales' Radius Technique ··· 190
Wales' Elbow Technique ··· 190
Sutherland's Interosseous Membrane Technique ··· 191
Sutherland's Hand and Wrist Technique ··· 192
Wales' Wrist Technique ··· 193

10
Techniques for the Viscera, 197

Barber's General Treatment of the Neck ··· 201
Barber's Treatment of the Eye Proper ··· 202
Barber's Treatment of the Lacrimal Duct ··· 203

Intranasal Technique ··· 204
Muncie's Technique (for Eustachian Tube Dysfunction – 1921) ··· 205
Miller's Technique (for Root of the Tongue – 2005) ··· 206
Chronic Cough Hyoid Technique ··· 207
Sutherland's Anterior Cervical Fascia Technique ··· 209

The Respiratory System

Asthma Technique from the 1938 Yearbook ··· 210
Wales on Asthma ··· 211
Crow's Treatment of Acute Asthma using a Tender Point ··· 212
Barber's Lung Technique #1 (Two-Person Technique) ··· 213
Barber's Lung Technique #2 ··· 214
Barber's Lung Technique #3 (Two-Person Technique) ··· 214
Barber's Lung Technique #4 ··· 215
McConnell on Diaphragm Doming ··· 216
Sutherland's Diaphragm Release ··· 216
Wales on Fascial Drag and the Diaphragm ··· 217
Wales on the Diaphragm ··· 217
Sutherland's Arcuate Ligaments ··· 218

The Cardiovascular System

Treating the Arrhythmia Point ··· 219
Unwinding the Pericardium ··· 220

The Gastrointesintal System

Fox's Treatment of Gerd ··· 220
Sutherland's Approach to Stomach ··· 221
Still's Stomach Technique ··· 221
McConnell's Duodenum Motion with Inhalation Technique ··· 222
Sutherland's Liver Release (Liver Turn) Technique ··· 222
Sutherland's Biliary Drainage Technique ··· 223
Mesenteric Lift Technique ··· 224
Sigmoid Flexure Technique ··· 225

The Genitourinary System

Kidney Lift ··· 225
Hazzard's Kidney Technique ··· 226
The Ureter and the Psoas Muscle ··· 227
Sutherland's Psoas Technique #1 ··· 227
Sutherland's Psoas Technique #2 ··· 228
Sutherland's Pelvic Lift ··· 229

11

Women's Health, 231

Wales on Pregnancy ··· 231
Wales on Postnatal Depression ··· 231
Wales on Dysmenorrhea ··· 233

12

Pediatrics, 235

Lippincott's Basion Technique ··· 235
Wales on Treating Children ··· 236
Wales on Treating the Newborn ··· 237
Wales on Treating Children's Sacrum ··· 238

13

Dr. Fulford's 'Putting It All Together,' 239

Fulford's Technique for the Lower Extremity ··· 240
Treatment of the Trauma or Shock Point ··· 241
Fulford's Technique for the OA and Atlas/Axis Release ··· 242
Fulford's Technique for the Sphenoid and Frontal Bone ··· 243
Fulford's Technique for the Pelvis – Part 1 ··· 243
Fulford's Technique for the Pelvis – Part 2 ··· 244
Fulford's Technique for the Scapula and Pelvis ··· 245
Fulford's Falx and Tentorium Release ··· 247

General Index, 249
About the Authors, 265

Introduction

This book is a compilation of osteopathic philosophy and techniques that are not currently taught in courses at osteopathic schools. In conducting our research, we accessed many old journals, books, and videotapes of the original generation of osteopaths, and had the good fortune to spend time with some of the older doctors, harvesting their knowledge before they passed on. The book is therefore a unique and extremely valuable collection of their techniques, as relevant and effective today as they were for patients in the past.

The task of modernizing the language used by the old masters in describing their philosophy and treatment methods has been a challenge. However, we have faithfully attempted to use modern day language and medical terminology to better explain the old doctors' invaluable and practical osteopathic principles and treatment methods. In doing so, we have tried to retain the osteopathic knowledge at its peak a hundred years ago and more. As you read this book, bear in mind how modern technology has changed and expanded our knowledge of human anatomy and physiology. No doubt in another hundred years our knowledge of human anatomy and physiology will have advanced even more.

To better understand how to apply each of the techniques and their underlying philosophy, we have provided a set of step-by-step instructions with associated photographs, and a clear description of hand holds and force vectors. If you understand the principles upon which the techniques are based, you can adapt them to your own style and physique.

We hope that by sharing this knowledge, our profession will be able to more effectively assist their patients in regaining homeostasis and maintaining a better quality of health and life.

This book may also be purchased from Eastland Press in digital format as an eBook: *www.eastlandpress.com.* Access to a website with video demonstrations of each of the 166 techniques may be purchased at ***https://www.osteomasterstechniques.com/product/video-access/***

—William Thomas Crow. D.O., F.A.A.O.

—Terence C. Vardy, D.O., M.App.Sc.

Acknowledgements

- Don Peska, D.O, Dean, and David Mason, D.O., Chairman of the Department of the Osteopathic Manipulative Medicine Department, Texas College of Osteopathic Medicine, University of North Texas Health Science Center—for allowing us to use the OMM lab to do the video and photography shoots.
- Kathy Broyles, archivist, University of North Texas Health Science Library – for access to the archives which contain the works, correspondence and other materials from Anne Wales and William Garner Sutherland.
- R. Todd Dombroski, D.O., Austin Henke, Alexander Jacobsen, Michael Almquist, Sean Hogan, and Tyler Trevino for their help in the production of the videos for this book.
- R. Todd Dombroski, D.O., Christina Ragland, D.O, Tim Pence, D.O., Jarrid Bernhardt, D.O., and Aaron Burket, D.O., for their help in the production of the photos used in this book.
- R. Todd Dombroski, D.O., for his very practical assistance in interpreting the techniques, and his valuable advice in translating old American medical language.
- Rob Gilliland for production of the website, eBook and other computer wizardry.
- Jason Haxton, A T. Still Museum—for his assistance with copies of the historical records of the profession.
- Stephen Webb, D.O., for reviewing the book drafts and for his valuable osteopathic feedback.
- Stephen McGowan, D.O., for his provision of the Anne Wales videos.
- We would also like to sincerely thank our wives, Janet Crow and Belinda Vardy, and our daughters and sons, Rachael, Ryan and Oskar, for allowing us the time away from our families to work on this project.
- We have both been blessed with many mentors and colleagues during our lives and osteopathic journeys. In particular, we would like to thank Drs. John Peckham, John Fox, Robert Fulford, John Jones, Alex Nicholas, Bryyon Lambert, Bill Kuchera, Herb Yates, Larry Jones, Robert Ward, Anthony Chila, William Johnston, Paul Kimberley, Wayne English, Todd Dombroski, Michael Kuchera and Elaine Wallace.

Source Materials

In connection with the various comments about the techniques described and illustrated in this book, we have quoted directly from the authors themselves, and have edited their statements for clarity and conciseness. Unless otherwise specifically noted, a list of our sources is provided below.

Anne Wales' comments are based on transcriptions of recordings of her made in Australia in 1978 by Stephen McGowan, D.O., and are reproduced here with his permission.

The Ernest Eckford Tucker material is drawn from his book, *Osteopathic Technic*, Clinton Press (New York: 1917).

Comments about the techniques of William Sutherland are drawn from "The Osteopathic Technique of Wm. G. Sutherland" by Howard A. Lippincott, published in the 1949 *Yearbook of the American Academy of Osteopathy*.

Comments attributed to Robert Fulford are derived from notes taken at his courses. The two places where he is quoted directly are so noted in the text.

Comments attributed to Ken Lossing were presented at one of his visceral courses and are printed here with his permission.

The Charles Hazzard material is drawn from his book, *The Practice and Applied Therapeutics of Osteopathy* (2nd Ed.), Journal Printing Company (Kirksville, MO: 1901).

The material on treatment of asthma is partially drawn from "Manipulative Treatment of Asthma" by Perrin T. Wilson, D.O., T. L. Ray, D.O., and Harry W. Gamble, D.O., in the Digest of Papers and Discussion presented at the Manipulative Therapeutic Section of the American Osteopathic Association at Cincinnati, Ohio. Published in volume 1 of the July, 1938 *Yearbook of the American Academy of Osteopathy.*

The Elmer Barber material is drawn from his book, *Osteopathy Complete,* Hudson-Kimberly Publishing Co. (Kansas City: 1898).

The William West material is drawn from his book, *Osteopathic Surgery: The Technique of AT Still Medical Operations in the Treatment of Disease,* Clifton Publishing Company (Centerville, IA: 1900).

The Carl Philip McConnell and Charles Clayton Teal material is drawn from their book, *The Practice of Osteopathy* (3rd Ed.), Journal Printing Company (Kirksville, MO: 1906).

The Curtis H. Muncie material is drawn from his article, "Hearing restored through the reconstruction of the Eustachian tubes" J Am Osteopath Assoc 1931;30:397-401, and his book, *Prevention and Cure of Deafness through Muncie Reconstruction Method* (7th Ed.), Muncie Institute for Hearing (New York: 1944).

The material for the "Root of the Technique" is based on a lecture presented by Edgar Miller, D.O., at a Sutherland Cranial Teaching Foundation Course in 2004.

The material for John Fox, D.O.'s treatment of GERD is based on personal interaction with him by Dr. Crow in 1996.

"Look Well to the Hyoid" is an address presented by G. W. Riley, Ph.D., D.O., and reproduced in the Digest of Papers and Discussion presented at the Manipulative Therapeutic Section of the American Osteopathic Association at Cincinnati, Ohio. Published in volume 1 of the July, 1938 *Yearbook of the American Academy of Osteopathy.*

1

The Philosophy of the Osteopathic Masters in their Own Words

Structure – the Basic Determinant of Body Function[1]

by Wilborn J. Deason, M.S., D.O.

Did anyone ever see an amoeba faint or a mule suffer from neurasthenia? Surely not. The exaggerated physiological reactions necessary to bring about such functional perversions would require a much more highly developed, and a far greater differentiated structural mechanism than either of these animals possess. One might as well expect a wheelbarrow to thresh wheat.

Function not only depends upon structure and structural relations, but it also requires a suitable or adapted structure, and differentiated or specialized function requires a 'more highly differentiated or specialized structure for its performance.'

The primitive and essential functions of protoplasm are performed by a relatively simple single-celled animal organism, but even here there are certain structurally different parts for the purpose of performing special functions. Passing to another stage, the colonial Protozoa, a beginning of cell differentiation may be noted, and still further, in the Volvicinia (algae), the outer cells of the group assume very definitely the beginnings of specialization. Here the outer cells take on the function of irritability, leaving other functions to other cells or cell groups of the now many-celled group, or metazoan. From here on one may follow Haeckel through many interesting stages showing how structure and function have developed together.

Spencer's definition of life as to continual adaptation of internal structure to external environment might suggest that there exists a constant demand for change, requiring that as new demands (or new functions) are required, the new or differentiated structure must be developed to meet such demands. This of course is true. As external conditions change, the animal to survive must migrate, hibernate, adapt or die. But this does not mean exclusively that function rather than structure leads in evolutionary development. It does mean, however, that those animals having the proper structure for performing the functions essential to life under a given environment will live and perpetuate their kind. It may also be

1. *The Journal of the American Osteopathic Association* 28, no. 6 (February 1929).

seen how function depends upon the structure.

This constant change and demand for continued change for maximum physiological economy renders a physiological normal or biological standard practically impossible to determine. Another biological law then becomes apparent, namely, that not only does function depend upon structure, but that structural-functional relationships must be maintained near to a constant balance so that a near normalcy of function or physiological balance can be maintained. This is the 'homeostasis of life'.

In the progress of evolutionary development, as differentiation continues to alter structure and to render certain functions more definite and different by demand, there arises a need for the control and balance of these various functions. Hence a very special structure—the nervous system—comes into existence as the software operating system for the body.

It should not be forgotten, however, that the nervous system is as much a part of the body as is any other differentiated body structure. While it has much to do in the excitation to action and control of practically all other body structures, it in turn is controlled by the body functions. The same environmental conditions related to a cell, supply of nutrition in the form of complex proteins, amino acids and oxygen, etc., and the elimination of wastes, are essential also to the function of nerve cells. Since so many centers of nerve control lie within the spinal cord, it may readily be seen why normal physiologic conditions in and around the cord are absolutely essential for normal nerve function.

Another biological theory applies, namely, that as differentiation of structure progresses, its resistance is decreased. In certain instances this is well known. The nervous structures of the eye, for example (following the just-mentioned case of the outer cells of volvox), become very highly differentiated, and are, perhaps, the least resistant of all body structures. The same is true of the ear, and in proportion, of the other special sense organs. Here again is another example, not only of the dependence of function upon structure, but of the fact that as special function requires a highly specialized structure, it suffers proportionately in its inherent resistance.

Had this process of differentiation continued indefinitely without some means of control other than that of the maintenance of physiological balance through the nervous system, perhaps only a few, and those only the far more simple species, could have come into existence. There was a requirement for some mechanism for an automatic body protection. This may have automatically and progressively developed as an additional or a primitive function of the simple cell. We might add to the other primitive functions of protoplasm that of immunity or self-preservation; for there is good reason to believe that this function, however it may be explained, has always existed. With all existing living organisms, the constant demand for the adaptation of internal structure to the external environment has encouraged the development of mechanisms suitable to increase resistance to systemic failure. This condition is ever present, and we often refer to this as auto-regulation or homeostasis. Such is the demand for such a function, that the various animal species simply had to develop it, or that particular species ceased to exist.

A resistant mechanism would, of course, not be confined to that which we know as gross structure, not even to microscopic structure, but to all biological reactions which would tend to increase resistance to internal and external physiological challenges. The development of special resistances or immunity to various body "poisons" comes naturally from stimulation or challenge, as the potential or determinant structure remains ever present.

Striking examples are afforded by the phenomena of immunity to attacks by micro-organisms, and to the action of poisons. Still more remarkable instances are those connected with the recovery of function or reproduction of tissue after injury or disease, or even complete loss of portions of the body.

This is but a brief summary, with all too poorly connected current understanding of the body's physiology, but it does suggest a line of thought that is worthwhile in the study of structure as a major determinant of body function.

SUMMARY

1. The cell constitutes the inherent structural and functional unit of the organism; and function is not only determined by, but varies with, the cellular structural mechanism.
2. Various cells have undergone certain processes of differentiation in the course of phylogenetic development of the species. Now in the higher forms certain organs are capable of more highly differentiated function as needed by the complex human organism and body systems.
3. The cell is to the organ as the organ is to the body. Each is dependent on the other.
4. The unity of functional relationship or the physiologic balance of function is a most important determinant in the overall maintenance of body health.
5. Every cell in the body bears a certain functional relationship to every other cell of that organ and to cells in other organs. Likewise, every organ bears a certain functional relationship to every other organ. It is this sum total of organ function that determines the body function as a whole.
6. The failure of any structure or group of structures having a common function may cause unequal balance and thus be detrimental to body health.
7. In the ever changing demand for adaptation, the nervous system, as a regulating mechanism, is constantly called upon. By virtue of its high degree of differentiation, this structure is likely to suffer or fail first.
8. Structure is affected by function. This is as true as it is true that structure determines function.
9. The balance of function or automatic regulation is the functional control of structure as affected by nerves and other structures.
10. The constant demand of function requiring continued adaptation of internal structure to external environment has developed natural resistance in all animal organisms.

This varies in degree from that of protecting against various poisons received to the regeneration of body structure from use.

APPLICATION

In organic sciences, there has been comparatively little accomplished by researchers in the application of biological principles to effective treatment intervention. Researchers in our universities are usually minimally interested in internal medical therapeutics. For the most part, they accept therapeutic tradition largely because too much effort is required to do otherwise. And yet one may say with little fear of contradiction, that they are possessed with little actual knowledge of pharmacology and allied branches, yet have great confidence in accepted internal medical therapeutics.

It was Dr. Still who first advanced a theory of the universal application of biological principles in the maintenance of body health and also as a method of therapeutic treatment in disease. Dr. Still was a student of the old school of biologists as represented by Spencer, Huxley, Darwin, Haeckel, and others. This I knew from personal association with him. In addition to his reading, Dr. Still was a keen observer, and had that rare ability of applying what he learned.

In considering the etiology of disease, Dr. Still always urged that we look first at the causes that maintain normal health and to reason from cause to effect. "Learn the normal," he urged, and "you will recognize the abnormal when you find it."

The anatomist of the old school studies body structure and applies his findings in surgery, but where and in what manner does he apply such knowledge in the actual practice of so-called "internal medicine" which refers to practically everything else in therapeutics?

The physiologist of the old school studies body function and has learned much. But here again, how much of this knowledge is actually applied other than in the remotest fragmentary manner in medical therapeutics?

Dr. Still's theory of osteopathy is primarily and basically a theory of the laws of structure and function as applied to the maintenance of normal health and immunity to disease. In this it resembles other great theories, such as Darwin's pangenesis, or Haeckel's theory of ontogeny and phylogeny. Osteopathy is a system of therapy only secondarily to Still's theoretical model.

In this respect and as a theory of therapy, osteopathy differs completely and distinctly from any and all other schools of therapy. Not one of the other therapies has, or ever had, even a hint of a universal basic theory founded upon biological fact.

The histologist of the old school delved into the realms of cellular life, and made some progress in correlating the microscopic anatomy with physiology. But here again, except in exceptional instances, made little or no advance in treating the problems of health and disease.

The pathologist of the old school learned much about the nature of tissue change as a result of disease, and of microscopic cellular change concomitant with disease. Incidental pathology it might be called, but what has been done to determine those cellular changes that bring about functional perversion, and which lead to the actual causes of disease, or of the causes of gross pathology?

The bacteriologist of the old school accomplished many truly remarkable advances in scientific knowledge pertaining to microscopic life. Many patient cases traced the undeniable relation of certain micro-organic flora to certain diseases. This is the brightest ray of hope to the student of internal medicine and of surgery, the micro-organic theory of disease, and likewise the vaccine and serum treatment have been grossly over credited. The medical profession, and because of extensive media propaganda, the general public, have naturally accepted most of such doctrine as absolute truth and call it modern science.

No problem has received half the attention from medical research as vaccine, serum therapy and allied subjects during the past thirty-five years, and yet how little has actually advanced therapeutically!

The application of many biological principles has accomplished truly remarkable advances in surgery. But surgery and internal medicine are wholly different. Surgery is more closely allied to osteopathy, both in theory and in practice, than to any other school of medicine. In fact, osteopathy is no less than surgery, but very much more. Osteopathy is the universal application of surgery in its broader sense, applied universally in therapeutics.

As a theory of the mechanism by means of which normal health is maintained, through structural-functional balance of natural body immunity and of therapeutics, osteopathy differs from all "Schools of Therapeutics" only in that it has its own distinctive teaching and application of the principles of the basic sciences. Osteopathic anatomy, osteopathic physiology, osteopathic pathology, etc., has made such progress that only the uninformed would deny their distinctive and definite existence. The time must come when this indefiniteness, this carelessness and haphazardness in therapeutics will cease.

The universal acceptance and application of biological law must ultimately be applied. No theory of therapeutics can be scientific which does not consider the biological causes which maintain health and body resistance. The osteopathic theory must, therefore, at some future time become fully recognized.

The Osteopathic Concept of Etiology[2]

by Carl P. McConnell, D.O.

The fundamental aspects of the body, whether pertaining to the physical or chemical, are intimately related and interdependent. This is true of all circulatory, nervous and chemical phenomena, of structural and functional relationships, and of structural continuity and functional unity. Physiology and biochemistry do not represent independent processes, but instead are part of a vital whole. Contingency is always manifest.

Dr. Still stressed the physical plane because it is both an indispensable and a neglected field. He was not though a stranger to chemistry. Furthermore, he realized the potential completeness of the body provided the structure is intact and diet and environment approach the norm. The properties of both bodily physics and chemistry are inherent. They are sufficient to maintain health, prevent disease and repair tissue, when structure is normal, function exercised, and food requirements met. Disorder or disease is present when the structure is perverted or when chemical supply is impoverished. Chemical impoverishment, however, is not always due to faulty supply. It is frequently caused by a disability of the structural mechanism.

It is a curious reflection on medical science and progress that no school prior to osteopathy viewed the body from a comprehensive mechano-physical standpoint. Though admitting that the physical is indispensable to the chemical, the physical body should be intact and exercised in order to 'promote and maintain health.' Physical restructuring is the essential work of the surgeon. The growth of surgery has been phenomenal; steadily encroaching on the field of the medical internist till it would almost seem that the internist's main forte is holding a diagnostic sack. This sack of knowledge is then often brushed aside at the operating table or autopsy.

The one-sided chemical viewpoint has not withstood the acid test of clinical results. If it had, surgery and osteopathy would not have made such remarkable strides. Chemotherapy

2. *The Journal of the American Osteopathic Association* 28, no. 6 (February 1929).

has simply attempted the impossible, somewhat similar to the "half-truth" of the "mental" school.

So it is not surprising that three important facts have been developed through osteopathic evolution. First, structure determines function. Secondly, natural chemical immunity is dependent on structural intactness. Thirdly, operative adjustment will set structure right.

The osteopathic concept of etiology is that the forces which change structure are of primary importance. These forces are innumerable, ranging from the inherited and congenital to the ever-present environmental. The effects upon structure are of infinite variety and variation. Although the simplicity of the essential, structure determines function, the discovery, analysis, correlation and application of the many factors require much firsthand information and experience. For there is no formula to follow or routine to indulge. General biological principles are the only guide, for the complexity of a given case is characterized by its individuality.

The structural reaction of an individual to his environment embraces every act of daily life. These structural registrations are just as much a part of the bodily condition as any other portion of the organism. They not only give definite clues to the health status, but they register the character of the environing forces. Furthermore, if they are not harmonious with the normal condition of the body, they lead to progressive dysfunctional involvement of nervous and circulatory functions. In order for them to be understood, one should be thoroughly conversant with both structural registrations and environing forces. If they are not harmonious with functional requirements, the structure is impaired both mechanically and chemically, and a pre-diseased state exists. Herein lays the osteopathic concept of etiology. It is a significant part of the natural history and progression of disease.

Thus, it is seen that abnormal conditions are not necessarily revealed by subjective and chemical manifestations. Although these are not to be ignored, they are only part of the clinical picture. Osteopathic science discovered the structural counterpart, and developed a structural etiology, pathology and therapy. This is a field as rich in manifestations as any other. Moreover, in view of the significance of structure, the importance of their discovery and evaluation cannot be gainsaid. That the chemical phenomena are important and relevant is beyond question. However, such changes are only part of the biological equation. They are factors to be considered, but only in their relationship to others.

The osteopathic concept of etiology has revealed an unmistakable new world of structural phenomena. It is a field hitherto unknown to exist. Osteopathic development has organized and classified this knowledge into a science. Pathologically, diagnostically and therapeutically this wealth of fact is beyond parallel. There is before the clinician a vast mass of structural signs and conditions to be elucidated; structural material bearing information on configuration, tone, elasticity and mobility, consistency and density, position and relationship.

This represents a wealth of facts that are not merely to be observed: they should be felt, and tactually appreciated in order to ascertain their important role. Thus a veritable new world of phenomena is placed at our command. This is the significant feature of osteopathic etiology. It gives the clue to etiologic forces, and no less points the way to recovery. It lessens the heretofore relative importance of chemical values. Not that they do not exist, but rather it also gives an appreciation to physical factors.

The physical field constitutes a universal plane of all body organs and tissues, which when damaged introduces and maintains functional disturbance. It requires experience, skill and judgment to interpret its signs.

Just like the field of blood, chemistry reveals both local and general phenomena to he who is able to read its meaning. Minutiae, initiative, and broad viewpoint are important.

Were it not for the inherent properties of immunity, repair and recovery, it is evident that the bodily mechanism would not be a vital and healthy one. It is equally evident that structural position and relationship are of prime importance, basically and essentially. Not that structure is merely confined to the principles of mechanics, but it also enters into the properties and functions of vital processes, no less in its way than the principles of chemistry. It is the interdependence of part to part and to the whole that makes the organism what it is.

That disabled structure impairs its inherent properties is just as certain as the effects of a deficient diet or inharmonious environment. In fact, environmental conditions are largely expressed through the structural mechanism. All of these are of basic import in the realm of etiology. Action and reaction are no insignificant terms as applied to the bodily processes. It means either normality or abnormality. In either instance the forces are registered on the structural pattern. Consequently, the structural pattern in view of its relationship to vital processes (in fact, being a part of them) is just as important and significant as the chemical one. In many instances, it is more important, for it is the vehicle of support for tissues and exchange of fluids and impulses. Both the structural and chemical are expressions of vital equivalents. The one on the plane of physiological physics, the other presenting the biochemical aspect. They represent respectively the two sides of a shield.

It is in this chapter of the early beginnings of disease that the osteopathic concept is so supreme, though at all stages of disease, with many possible exciting and complicating factors, the structural status retains its underlying importance. It is a field that has heretofore been overlooked. The early beginnings of disease, the predisposing factors, the pre-diseased state of circulatory stasis and afferent inhibitions that lead to organic impairment and lessened resistance, is of greatest importance in not only obtaining a true perspective of disease history, but also in the field of prevention. It constitutes a biological chapter of the utmost significance. It adds materially to our understanding of immunity.

The import of structural conditioning and of surgery has long been recognized. The osteopathic concept does not contradict these same principles. In fact, it carries them out logically to the very minutiae of all tissues, and to a detailed mechanical degree that is harmonious with their functions. It consistently fills a heretofore physiological gap in the etiologic field.

The practical application of the osteopathic concept is fraught with many difficulties. The same is true of the principles of surgery. Practical application demands much experience and close study of the living subject. Living physiology is extremely varied. To attain sound clinical sense requires close application of all diagnostic methods, of which palpation is second to none in value. The feel of the structure, its temperature, tone and consistency, its elasticity and resiliency, and its alignment, comprise a vast world to the clinician who is able to interpret it. The various structural registrations are vital reactions, no more nor less. If he is able to interpret his findings, analyze and correlate them, and then evaluate them diagnostically, he possesses a method and skill that is invaluable.

Then what is of equal value to this etiological concept and diagnostic method is that the therapeutic indication is consistently based on the pathology. There is no gap to be bridged between etiology and therapy. The fields of osteopathic science comprise a consistent whole. The same principles of viewpoint and application are enlisted. The feel of structural tissue, revealing its status of consistency and position, is equally important in etiologic elucidation, pathologic determination, and therapeutic application.

There is no question that discordant environmental reaction is an important cause of disease. The effect on structure and dependent function is well known. It results in an imbalanced state of muscular tension, skeletal abnormalities, and a slumped posture. This means lessened tone of the tissues, strained ligaments, osseous mal-alignment, and displaced organs. The effect upon circulatory channels and nervous courses is one of obstruction and impediment, leading to organic disorder. A distorted organism means a crippled mechanism. Although adaptation and compensation are dependent upon genetics and margins of safety, nevertheless reserves and resistances are proportionately lessened and impaired. The osteopathic lesion distinctly predisposes to infectious sites and toxic states.

Why should the organism be primarily considered (and oftentimes entirely) from the standpoint of chemistry when its vehicle is a physical one? Recognizing that the chemical constituents and their properties are indispensable, why neglect the equally indispensable physical arrangements? Especially in view of the fact that the body contains the attributes of both a vital and physical mechanism.

Associated with structural intactness is natural chemical immunity. Arterial supply and nervous impulse are beyond doubt controlling forces. Either may be disordered by physical derangement, marking the early beginning of disease. Freedom of mechanical structure, rational diet and right living constitute the requirements of normality for the combined physiology and biochemistry of the vital organism. Changes in the physiochemical system affect the energy relationships, of which adaptation to environment is a critical part of the living process.

Treatable Diagnosis of Osteopathic Lesions[3]

by Russel R. Peckham, D.O.

The field touched on by this discussion will be limited to local conditions involving only the relationships of one segment with its immediate neighbor. Posture, anomalies, constitutional pathology, exceptional or unusual conditions, methods of lesion production, manner and predispositions to lesion production, and other related subjects of great importance to the consideration of lesion conditions will be omitted by intent, in order that the attention may be directed to the determination of just what that lesion requires by way of manipulative treatment. Space will not permit discussion of the physiology and perverted physiology which occasion the symptoms of a "lesion." Such discussion would be redundant, since the profession has become well-grounded in these basics through the excellent work of Dr. Louisa Burns and others.

This paper will deal with those phenomena which with reasonable constancy appear coincident with, and follow, the occurrence of an inter-segmental articular lesion of the vertebral column. An endeavor will be made to evaluate findings in a manner permitting application, and if possible, prevent misapplication.

The discrimination of the proper values to be given to different findings, and

3. *The Journal of the American Osteopathic Association* 28, no. 1, part II (September 1928).

interpretation of the phenomena, is the measure of the ability to diagnose lesions.

The basic causes of articular dysfunction should arise from exaggerated physiological or pathological disturbance to some or all of those tissues which comprise the joint, or are related to its functions.

These functions are support and movement, and it is to the tissues which have to do with support and movement that attention should turn.

First, the tissues of support:

- Bone with its specialized coverings
- Ligament, of at least two types, fibrous and elastic
- Muscle, in so far as it is at times a tissue of support

Nerve reflexes are included in this neuromuscular unit of function. Variations of osseous structure, such as atrophy and hypertrophy, are important inasmuch as they affect apparent relationships.

Hypertrophy of the type which produces lipping, must be borne in mind in consideration of limited movement. The periosseous tissues covering the opposed articular surfaces, hyaline cartilage and synovial membrane, are likewise subject to a variety of changes, e.g., inflammatory changes of the acute type, edema, and on through successive changes to hypertrophy and hyperplasia. Erosion, adhesion and atrophy are frequently encountered.

That some of these changes are always present in older lesions and in lesions of recent production, there is no doubt. Likewise, there is no doubt that such changes do in part account for the syndrome of phenomena called "lesion." The roentgen ray (X-ray) will often demonstrate these changes and it must be admitted into the diagnosis.

Edema of these two tissues covering the articular surfaces should and does make free movement difficult. Thickening of these tissues and adhesions or erosions may give the appearance of malposition and does affect and limit movement. Thinned cartilaginous surfaces may handicap movement by mal-positioning the fulcrum for force application.

Thus may the tissues of support through hypertrophy, hyperplasia, atrophy or edema produce limited movement of an articulation or give the appearance of mal-relationship of the osseous structures.

It is probable that the condition of the ligamentous structures serving an articulation of a vertebral segment becomes the most important single tissue in concluding a treatable diagnosis. These tissues are the movement limiting structures, and as such determine the nature and extent of possible movement permitted for that joint.

These ligamentous structures will here be classified under three headings: weight supporting, tension supporting, and capsular.

This classification is used for the reason that all three are subject to the same pathological changes, and that it is in these three structures that most of the pathology is present.

1. Weight supporting—in reference to the intervertebral disc, so designed and constructed of fibrous and elastic tissue and fluid that it is capable of supporting great superimposed weight, and of receiving forces from a constantly varying direction, and of shifting its medium for support without difficulty as occasion demands. It is to be borne in mind that the material of which the disc is made is the same that comprises the other two types of ligamentous tissue, and therefore is subject to the same processes of pathology.

2. Tension supporting tissues—the fibrous bands of ligamentous material related to each joint, which hold the bones together, and importantly limit each type of movement at some certain point. These ligaments are called supporting ligaments, and are practically incapable of stretching. They do not stretch unless the strain greatly exceeds that intended for that joint. These bands consist almost entirely of gray, fibrous tissue. Forced relaxation, if maintained, might elongate them.

   More frequently, and the usual change occurring in them, is the ordinary infiltration of fibrous cicatricial (scar) tissue as a result of irritation or inflammation. Such infiltration thickens and contracts these bands and decreases the normal movement of the joint served.

3. The elastic or capsular ligaments. These thin elastic ligaments complete the joint cavity, and serve most in that they prevent the escape of synovial fluid. Being elastic, they tend to shorten as far as attachments permit.

   They are never normally strong enough to accomplish change in osseous relationships through their elastic contraction power. Neither are they normally strong enough to limit or impede the movement of the joint. They are subject to the usual changes as the result of irritation to be expected in all structures of mesodermal origin, i.e., fibrosis.

All of the structures of the ligamentous group are of the same general class of tissues and develop similar pathology under similar conditions of functional embarrassment. These changes cover a rather long succession of developments, among which the essential ones in this discussion are edema, leukocytosis, fibroblastic infiltration, infiltration of fibrous tissue, and finally cicatricle (scar) contraction and shortening and stiffening of the ligament itself.

Let it again be remarked that the disc consists normally of proper proportions of fibrous and elastic tissues and fluid. Should there develop a disproportion of these tissues, with excess of the fibrous type, the effect would be obvious. More than that, should the excess fibrous tissue, as infiltrated fibrous tissue does always, and everywhere if possible, contract with time, it is obvious that the actual reduction in volume of the weight shifting medium of the disc might occur.

Just what the total change within these ligamentous structures is cannot be completely described. Perhaps fibrous tissue replaces elastic. Surely the total amount of fibrous tissue increases, and surely such increase limits the movement of the joint in one or more of its mobility possibilities, either through disc involvement, lost elasticity of capsular ligaments, or through stiffening and shortening of the supporting ligaments.

Neuromuscular Mechanisms

A joint designed for movement requires some dynamic force to move it. This force is supplied by the neuromuscular mechanism. Very limited space will be given the subject here.

The conditions of muscle will be grouped into three classes:

1. Hypertonic musculature, refusing the normal readiness of joint movement, may result from exaggerated nerve stimulus, intra-toxemic states (infection, fatigue toxins, etc.); from mechanical stimulus such as derangement of the attachments of the muscle bundles; and the condition of physiologic contraction voluntarily induced by the patient. These limits of movement may be readily overcome by applying force which exceeds the force of the hypertonicity.

2. Fibrotic musculature, which limits joint movement simply because the muscle is denied its normal measure of relaxation by the presence of the accumulated fibrous tissue. There may be some decrease of muscle fiber. This is the type of muscle condition resulting from a long-standing low-grade inflammation. It seems certain that most of these are accentuated and accelerated by the presence of low-grade streptococcus constitutional infection.

3. The atrophic fibrotic type, less rapid in development and the result of atony and replacement of active parenchyma with fibrous tissue. The only importance for the separate classification is that of prognosis as to the functional recovery of the joint.

Short Discussion of Neuromuscular Physiology

It is a well-received law that the muscles of the specific function of some joints receive the major nerve stimulus, reflexly, from sensory nerve endings related to that particular joint. Further, that muscles serving a specific function, such as side-bending, receive reflex stimulus from sensory nerve endings stimulated principally by that type of movement.

It is for this reason that the small muscles of the vertebral column respond so accurately to irritations of the articular structures in the presence of a lesion. It also explains the fact that small specific groups of muscles, those related to some specific type of intersegmental motion, demonstrate symptoms of hyperirritability and dysfunction when that particular type of movement is involved in the lesion. Thus, when rotation to one side is invalidated, the small specific group of rotators of that segment develop tenderness, hypertonicity, and later atony or fibrosis.

To be more explanatory of this point, it is necessary to review briefly the neuromuscular mechanics of maintenance of position, and the initiative and consummation of new intervertebral movements under normal conditions. When a movement is initiated, two sets of muscles related to that motion begin to work: those which move, and an opposing group, which prevent jerkiness and exaggerated motion. A large part of the action is reflex through the cerebellar and cord reflexes. The stimulus arises chiefly in the structures which are moving, and as changes in pressures on supporting structures, tension on ligaments and muscles occur co-incident with the changing position, different degrees of stimuli arise from different structures and surfaces. Likewise, different muscle groups, through their nerve reflex arcs, successively act for maximum efficiency in the completion of the movement. It also follows that when a fixation of a joint occurs at any point in its movement, the stimuli arising from the joint unit are being distributed largely to some muscle groups, related reflexly as described above. With cessation of movement, the origin of stimuli is not stopped entirely and may be increased by the inflammation resulting from the lesion condition. Thus the muscles are subjected to continuous activating stimuli, and hypertonus, inflammation, tenderness and pain may appear.

It may be said that the tenderness associated with a lesion should be related to one of the muscle groups described above, or the attachments of those muscles, supporting ligaments put on tension, or attachment of those ligaments. The difficulty of locating these small structures accurately suggests the possibility of placing too much importance on the findings of tenderness. The principal value of the finding of tenderness in most lesions is that it generally signifies the locality of disturbance.

Pain

The significance of pain in the diagnosis of lesions is slight. These paragraphs will not include discussion of visceral reflex segmental disturbances, since these reflexes do not seem to determine the type of lesion, but rather predispose to a lesion through general irritation to the segment, or group of segments.

According to recent physiology and anatomical studies of the central nervous system, only one type of sensory nerve ending is capable of receiving an impulse of pain. These nerve endings become stimulated by such irritants as may endanger the life of the tissue in which the endings are resident. These are called naked nerve endings. These nerve endings are found in nearly all tissues of the body. It is probable that ordinarily these nerve endings are not responsive to any of the conditions in absolutely normal tissues, and become activated only in the presence of injurious tissue conditions in their resident structures.

Hence, since the condition of 'lesion' may involve all the tissues related to a segment, and since these nerve endings are copiously distributed in the synovial membrane and periosteum, and in lesser degrees in the other tissues of the joint including muscle, pain may arise from any condition in or around the joint. That is, pain may arise from disc, periosteum, ligament attachment, muscle or muscle attachment, synovial membrane or even the hyaline cartilage. In this matter we call forth the law of referred pain, because not all of the tissues of the joint unit are of the same degree of sensitivity. Thus, disc involvement might be referred to and interpreted as arising from the articular surface of a facet. Ligamentous involvement might readily be referred to and interpreted as arising from some muscle group. The point here to be noted is simply that the symptom of pain is not in any measure a valuable diagnostic symptom of the lesion, subject to wide error, and frequently actually misleading.

It is only safe to assume that an involved joint will distribute most of its actual and referred pain to the same segment, and the greater portion to the lateral half of the segment in which the pathology is located, and hence from which most of the irritation arises.

The progress of diagnostic methods has gradually but certainly developed a better understanding of the actual condition in a lesion, and with this better understanding the importance of "relative position" as a diagnostic factor has greatly diminished.

There was a time when the diagnosis of lesions was made almost entirely by the relative position of the involved segments, usually by examination of the spinous processes. Later, students of the subject began to question themselves regarding the relations of the other portions of the bones involved. Later still, interpretations of tenderness received considerable attention. Fortunately, the more recent students are devoting the greater part of their thought to the general pathology around the area involved; and with these studies have come a better understanding of the limited movement of lesioned articulations. Relative position still has its place in diagnostic procedure, its importance being to determine position. Knowing the position in which fixation has occurred furnishes indication for treatment only in so far as it precedes the next step in diagnosis, that of discovering wherein the fixation lies.

It must be definitely understood that accomplishing proper alignment may be a widely different thing from relieving the pathology of the joint. Moreover, in many instances forcing complete alignment would add greatly to the pathology present.

A Treatable Diagnosis

Such a diagnosis must consist of two general conclusions.

The first should inform the physician as to the relative position of lesioned segments together with the type of limited movement present. This simply means what the nature of the mal-relationship is, and what type of movement is stopped, thus refusing the articulation permission to recover proper position.

The second conclusion must inform the physician as to the quality of the limited movement. The quality of limited movement indicates the general degree of pathology of the articulation. With these two opinions formed, the technic for adjustment is a foregone conclusion. We will now consider these two factors in more detail.

Discussion of "relative position" would be of little value in this paper. All osteopathic literature contains much regarding this point of diagnosis, and though there are numerous contradictions in explanation and differing manners of description, it remains true that most practitioners have a classification which suffices for them. That of which the following makes mention may be applied to any classification of lesions whatsoever. To avoid confusion, "relative position" is taken for granted, as being understood.

Type of limited movement as a factor in diagnosing lesions must receive careful analysis. It has been the experience of all practitioners that the same condition of lesion, that is, a lesion having the same general picture as to position, tissue response to palpation, location, etc., as another, may require a different manipulation for adjustment. If the type of limited movement is determined before the manipulation is chosen, specific manipulation may be indicated for that limited mobility type. That such a predetermination is of vast importance any experienced physician will agree. It is at just this point that determination of relative position is inadequate information to precede manipulation.

In examining for limited movement, lesions will be encountered in which movement in any direction is impossible, or so nearly absent that delicate palpation will not discover it. Such a condition should be considered an ankylosis until conservative treatment develops palpable motion of the articulation. There are joints without ankylosis with fixation so closely approximating it that palpation may not demonstrate any movement. This condition will, however, respond to continued treatment. Treatment is therefore indicated pending positive contra-indication. There are comparatively few local lesions in which ankylosis is present. These lesions do demonstrate variable degrees of limited motion. This limited motion is of specific types.

An intervertebral articulation has different movement directions. It may be bent forward or backward. These motions may be accomplished without involving other types of movement. It may be side-bent. Side-bending does, however, early in its movement, include some other movement: rotation. And if the side-bending is pronounced, flexion or extension becomes likewise involved. Side-bending is not a simple movement, but rather a complex one with complementary rotary and flexion or extension movements included. However, the rotation may be the essential or most pronounced type of movement, the others abetting the primary movement. The same process may be described in relation to the rotation movement. Rotation might be the primary motion, but side-bending will often be associated, and if the motion is exaggerated, will include forward or backward bending.

From these facts we may conclude that limiting any one type of motion will affect in lesser measure the other possible movement planes. This small point is the crux of the problem of investigating limited motion. Examination of numerous lesions with this idea in mind will disclose the fact that lesions having the same relative position are maintained in that position by obstruction to entirely different types of movement. In one, realignment may be opposed because the articulation cannot side-bend; and in another presenting the same picture in all other respects, recovery of position is prevented because rotation is obstructed or prevented. In a third, because flexion is impossible; and the next, because extension is not available. Bear in mind that with the exception of this specific factor of limitation of a particular type of motion, the lesions may appear identical.

The particular thing which any particular lesion needs is a release from the specific limiting factor. Therefore, whatever manipulation is used, it must be one which emphasizes and forces the motion which is restrained.

Often the same manipulation may be used for an area, regardless of the specific factor of the lesion, if it but be remembered that in the application of the manipulation, care and specific direction must be superimposed upon the regular manipulation to correct just that obstruction which is really requiring assistance and normalization.

In examining for this limited movement, it will be found that most lesions do give some movement in all directions but one. All movements will be decreased somewhat, because the movements are complex, and fixation of any one type of movement will affect the freedom of all the others in some degree. Still, the absolute stoppage of one type of movement remains predominant. Experience shows that with relief of this one type of movement, the others recover spontaneously. Occasionally two planes of movement are involved and sometimes more. It seems probable that if more than two planes are actually normalized, all palpable restricted movement disappears.

Treatment without this careful examination of the lesion may produce three results.

1. The technic selected may be the exact manipulation needed for that lesion. The results would be good.

2. The technic might not be specific and adjustment would not result.

3. The force and general direction of force might be great enough to accomplish realignment of the malposition through forcing or exaggerating some of the other types of movement. This situation is not so uncommon in the experience of the best of technicians. Most physicians have frequently had to deal with increased symptoms, and more limitation of motion than before the treatment was applied. Exaggeration of a type of movement not primarily found limited in the lesion when overcoming the limitation generally results in a fixation of a movement not involved before. Hence, as was suggested earlier in this paper, accomplishing realignment is not always reduction of the lesion. Such realignments simply multiply the pathology of the joint.

The second conclusion to be drawn in developing a treatable diagnosis is concerning the quality of the limited motion. Determination of the quality of the limited motion should inform the physician regarding the stage of progression of pathology in the tissues involved in the lesion.

The Osteopathic Philosophy of Carl Philip McConnell and Charles Clayton Teall[4]

Osteopathic etiology and pathology constitutes the most interesting chapter of osteopathic science. The primal divergence of the osteopathic schools from previous systems is to be found in the osteopathic interpretation of disease causes and processes and not in osteopathic therapy as some may think. Osteopathy makes claim to an independent school because it possesses a distinct etiology, pathology, diagnosis and treatment. Thus osteopathic practice is not a mere method, but instead a system, a school, a science.

At no period of medical history have physicians of the older schools felt more keenly the futility of medical methods and the lack of an all-embracing principle of medicine than at the present. A recent writer (Sajous—The Internal Secretions and the Principles of Medicine, Vol. I, 1903) who claims to have discovered a principle that encompasses the entire field of medicine, says: "We found, we may say, that the backbone of medicine was the absent factor, and that if the patient labors of so many great minds had not proven as useful in the development of practical medicine as they should, it was because they lacked such a fundamental framework to afford a fixed nidus for each discovery, wherein its true relation to other discoveries would at once become evident."

Since the conception of osteopathy its fundamental framework has not changed one iota as to principle, although the application of the principle has been greatly elaborated. When Dr. Still proclaimed that "the rule of the artery is supreme" he gave utterance to a basic physiological truth. But when he demonstrated that osseous and other anatomical-mechanical lesions disturbed the artery and caused disease, and that readjustment of the anatomy cured the disorder, thus allowing the physiological to potentiate and revealing that the living body contains all the attributes of a vital and physical mechanism, did his teaching contain the germ of a comprehensive philosophy, and thus provide osteopathic science with a "backbone" and a consequent fixed nidus for all existing facts and future discoveries? It should always be emphasized that mechanical readjustment of the component parts of the vital body is the eternal keynote of the osteopathic school of healing.

The Osteopathic Lesion

Broadly speaking a lesion is "any morbid alteration in a tissue whether attended by a recognizable structural change or not; but especially a change in which the continuity of some of the tissue elements is broken in upon." (Foster—Medical Dictionary) There are several kinds of lesions expressing the tissue involved, character of degeneration, locality of same, etc. But upon analyzing the medley of arbitrarily defined lesions, the fact will be evident that much of medical etiology and pathology has not been logically and consistently sifted and arranged; and, moreover, it will be found the cause of many diseases is unknown.

Herein arises the great significance of the osteopathic lesion, for the lesion alters the very governing and controlling tissues of the body, viz., the nervous tissue and the vascular channels. Hulett (Hulett—Principles of Osteopathy) defined the osteopathic lesion as "any structural perversion which by pressure produces or maintains functional disorder." The constant maintenance of the structural perversion will, also, cause organic disease, although it is granted that functional disorder must necessarily result prior to any organic change.

4. Carl Philip McConnell and Charles Clayton Teal, *The Practice of Osteopathy*, 3rd ed. (Kirksville: Journal Printing Co., 1906).

The osteopathic conception of a lesion, functional and organic disorder caused by pressure from disturbed structures, does not bring us into an absolute new field. Medical literature of all ages contains references to diseases caused by pressure of tissues on nerves, blood vessels, or other channels. But the osteopathic idea is an absolutely new one in the application of this principle universally. It simplifies and makes uniform the arbitrariness of present semiology.

Thus the osteopathic idea that many diseases originate, primarily, from anatomically mal-aligned, mal-positioned, or mal-related tissues, causing a blockage of vital processes, immediate or remote, is a theory inclusive of disturbances to all tissues. This principle is fundamental and is supported by the physiological truth that uninterrupted vital channels preserve health; moreover, clinical and experimental data, as will be shown later, substantiate this fundamental. It at once places interpretation of a lesion in an entirely new light from preconceived concepts, and is analogous to and co-extensive with etiology and pathology.

Etiological Factors: The osteopath believes in the potency of inherited and environmental influences. There can be no question that a few diseases and certain disease tendencies may be inherited. The principle feature, however, from the standpoint of heredity, is that various organs and tissues have less vital resistance. These should not be confused with congenital weaknesses and diathetic tendencies.

Environmental influences are very important factors. One's surroundings and daily habits in the home, shop, or office count for much in the aggregate. Food, drink, air, rest, sleep, clothing, exercise, mental attitude, etc., all count for much in the sum total of health, and consequently ill-health may be traceable to their abuse. In fact, all hygienic and sanitary measures are duly considered by the osteopath. Various abuses, over use, and disuse of the functions will certainly be followed by physiological discord.

The germ theory contains much truth, but in the very large percentage of cases where the micro-organism is a factor, its significance is only of secondary consideration. Usually the micro-organism plays the role of an exciting and determining factor; before it can multiply and grow there must be a field that is first nutritionally disturbed. Nutrition of the tissue is the one great point always to be considered. The constitution of an individual is the pivot around which predisposing, environmental, and exciting factors of disease center.

Health represents the integrity of the artery as well as a maintenance of that master tissue, the nervous system, and anything that produces or influences, directly or indirectly, a disturbance of physiological functioning borders on the pathological. Hence the osteopath recognizes many of the common medical causes of disease, but reserves the privilege of rearranging their relative positions, for the osteopathic cause of diseases greatly modifies their value.

Osteopathic etiology distinctively emphasizes structural derangements and perversions. Of first importance is the osseous lesion. This lesion is represented by any abnormal change of position or relation of the many bony constituents of the body. The framework of the body is subject to not only any and every physical violence as with any mechanism, but moreover being the corporeal foundation of a vital mechanism, is subject to both direct and indirect biochemical changes and influences.

Thus the osseous lesion is caused (a) by trauma, e.g., strains, falls, blows, etc. (b) indirectly by atmospheric changes, over and violent exercise, etc., through the medium of muscle changes (c) by nutritional effects disturbing the elements of bony tissue (d) compensatorily and reflexly through the media of body distortions and muscular irritability or debility, e.g., an innominate lesion may be compensatory to a lumbar curvature, dietetic errors may cause dorsal muscular irritation and contraction, and produce a constant osseous lesion which in turn may result in chronic indigestion.

The pathological changes in the osseous lesion are commonly one of structural derangement, deviation, or complete displacement. The vertebral segments are of primary consideration owing to their important relationships to the spinal nerves, spinal cord centers and sympathetics; the ribs owing to the close sympathetic and spinal nervous relations, and then other osseous tissues, such as the innominate, clavicle, etc., depending upon their importance to contiguous vessels, nerves and organs. It should always be remembered and emphasized that mechanical changes of the anatomical structures are the primary essential in osteopathic etiology. This is the one great insight of pathological variations from the distinctively osteopathic conception, which the osseous lesion typifies. Consequently, the osseous lesion factor is actually a luxation (complete, or partial, even to a very slight degree), or malalignment of the bony constituents, which by virtue of their physical malposition impinge or irritate contiguous tissues.

Second in importance is the muscular lesion. The muscular lesion may be an actual dislocation of either muscle or tendon, but rarely. Commonly it is a contracted, tensed, or contracted muscle. The muscle, also, may be diseased either from primary or secondary sources and thus be an etiological feature.

The muscular lesion is caused (a) by direct or indirect violence the same as the osseous lesion (b) by atmospheric influence (c) by reflex irritations (d) by compensatory changes (e) by disease causing hypertrophy or atrophy, and (f) (which is of the most frequent origin) secondary to osseous lesions, being the result of impingement to the muscles' nervous control. The tensed or stretched muscle results from a separation of the points of origin and insertion.

Herein, as with the osseous lesion, the fundamental osteopathic concept is the resulting affection due to the physical encroachment, directly or indirectly, of the muscle tissue upon vascular channel or nerve fiber.

Muscular contractions, displacements, and tensions play a most important part in acute disorders, although muscular lesions that are secondary to other lesions are usually taken into account when treatment is given. Muscular lesions affect (a) blood and lymph vessels and (b) nerve fibers. Muscular contractions, especially, impede mechanically the return of the venous blood to the heart. The lesions to the nerves may be manifested in innumerable ways, depending upon the location of the muscle and the function and distribution of the nerve affected.

Then there is the relaxed, overstretched, and atonized muscle. This condition results as a secondary effect to mechanical strains, these being so severe and constant as to cause direct stretching and possible tearing of the muscle fibers. This should be distinguished from the exhausted or debilitated muscle, e.g., as found in neurasthenia and anemia.

Diagnostically, there are (a) contractions of more or less area, symmetrically, due to atmospheric changes (b) the deeply seated contractions involving a very small area, caused by vertebral and rib lesions (c) contractions due to reflex disturbances (d) contractions caused by postural effects and deformities (e) contractions from spasms of the blood vessels as a result of nervous irritations (f) contractions due to toxicity of the blood. All of these characteristic muscular lesions give a direct hint as to both etiology and prognosis.

Third, the ligamentous lesion is usually of secondary importance to the osseous lesion. There are two features that should be noted in particular when considering this lesion, first, thickenings and adhesions, and, second, relaxations.

The tone and integrity of the ligaments cannot but be of vital concern to the stability, suppleness, and adaptability of the bony framework in all physical movements. No matter how slight the osseous lesion may be, the ligament must of necessity be involved. The osseous derangements are either a source of irritation to the ligamentous tissue, resulting in congestion and inflammation and hence thickening and adhesions; or else the ligaments are so strained and tensed that in time atony occurs. Probably, in a fair percentage of atonized cases the first disturbance to the ligament was one of irritation and congestion, and then from long continued involvement, irritation was supplanted by debility.

Consequently, the primary consideration of the ligamentous lesion from the etiological standpoint is the character of the tissue (ligament) changes. This also gives us a direct hint that is of the utmost value in prognosis. The independent displacement of a ligament is rare, thus ligamentous lesions from the viewpoint of purely physical displacements are secondary to, if not an actual part of the osseous lesion. Ligaments, when displaced or tensed, readily impinge or irritate contiguous tissues, but the original cause of the structural perversion is commonly the osseous lesion. Hence, whatever factors enter into the production of the bony lesion will at least indirectly produce the ligamentous lesion.

Fourth, the visceral lesion is frequently overlooked as being of as much moment as an osteopathic lesion. Visceral displacements acting as a source of functional and organic annoyance on the physical plane (structural perversion which produces and maintains pressure) alone, are not in the least uncommon.

Any or all of the abdominal viscera, or even the organs of the thorax, may be displaced (physically) pathologically. Actual displacement of the viscous is a prolific source of distinct disorders and many obscure symptoms. It is true the organs are most frequently displaced from indirect causes, but nevertheless the actual physical malposition is in turn a primary cause of still another train of symptoms and diseases.

Visceral lesions are caused by (a) vertebral lesions (b) postural defects (c) direct violence (d) nutritional disorders (e) childbirth (f) unhygienic measures (tight lacing, heavy skirts, etc.) (g) congenital weakness.

From the displaced heart due to valvular and debilitating influences to the displaced liver, the stomach, the kidneys, the intestines, the ovaries, and the uterus, may arise a source of direct or indirect irritations, a train of apparent or masked symptoms, or a group of nutritional disturbances that include an extremely important chapter in etiology. Moreover, not only may one organ alone be involved, but several may be displaced or prolapsed as a whole as in splanchnoptosis; and even these in turn may be the direct cause of further organic displacements as the abdominal viscera prolapses upon the pelvic organs. Here is a very fruitful field for the diagnostician, for to separate cause from effect requires keen perception, an acute sense of touch, and above all, most careful weighing of all the factors that enter into the maze.

Fifth, the composite lesion is not always recognized as an extremely important osteopathic factor. By composite lesion is meant a structural lesion that primarily includes the osseous, muscular and ligamentous tissues as a whole. This may be termed a lesion en bloc or en masse.

Composite lesions are of exceedingly frequent occurrence. Indeed, many composite lesions are overlooked, and instead of treating the en bloc disturbance as a consistent whole, the component factors are treated separately with no concern or attention to the whole.

Postural defects are excellent examples of the composite lesion. The various curvatures, the tilted pelvis, etc., are representative of the composite lesion. Etiologically, pathologically, diagnostically, and therapeutically, the contour of the spine and ribs, the relation of the innominates to the sacrum and spine, and the symmetry of the body generally should be recognized and appreciated. The relation of the part to the whole and of the whole to the part are of vital etiological concern. An incipient curvature may be easily overlooked, a pendulous abdomen neglected, and a slipped innominate pass unnoticed wherein as a result the entire vertebral column is mal-aligned in relation to the normal physiological curves or to the body's perpendicular line of gravity.

Frequently, attempts are made to correct individual lesions when attention should be directed to the composite lesion and vice versa, e.g., a displaced rib is usually dependent upon a corresponding vertebral lesion, and thus the transverse plane or section of the body should be considered as a whole. A single lesion may be dependent upon a composite lesion or a composite lesion dependent upon one or more single lesions. A slipped innominate or a disordered hip joint may bring about a strain to a greater or less section of the spinal column, or a twisted vertebra may cause a curvature. On the other hand, postural defects may cause a strain at its maximum focal point, resulting in overstretching and relaxing of ligaments so that an osseous lesion results, or a spinal curvature cause an innominate displacement. Thus there is a constant establishing of equilibrium, physically and physiologically, through the medium of compensation. But at some phase of the change there is apt to be pathological phenomena resulting, and very frequently physiological harmony is not re-established but instead irritation, debility and other disease symptoms are constant effects until relieved.

Consequently, osteopathic etiology is many sided and complicated. To know whether an osseous, ligamentous, muscular, visceral, or composite lesion is primary or secondary, compensatory, reflex, predisposing, or exciting, requires a command of theoretical knowledge backed by much actual clinical experience.

In noting the above distinctive osteopathic etiologic features, the student should not lose sight of the constitutional status of the patient which may be modified by inherited, congenital, diathetic, and environmental influences, all of which go to make up the predisposition of the individual, and has an important relation to osteopathic factors. Then it should be recalled that disease processes may be of insidious progress, and the products and effects of pathologic changes cumulative.

Osteopathic Pathology

In the etiologic study the osteopathic characteristics have been designated structural mal-adjustment, although at the same time not losing sight of the fact that the body is not only a physical mechanism but also a vital mechanism. Structural perversions characterize the osteopathic distinction when dealing with the physical body, and remembering the vital or biochemical mechanism, mental attitude, diet, hygiene, etc., are not to be forgotten. To retain or attain health, thorough appreciation of both the physical and vital mechanism should be kept in view, for there is both an independent and dependent interaction on the part of each. The living body being an entity premises a system of therapeutics both physical and vital that acts in direct accord and harmony with physical laws and physiological functioning.

Osteopathic pathology deals with the distinctive osteopathic lesion as a factor in production and maintenance of disease. Then the province of pathology is, firstly, to determine whether the lesion is in reality an etiologic factor. Secondly, the immediate character of the lesion disturbance. Thirdly, how organic life becomes involved.

Inspection, palpation, clinical results, dissection and laboratory experimentation include the methods employed to prove that the lesion is of practical consequence. That the lesion is an etiological factor can be known only through clinical and experimental proof. The immediate character of the lesion disturbance can be determined by dissection, and how organic life becomes involved requires the summation of histological, physiological and pathological data.

The following outline assumes that the reader is familiar with anatomy, physiology and pathology. Osteopathic pathology does not add to medical pathology, but is an absolutely new pathology in all of the present known numerous details. Osteopathic pathology interprets much of clinical pathology anew. Furthermore, it presents absolutely new data that is exclusive, but germane to the present general medical and surgical fields.

Nervous tissue and arterial blood are the master tissues, the controlling and governing factors in health, and disturbances of these tissues are necessarily the cause of ill health. The rule of the artery and the control of the nerve must continue uninterrupted in order that physiological functioning remains intact. The body should be looked upon as being complete, no more or less, each tissue and organ essential to the whole, and the organism as a whole essential to every part. This is fundamental and germane to a living structure, and hence disturbance to the governing and controlling tissues, the nerves and vascular channels, must necessarily cause a break in the concatenation and disease must logically follow.

Thus, in the osteopathic pathology, we look to those influences that primarily disturb the nerve or artery, study the disease process or extension from inception to effect and from primary lesion to morbid results, and note action and interaction of tissue upon organ and organ upon organ.

That all parts of the body are in intimate and dependent relationship each with the other through the medium of the nervous system is a well-known fact based upon histological and physiological grounds. The neuron being the physiological unit implies that any disturbance to the cell quickly disturbs any or all of its processes. It may be said that "nervous tissue is dependent for its integrity upon two things, blood supply and trophic influences. The nerve cell is solely dependent on a proper supply of blood, and dies when this is withdrawn. But the nerve fiber is more dependent on the trophic influence of the cell, of which it is a prolongation. It dies when cut off from the cell, but it can get along for a time with but little direct blood supply. On the other hand, if the nerve fiber is injured it reacts on the cell, leading to a partial but curable degeneration of the cell body." (Dana—Text Book of Nervous Diseases) Here is the immediate pathologic key to many diseases. Whatever cuts off or obstructs the artery leading to the cell is a primary etiologic factor. This then leads to degeneration of protoplasmic processes and axon. It should be carefully noted that if the obstructed blood vessel is one to the nerve fiber, only the resultant partial injury to the cell is curable.

When an axon degenerates the retrogressive process involves not only the main axon, but also its terminals, together with the collaterals belonging to it with their terminals. (Barker—Reference Handbook of the Medical Sciences, Vol. 7, 1904) This is an exceedingly important link in the explanation of osteopathic lesion. Moreover, degenerations of a secondary character may occur in those systems of neurons which are more or less dependent upon the peripheral sensory neuron system for their impulses. (Delafield & Prudden—A Handbook of Pathological Anatomy and Histology). This is equally true with the central motor neuron, or any neuron. It shows how far-reaching is a degenerative process, and also how far-reaching its effects may be. It further makes clear that nerve intactness is directly and absolutely dependent upon a normal circulation; and that it is self-evident any blockage to either blood vessels or to neurons will vitally affect those tissues that govern and control the life processes of the body.

The above is presented so the student may see how osteopathic spinal lesions, if deeply seated and effective enough, can involve remote tissues and organs. No one will doubt that fractures and complete dislocations of the spinal column will seriously affect visceral life, or that a prolapsed kidney will be a cause of nutritive disturbance, or a displaced uterus the cause of ovarian congestion, or a dislocated hip the cause of atrophy of the leg muscles. It has remained for the osteopath to offer proof that slight misplacements of the vertebrae or ribs, incipient curvatures, postural defects, slight deformities, and unsymmetrical bodies are of sufficient etiological importance on the physical plane to affect neuron integrity and obstruct artery courses, and thus organic life.

The question at once arises, what is the immediate or direct effect upon blood vessel or nerve of the osseous, ligamentous, muscular, visceral or composite lesion? The osseous lesion will be initially taken as a distinct type. The direct effect is usually one of hyperemia or ischemia, generally the former. As physiologists and clinicians observe irritation commonly precedes debility. In the vertebral and rib lesions, the effect is to exert direct pressure upon the spinal nerve at its spinal foramen exit, or on the sympathetic chain directly contiguous to the heads of the ribs. This causes congestion, inflammation, ecchymosis, and degeneration of the nerve fiber, followed by macroscopic and microscopic changes as connective tissue proliferations, arterial scleroses, etc.

Thus the cells sensitive to altered vascular changes are directly and remotely affected, and disease characteristics dependent upon structure and function of tissue, and degree of irritant, are evident. This can vary, in degree only, with the muscular lesion that irritates sympathetic life, or the composite lesion that deforms or perverts structure en masse.

But is the physical noxa as potent an etiologic factor as the chemical or bacteriological? Adami (Inflammation, Allbutt's System of Medicine, Vol. I, 1898), informs us that whether an irritant is physical, bacterial or chemical, no satisfactory distinction can be founded on the duration of the irritation. A local irritation of the nervous system may lead apart from direct reflex action, to changes of nervous origin in the region of the injury, and in the reflexes affecting associated regions, and the higher centers. Through them the system at large may become affected by paths that are not always easy to trace. Again he says that centrifugal impulses alone, apart from any local injury, may originate a succession of phenomena of inflammation in a part. And in all probability a nervous and central origin must be ascribed to some, at least, of the sympathetic inflammations seen to occur in areas supplied by the other branches of the nerve supplying a part primarily inflamed. Again, this is evident in areas supplied from the same region of the brain or cord as the inflamed organ.

Other inflammatory changes, of course, may occur independently of centrifugal nervous influences, and the vessels react independently of central influences.

This presents a situation postulated thus:

1. The body follows definite structural relationships and is influenced by mechanical arrangements in its morphology.
2. The integrity of tissue depends upon structural freedom of nutritive courses.
3. The above predicates a structural etiology as exact and precise as structural relationships are important to nutrition.

What proof then of the foregoing have we to offer?

Firstly, the clinical proof. Clinical results have been obtained in tens of thousands of cases that include disease of various types and lesions, and of all sections and organs of the body. The art of osteopathy has been perfected in many of its details, based upon actual experience and splendid results. The cure of the patient is paramount to all other considerations, and whereas the osteopathic school has been shown a superior system, it logically follows on a priori grounds that relief and cure of suffering is of the first and final importance.

Were it not for clinical results no new system of therapeutics could withstand criticism and calumny and finally triumph and be publicly, legislatively, and scientifically recognized.

Secondly, the autopsy proof. Many dissections have been made and autopsies held with the view of discovering the character and the potency of the osteopathic lesion. This very important work has borne out the osteopathic theory of disease. Vertebral and rib displacements have been noted, corresponding ligamentous tissues thickened, associated nerve tracts and vascular channels disturbed, and finally the related organ found diseased. (Clark—Applied Anatomy)

Thirdly, the experimental proof. Experimental proof appeals, logically, to the scientific mind. This proof (McConnell—The Osteopathic Lesion, Journal of the American Osteopathic Association, Sept. and Dec., 1905, May and August 1906; Burns—Partial Report of Experiments upon Visceral Reflexes, The Osteopathic World, Aug., 1905; Pearce—Some Laboratory Demonstrations of Osteopathic Principles, The Osteopathic Physician, November 1905) has not been extensively developed, but what has been accomplished is worthy of attention, conclusive as far as attempted, and no doubt the near future will present substantial additions.

Experimental investigation has been successfully carried out upon dogs, cats, rabbits, and guinea pigs. The experiments conclusively proved that not only spinal inhibitory and stimulatory manipulations (mechanical) were productive of immediate physiological changes in the viscera, but that the structural anatomical lesion or noxa was an important factor in the etiologic field. Pathological changes in several organs directly followed the artificially produced vertebral and rib lesions, showing beyond doubt the reality and effectiveness of the osteopathic lesion. This emphasizes the point that centrifugal impulses originate an inflammation in a previously healthy and uninjured tissue or viscus. And as "inflammatory phenomena may be sympathetically developed in regions innervated from the same area in the brain or spinal cord", it remains to prove the actuality of vertebral and rib lesions, i.e., structural perversions, really affect contiguous nerve courses and vascular channels. This has been demonstrated in laboratory experiments and at the autopsy. Consequently the vertebral, rib, or other lesion may be an important etiologic factor either to the nerve strand from cord or brain to viscous, or from viscous to cord or brain.

Dr. Still says in his *Autobiography* "that all nerves depend wholly on the arterial system for their qualities, such as sensation, nutrition and motion, even though by the law of reciprocity they furnish force, nutrition and sensation to the artery itself." It matters little in this outline whether or not the obstruction to nervous integrity is by way of an impinged artery or by direct pressure, or both, for the primary consideration is the noting that the osteopathic lesion is a real and potent factor of disease. Sajous (Internal Secretions and the Principles of Medicine, Vol. 1, 1903) informs us that "a neuron is directly connected with the circulation (via neuroglia-fibers) by one or more of its dendrites, which serve as channels for blood plasma". A neuron receives its nutrition directly from the general circulation, and from the axon the blood passes into a lymph space connected with a vein. Thus, in reality a part of the circulatory system is that of the entire cerebrospinal system.

It has not been the purpose of this section to go into details, but rather to follow logically an outline of osteopathic etiology and pathology. The various details will be found in the osteopathic works on principles as well as in the experimental articles referred to. It should be understood that the osteopath believes thoroughly in vis medictrix naturae, whether the indications are for stimulation or inhibition, or for the basic readjustment. Generally speaking, however, therapeutic philosophy resolves itself (ultimately) into the principle that a cure depends upon giving an impetus to impaired, habitual and latent forces. In the osteopathic field this implies fundamentally adjustive manipulation, whereby the resultant impetus or physiological stimulus is initiated.

In a word, osteopathy premises that the body is a vital and physical mechanism subject to derangements, structural alterations, functional changes, as results of violence on the mechanical plane, as well as disturbances on the psychic and the biochemical planes. Hence, Osteopathic philosophy is inclusive of preventive, palliative and curative measures.

The Osteopathic Philosophy of Ernest Eckford Tucker[5]

The science of osteopathy is the most exacting technical study in the world. The practical side of osteopathy is its technique. The spirit in which it should be approached is that of technical training.

Good exponents of the science state that it requires not less than a year to be at all confident in the matter of diagnosis alone, except in the more obvious disorders. That is, it takes a year to make a good beginning in diagnosis, the first step in osteopathy. To develop a matured and efficient technique is a matter of years or a decade.

Without adequate diagnosis, much can be done for a patient by stretching, passive motion and stimulation, the so-called general treatment, but this is not osteopathy. With the adequate diagnosis, some means can usually be found, even if slow and uncertain, to affect a restoration. But this is not true osteopathy. With adequate diagnosis, some means can usually be found, even if slow and uncertain, to affect a restoration. But this is not true osteopathy.

True osteopathy consists of adequate diagnosis and adequate technique. Adequate diagnosis consists of thorough and practiced knowledge of the structures of the parts

5. Ernest Eckford Tucker, *Osteopathic Technic* (New York: Clinton Press, 1917).

of the body, a trained perception of touch and muscle sense and other senses used in physical examination, and a trained imagination. Adequate technique consists of thorough and trained knowledge of the movements, tensions of ligaments and muscle, limitations to motion, changes of motion, leverages, etc., of the parts of the body. Also required is a trained muscle sense and a well cultivated mechanical instinct. This is the perquisite for an osteopathic foundation. To it must be added the mechanics of lesions, the principles of technique, and some training in actual forms of technique that illustrate these principles. If at all possible the student should be made acquainted with some of the different forms of technique developed by different physicians.

This is not a thing to be acquired in a term or from a book. All of the time spent in the school is not too much to devote to the subject. It requires also personally supervised and criticized individual instruction. This may seem severe and exacting. I venture to say, however, that the majority of experienced practitioners in the field will say that not less, but rather more than this, should be required.

Why Exacting

There are three reasons why the science of osteopathic technique is so exacting if it is to be at all efficient. The first is that it deals with structures covered by skin and muscle and often fat. Among these structures it is necessary to locate disorders, and having located, to define them in all possible ways. Having located and defined the lesions, to devise some logical technique of correction, using such few and narrow holds thereon as nature affords. The second reason is simply that the health, happiness and life itself of human beings depends on the skill that can be exercised in that narrow field.

Our sole immediate contact with disease, the one thing that makes the rest of the knowledge that we have acquired effective at all, is this one thing—technical skill. The third reason is that the sense of touch and the muscle sense are but feebly developed in human beings.

Still's Technic

Dr. Still in training himself for the work of his life used to carry the bones in his pocket, where his hand could feel them, forming thus a sense-of-touch picture of them. Hour by hour he experimented with them until he had formed a moving picture of them in his mind. He also spent months and years in dissecting the bodies of the Indians, preserved in salt. The amount of time and concentration that he put into making mental pictures of the anatomy of the living body may be surmised from the fact that when he was seventy-five years old he still "camped in the liver" for a week or a month. He daily explored, as a research worker would explore, recesses in the human anatomy. Perhaps forty years were thus spent before he came before the world with his discoveries.

A very large part of the training that he gave to his immediate pupils, in the early days of the science, was in the practical subject of technique.

History

Much of the technical training of Still survives in the profession, spreading hand-to-mouth as it were. The profession, however, and the schools have made no special effort to preserve it. They have not always kept clearly in view the exacting nature of the training necessary for true corrective work. They have been exceedingly busy the last decade in absorbing, digesting, and adapting to osteopathic philosophy the accumulated medical learning (all, that is, except experimental medicine), and in meeting pre-existing medical standards in every way. This was perhaps a necessary phase of the evolution of the science and the profession. Technic, however, has remained an art, an individual and an empirical matter. There has been neither a model in the medical world, nor a great leader among ourselves. The phrases such as "Find it, fix it, and leave it alone," and "Ten-fingered osteopathy," have been rallying calls for the purity of osteopathy, rather than for the development of technique. And yet osteopathic technique is the only medium between our scientific knowledge and the diseases it should benefit.

New Rallying Call

A new rallying call is needed for the profession: "No osteopathic physician is any better than his technique." The profession as a whole is no better than the standards that it sets in this, the practical side of its work. As the twig is bent the tree will incline, so the proportion of time spent on this subject in the schools will determine largely the amount of attention it will be given by physicians.

Popular Conceptions

There is another excellent reason for putting stress on technical training. That concerns itself with the parasitic imitators of osteopathy.

First, note that the philosophy of the matter is extremely simple. Moreover, those simple rallying calls of our past have emphasized the simplicity of pure osteopathy, and rightly no doubt. Note then that much can be done by perfectly obvious methods, and perhaps every case can be helped to some degree by measures dangerously simple and obvious. The field is broad for the most superficial methods, so long as they simply stimulate or "get motion"; and many there be that wander therein. Lastly, note that the exacting nature of the technical requirements for true osteopathic work are by no means obvious to patients or to general public. The public wonder, therefore, whether it is worth the fees charged for it. Add all these together and let them get planted in the public mind, and we have the reason for the easy success and popular acceptance of the shallow imitator, and a condition leading rapidly to the sinking of genuine osteopathy.

Says Dr. Fleck: "The corrective principle is so potent that anybody practicing it on even a hit-or-miss basis is sure to get some sort of results and so can get away with it." Our proper answer to the illegitimate practitioner and the fakir is to lay increasing emphasis on the technical training requirement for doctors of osteopathy, in schools and in publicity, until it has become generally understood.

Ideals

The ideal training in technique would be one that began with the first day in school and continued till the last. Knowledge of anatomy is presupposed before study of technique can begin. It should be put to immediate use, the very day it is acquired, in relation with the sense of touch, the sense of measurement, the muscle sense, and in forming a living and moving picture of all the parts of the body. In this way the real object of the study is in view from the first. The study of anatomy for osteopathic students also should begin with the part where osteopathic thinking begins—with the spine.

The student mind will take on the average just what is given it and no more—usually a little less—and in just the form in which it is given. This the student will try to utilize in therapeutics in the most obvious sort of way. There is little initiative in the average human being, and in any case it is unfair to demand it and rely upon it. It is therefore an ideal of technique that the parts of anatomy as they are studied should be immediately referred to the living body where alone the knowledge is useful. They should be outlined on the surface and practice, so outlining should be provided. Practice should include locating them by the sense of touch with the eyes blindfolded. The sense of measurement should be cultivated by measurements first with tape line, followed by examination with the fingers to verify the tape line examination. This should be done in erect and flexed position.

The senses of touch and measurement being as a rule so weakly developed in human beings, it should be the constant endeavor to educate them to a state of osteopathic proficiency. Psychology tells us that some persons are eye-minded, some ear-minded, some touch-minded—the latter vastly in the minority. This sense then suffers an actual handicap in a curriculum that consists so largely of reading, of pictures and of lectures. Being so weak in civilized beings, this sense is subject to bizarre variations. Dr. White tells how he discovered by accident that things felt larger to his right hand than to his left. I have noted extreme variations between different osteopathic physicians in their interpretation of certain conditions. In justice to the student, these anomalies should all be discovered and normalized or discounted. Training that should develop tactile sensitivity should also provide a minimal normalized level of this sensitivity in the graduated osteopathic physician.

So numerous are the elements that go into a perfect technique that they should be taken up one at a time and woven gradually into the composite sense of technique.

Those who leave the osteopathic schools bearing the credentials of the profession take its reputation in their hands. It is the right of those who have labored to build that reputation to insist that those into whose hands they put this reputation shall be sufficiently well trained in the distinctive osteopathic subjects to be able to uphold and advance the cause of osteopathy.

First Principles

The first principle of Osteopathic technique is not to hurt the patient. That this is at all times difficult and sometimes impossible will be admitted, since quite some force must at times be used, since the structures are held together by high tension. For their protection, nature has provided nerves that are quite sensitive to any threatening force, and also they are at times quite sensitive from the abnormal state they are in. But this too must be evident, that it is at all times impossible without such a technical knowledge to use only the minimum force. Also to use it without awkwardness to the actual mechanical factors in the case. Without this knowledge, there is sure to be a very great amount of unnecessary pain and a great exaggeration of the really necessary treatment pain.

For this reason, experience in being treated is also a necessity in the preparation for osteopathic work, in order that the practitioner may be able to see from the patient's point of view. I find that I am always more gentle with my patients after I have been myself recently treated. But familiarity breeds contempt. Not ourselves feeling the pain, and the patient feeling that it is "up to him" to endure what he believes to be necessary. We all can allow our methods to grow more and rougher, intent only on the effort at correction and not on the feelings of the patient.

And the second principle of osteopathic technique is not to hurt the patient. For in order to cure it is necessary to retain the patient. For every case that is lost to the profession through failure to cure, there are many lost through roughness in handling, through pain caused by the treatment. A great many practitioners, in order not to hurt, ignore the correction of lesions, or largely ignore it, and resort to simple stimulation. They at least retain the patients longer, only to lose them eventually through failure to cure, or through too great a cost of the treatment. Some also follow the "general treatment" method, through failure or ability to make diagnosis of mechanical disorders. It is safe to say that but for these two failures the profession would by this time have been immeasurably farther along the road to general acceptance. Both are failures in technique.

The third principle of osteopathic technique also is not to hurt the patient. The success of technique depends on the relaxation of the patient, and this becomes impossible if fear or motor reflexes are excited by pain. It was Dr. Harry Still who used to remark facetiously that if the patient could relax sufficiently, he could move any bone any distance. When God punishes us for our sins, it is not His punishments, but our resistance that hurts. So is it in the corrective work. With a proper technique the only pain that the patient need suffer in the majority of cases is such as comes from his own resistance. To secure that "relaxation" is the first art of the practitioner. If there be contractures, then these must of course be relaxed. But the voluntary contractions are always to be obviated. The success of a proper technique is in direct ratio to success in this. First there are the mechanical instincts of the body which oppose force with force. To offset this, the practitioner must endeavor to secure relaxation by gentleness, and must win confidence with evidence of care. Conspicuous carefulness and impressive caution are all within the limits of positive and convincing work. With an assured technique this is not difficult. It is the bungler who excites the patient's resistance. But often some definite training of the patient's muscles in the art of relaxing is necessary.

And the fourth principle of osteopathic technique is the same—not to hurt the patient, and not to increase his nervous excitement by fear. There is such a thing as disease-fear. This is the fear of the subconscious mind when a state of disease exists in the body. Although sometimes this very fear enables the patient to yield to and endure things that it would be impossible to yield to in a state of self-confident health. Yet also it may act to magnify the ill results of ungentleness on the part of the physician. The nervous system is always in a state of excitement in disease. The immediate shock of correction may at times be unfavorable.

The nerve strain from a continuing lesion is always greater than the shock of correction, provided correction is actually obtained. It is better to correct with shock if necessary than to allow the lesion to remain. But there is no excuse for making any more shock than is absolutely necessary at any time.

It is usually desirable to make the first treatment as light as possible, an educative sort of a treatment. To the patient visiting a new doctor and trying a new form of treatment, this will seem heavy in any case. It seems wise to explain to the patient that there is likely to be some soreness or stiffness from the first manipulation of the deep tissues of his body. To explain why—just as there is likely to be stiffness from the first day's skating or any unaccustomed form of exercise. Following treatments may be made heavier as needed, and "little soreness from the treatment itself is to be looked for after the second or third treatment."

Etiology Of Lesions And Principles Of Technique

With the description of the sacroiliac lesion before us for illustration, it is possible for us to consider the etiology of lesions and the principles of technique. To some extent the conditions of the sacroiliac lesion are true of all lesions—that are of all primary, direct or traumatic lesions—as distinguished from warp or habit lesions. The contrast between these two and a more detailed description of individual lesions will be given later. The general principles only will occupy us now.

Primary lesions are due to a sudden straining of an articulation beyond its normal range of motion so that it is unable to return spontaneously. There is then found to be a double deviation, a deviation in two directions—from mid position, as though having reached the limit of normal motion—and being strained farther—it turned in some abnormal way. In such position the articular surfaces are no longer parallel, but assume an angle to each other. Some part of one side then engages against the opposite surface, and makes a dent, so that when released it does not slide back normally. Under the tension of the stretched ligaments, one side assumes an even sharper angle, restrained by the dent it has made. The ligaments, radially disposed, permit this abnormal motion, and even provide for the secondary deviation. In the resulting position the fibers of this ligament are not necessarily all stretched, but possibly only a few of the fibers are stretched, the rest relaxed. The factors in lesion then are motion beyond normal under high tension, assuming an angle and indentation of a surface by a projecting portion.

There is also high tension of part or all of the restraining ligaments, and in partially returning toward normal, the assuming of a position still farther from normal. The principles of technique here described apply to all such lesions. They are necessarily mechanical principles, and are exceedingly obvious as principles, though not so easy in application as they are of understanding.

First, it is necessary to have tension or pressure or fixation on both of the bones involved in lesion, as is found on both the sacrum and ilium.

Since, however, it is rarely possible to take hold of the two bones, and in most cases is impossible to get effective hold of either of them, as in the dorsal and lumbar spine, it is therefore necessary to use other factors. These are positions in which there is ligamentous drag on the one, through the weight of the body, and motions in which all of the joints are at the limit of their motion, between the lesion and the point that can be taken hold of. This principle—that joints must be at the limit of their possible normal motion before corrective force can be transmitted through them or made effective on them—is the point that seems to me most neglected, and to be responsible for most of the failures in technique. As, for instance, it is necessary to have all of the joints of the spine and of the shoulder at the limit of their motion before tension can be transmitted through them to the sacrum.

Third, it is necessary to so direct this tension or pressure so that it comes to a focus at the point desired. As in breaking a stick held in the two hands, it is possible to break it in the middle or near either end by differently adjusting the force of the two hands. So it is in directing the force of correction.

For instance, in the first technique described for correction of an anterior sacral lesion, if the pressure of the left arm is over the middle of the crest instead of over the anterior superior spine, the effect is not to cause gapping of the lesion, but to cause increased pressure over the point in lesion. The technique then takes effect at the last lumbar joint. If the spine is flexed, the effect of rotation of the shoulder backward is to cause strain at the apex of the posterior curve rather than at the point desired.

Fourth, it is necessary to direct the force to release the engaged part from its indentation against the opposite surface. This is similar to pressing down on the anterior superior spine where the articulation is gapped open in the back, the front edge therefor being the fulcrum. To do this it is usually necessary to use one part of the articulation as the fulcrum to move the other part. In a rotated dorsal vertebra, for instance, the engaged side is the side toward which rotation has occurred. In a spine rotated to the right, the articular surface on the right is caught in flexion, and the left side extends alone, producing secondary rotation to the right. To release this lesion, it is necessary to carry the left side to the limit of its motion, and with that limitation as a fulcrum, to gap open and release the engaged part.

Fifth, with all articulations at their limit and the leverage adjusted, a quick spring is much more effective than steady force. It needs only a fraction of the force, with less danger of injury to the soft parts, and gives a cleaner and more perfect correction. This is because the parts engaged are elastic. The quickness of the spring should be in proportion to the elasticity. It is also easier to apply just the right degree of force, calculated beforehand, in the quick spring than in steady pressure. A quick and shallow springing motion does not go so far beyond the instant of actual correction as a steady force, because in the latter it is impossible to calculate the moment of release, and so to check the corrective force.

Meaning of the "Pop"

The instant of correction of a lesion is usually indicated by a "pop." This is not always the case. Also the pop may signify the making as well as the correction of a lesion. Let us examine the mechanical factors in the "pop." In the lesion we have articular surfaces at an angle with each other, and some edge of one surface engaged against the other surface. This makes an indentation or a wrinkle of the tissue, by which it is held as a lesion.

But this means that whereas at one point there is compression, at another there is separation.

A vacuum or at best negative pressure, "suction" as we would call it, is a potential vacuum. What fills this potential vacuum? The tissue of the joint we will remember is elastic. It is compressible, but it is also expansible. Gas or fluid may collect there under the differential pressure, but also the tissue may expand to fill the negative space. All of the bony tissue involved is under high pressure from the stretched ligament, whose elastic tension holds them in their false position. As Dr. McConnell discovered, if all of the ligaments of a joint be cut, the lesion will correct itself. When, therefore, under the sudden spring of the corrective force the engaged point is released, the readjustment takes place under all of these elastic forces. The "pop" is in proportion to the suddenness of the release and the degree of elastic tension of the ligaments and of the elasticity of the tissues compressed.

These principles of correction may be thus summarized:

To transmit force, articulations must be at the limit of their motion. Effort must be properly focused on the lesion. It must be so directed so as to release the engaged points. One side of a joint is used as a fulcrum for the other. Elastic spring is used to overcome the elasticity of parts.

Many physicians carefully avoid the "spring" technique, finding it painful and giving a shock to the patient. They use a technique that involves so stretching the ligaments that release comes spontaneously. If cutting off all of the ligaments allows a lesion to correct itself, so will sufficient stretching of them achieve the same result?

Meanwhile the patient profits by the stimulation that comes from the stretching. The choice here is between the radical technique with positive results and the gentle technique with much greater expenditure of labor, but less pain to the patient, and less immediate results, with greater danger of recurrence. Probably a combination of the two is best. Our purpose at present is to build a mental picture of the mechanics of lesions and their correction, for which purpose the radical technique is described. Different description of the gentle technique is not necessary. It consists in a gentler modification of the radical technique. The principle of this gentler technique is like that of moving a heavy barrel, by very slightly tilting one side and then rolling it.

With a clear picture of all the leverages, with a practiced control of all tension, and with persevering practice, this gentler and more ideal technique may be mastered.

The Osteopathic Philosophy and Principles of Anne Wales, D.O.[6]

Most of the time we talk about osteopathy in terms of articular or skeletal dysfunction.

Osteopathic articular dysfunction, being primarily an unbalanced tension of the ligaments with strain as the usual cause, is corrected mainly through the agency of the ligaments themselves. The natural tendency of the body is to revert to normal when the balance is restored and the factors preventing the return are removed. It will be noted that as a rule, gliding separation of the joint surfaces is used to tense the ligaments in vertebral, sacroiliac, carpal and tarsal dysfunctions.

Fulcrum leverage for disengagement is employed in dysfunctions of the long bones, combined with exaggeration of the dysfunction position in those of the extremities. The principle of fascial treatment is to lift the fascia at its more dependent part, the patient cooperating. Dr. Sutherland's technique seems a radical departure to most of us. It avoids the familiar thrusting and popping of joints. However, it is based upon the fundamental principles of osteopathy as conceived by Dr. Still, and accords with his admonition that osteopathic technique should be gentle, easy and scientific.

It's something beyond what begins the strain, and the result is in the skeletal mechanics, and which is not resolved during sleep or action. We collect these things every day in our waking moments and in our various activities. Most are resolved by the positions we take during sleep, and what doesn't resolve gets reorganized when we wake up and get about our business. Action calls for the 'normal' from the body, so the thing that doesn't respond to that call is an osteopathic lesion or a strain in the mechanism. That's what we treat. It's the thing that hangs on and hangs in there, not the thing that brings it on. But it's useful to

6. Transcription of videos provided by Stephen McGowan, D.O. (Australia).

understand that this ligamentous articular strain, membranous articular strain or vascular mechanism strain, or whatever we call it, is an osteopathic lesion. We use the word lesion more than the orthodox medical literature does so there's been a lot of criticism about that in the past. But it's still useful to have one word that says what you're talking about. I liked it when Will [William Garner Sutherland] gave this other terminology that described it as a mechanical problem in a mechanical mechanism, and that the mechanism resolves the problem if you balance all its parts in action. Everybody at that time was trying to put into words what Will meant by the increased tension which unbalanced the joint, because by the time you find it, it's stuck there like a bureau of drawers is stuck in its slot. How you realign the bureau drawer is to take it out of that position, realign it, and push it in. Well, that's about all you're doing with these joints, but you have to know your anatomy in order to know how to use this balanced state to release the strain in the mechanism.

Now with a bureau of drawers, if you just tried to push it in you'd keep making a dent that makes a groove in the alignment. You have to realign it before it can go back into its track. But you know, it's not fashionable to think mechanically or to talk mechanically and that's why we're 100 years old and still working on the frontier.

To say the most neutral position is to say the balanced position. You may describe the same thing in another way. The thing which I was still working on and to grasp is what is this "beautiful balance"? All the tensions have been reduced to the absolute minimum in this neutral position of balanced tension. It's the function of the ligaments to move the bones. Muscles also move the bones, but in the first place the shape of the articular surface governs the motion that occurs at a particular joint. Then the ligaments that are around that joint and hold those bones together are arranged so as to permit the motion in the joint. The limiting factors are the anatomical limits, which prevent the joint from moving other than it should. The muscles which are related to the motion at this joint have a tone which creates a further limit on the excursion. They are the agents of voluntary mobility. They are part of the neuromuscular system which moves the skeletal system according to what the person decides to do.

When muscles have the framework within which they function, their origin and insertion in the skeletal framework, changed sufficiently so that the distance between the origin and insertion is shortened, then the muscle or muscles will contract. If the distance between the origin and insertion is lengthened, they will lengthen as they become fibrotic. They can't contract. We address the mechanical problems in the skeletal system as a mechanism in order to make it possible for the neuromuscular system to be at ease.

Now in today's world, and in much of the custom of the osteopathic profession in the past, there has been much said about preparation for the technique to resolve the joint situation. So it was called 'soft tissue work' to relax the muscles. The thing that relaxes the muscles is to change the framework within which they work. But this is the message you're going to take into the future. This tension is in the ligaments which are always tense, and which are non-extensive. They don't stretch, so the positional relationship between the bones at the joint creates the lesion, the ligamentous articular strain, the membranous articular strain. The strain is in the ligaments and in the membranes and in the fascia. I can't tell you how long it took me to understand what Dr. Sutherland meant when he said that, but I think I've got it.

So you balance the tensions in the direction of ease, in the direction of neutral, where all the tensions are reduced to an absolute minimum. This is when the ligaments have their natural power back to move the bones into their normal relationship. But what I don't quite see is how that happens. So I'm not going to talk about what I don't see clearly at this moment.

This balance point, this neutral point, is the fulcrum. You find the fulcrum where you find it. At the moment, you're making your diagnostic survey and that's a working diagnosis for finding the point from which to administer the treatment. When the ligaments move the mechanism from its strained relation you resolve the mechanical problem and the fulcrum gets back to another place, another shift.

The powers within the patient's body are more powerful for the correction of the lesion than anything which you can bring to bear upon it from the outside. So what are powers within the patient's body? Respiration is one of them. The reason for this is power, because the diaphragm is going up and down in the cylinder of the trunk. It's a fascial septa with muscles in it, and of course I was delighted to hear Dr. Willard [Dr. Frank Willard, Ph.D. anatomist at University of New England College of Osteopathic Medicine] say that all the muscles are in the fascial envelopes. Consequently, since the fascia is part of the skeletal system when the muscles change their shape, they pull and act upon the bones of the skeletal system. But in the vertebral column the anterior longitudinal spinal ligament is the mainstream of the trunk. It's attached to the basal process of the occiput at the top and to the body of the sacrum and some sacral vertebra at the bottom, and to all of the vertebra in front and the annular fibrosis in the vertebral discs. The posterior longitudinal spinal ligament in the front of the spinal canal belongs to this column of vertebrae, called the "spinal organ".

The vertebral bodies with their discs, and with their anterior and posterior longitudinal ligaments, are the central core of the anatomy of the trunk. Mabel Elsworth Todd [author of *Thinking Body*, 1937, reprinted 2008] makes a point of that as a tension spring. A line of gravity making contact at the junction of the curves. Everything ventral to the line of gravity is essentially tension and everything dorsal to it is compression. So we bipeds are walking around our two feet in a vertical posture and it's like a tripod. The center of gravity is in front of the sacrum behind the hip joints and that is the center of the tripod. This third leg, the spinal column, is thrown up over the other two. This modified sphere is on top of it. So we have a midline, and a pair of lateral structures illustrated by the ribs.

When Dr. Willard said that, it caught my attention, as he was giving us anatomy slides on the upper extremity. He said the whole of the upper extremity is just plastered onto the sides of the body, one on either side. It's attached to the nuchal line on the back of the occiput, and everything that goes into the mechanics of this upper extremity is there on top of what's underneath. This extends all the way down to the pelvis.

Dr. Sutherland spoke of the core link between the cranial bowl and the pelvic bowl. He was talking about the spinal dura mater which connects the occiput and the sacrum. This vertebral column or column of vertebral bodies, however you want to say it, is a ligamentous articular mechanism and the crura of the diaphragm is attached at the level of the upper lumbar vertebrae to this anterior longitudinal spinal ligament. Every time the diaphragm goes up or down it moves the anterior longitudinal spinal ligament, and that is the midline of the boney part of the appendicular skeletal system. The bones need their joints held together by ligaments. There are tendons and fascia. All the fascia mechanisms ultimately attach to the boney skeleton. So that's why we're osteopaths. That's where you start.

When the physicians come in different sizes, you then think about how the individual physician is related to the individual patient. There are some things which Dr. Sutherland used and taught that I cannot use effectively. So I work with the principles that he taught in my own way. I think that you could use my own "way" to your advantage. It never hurts to learn as many different ways of doing things as possible. Some other osteopaths say "All you have to do is this", and incorporate two or three things in one maneuver. But I can't do that. So it eventually emerges that we're talking about the same thing, only I do it in steps. It's possible to incorporate some procedures in one operation that includes all the steps, but that's not the way I work.

Lippincott's Statements on Dr. Sutherland's Philosophy[7]

Osteopathic lesions are strains of the tissues of the body. When they involve joints it is the ligaments that are primarily affected. So the term "ligamentous articular strain" is the one preferred by Dr. Sutherland. The ligaments of a joint are normally in a state of balanced reciprocal tension, and seldom, if ever, are they completely relaxed throughout the normal range of movement. When the motion is carried beyond that range the tension becomes unbalanced. The elements of the ligamentous structure, which limit motion in that direction, are strained and weakened.

The lesion is maintained by the overbalance of the reciprocal tension by the elements which have not been strained. This locks the articular mechanism, or prevents its free and normal movement. The unbalanced tension causes the bones to assume a position that is nearer that in which the strain was produced than would be the case if the tension were normal. The weakened part of the ligament permits motion in the direction of the lesion in excess of normal. The range of movement in the opposite direction is limited by the more firm and unopposed tension of the elements which have not been strained.

Principles of Corrective Technique

Since it is the ligaments that are primarily involved in the maintenance of the lesion, it is they, not muscular leverage that are used as the main agency for reduction. The articulation is carried in the direction of the lesion, exaggerating the lesion position as far as is necessary to cause the tension of the weakened elements of the ligamentous structure. This is equal to or slightly in excess of the tension of those ligaments that were not strained. This is the point of balanced tension. Forcing the joint to move beyond that point adds to the strain which is already present. Forcing the articulation back and away from the direction of the lesion strains the ligaments that are normal and unopposed. If this is done with thrusts or jerks there is a definite possibility of separating the fibers of the ligaments from their bony attachments. When the tension is properly balanced, the respiratory or muscular cooperation of the patient is employed to overcome the resistance of the defense mechanism of the body to release the lesion. If the patient holds their breath in or out as long as possible, there is a period during the body's involuntary efforts to resume breathing when the release takes place. In appendicular lesions, the patient holds the articulation in the position of exaggeration, and the release occurs through the agency of the ligaments when or just before the muscles are relaxed.

---

7. Howard A. Lippincott, "The Osteopathic Technique of Wm. G. Sutherland," in *Yearbook of the American Academy of Osteopathy* (Chicago: 1949).

There are exceptions to the general principle of correction of exaggerating the lesion position. The disengagement method, with the rib technique as an example, uses a fulcrum upon which leverage tends to separate the bony surfaces and tense the ligamentous connections. This method is combined with exaggeration of the lesion position in treatment of the long bones of the extremities. Under some circumstances, it is unwise to add tension to the involved ligaments, as in the case of a severe strain of recent production. In that event the pain will be increased under exaggeration and the correction is made by holding the more distal bone in the direction of its normal position while the patient participates by gently and slowly moving the proximal bone toward its proper relationship.

This is known as "direct action" technique. It is used in the postural sacroiliac or iliosacral lesion in which the irregularity of the auricular surfaces prevents a wide range of motion, especially on the axis through the second sacral segment.

The participation of the patient in this technique is a matter of importance. If the physician holds the bone which is in lesion, and the patient moves the one upon which it is 'lesioned,' there is less likely to be undue strain placed upon the ligaments than if the physician exerts the force necessary to accomplish a reduction. Considering the lesioned bone as the 'bolt', and the one proximal to it as the 'nut', it is a better mechanical principle for the physician to hold the bolt and allow the patient to turn the nut than for the physician to turn the bolt. The physical equipment needed for this technique is simple. An osteopathic table, a stool and a chair are the main items. The stool should be a minimum height of twenty-one inches or in modern day 'adjustable' for use of this work. Of greatest importance, however, is the mental equipment of the physician, his ability to visualize the structures concerned in the lesion, and the "keen tactile sense common to osteopathic physicians".

2

Techniques for the Head

Tucker's Posterior OA Technique

PHYSICIAN: Standing at the head of the table
PATIENT: Supine

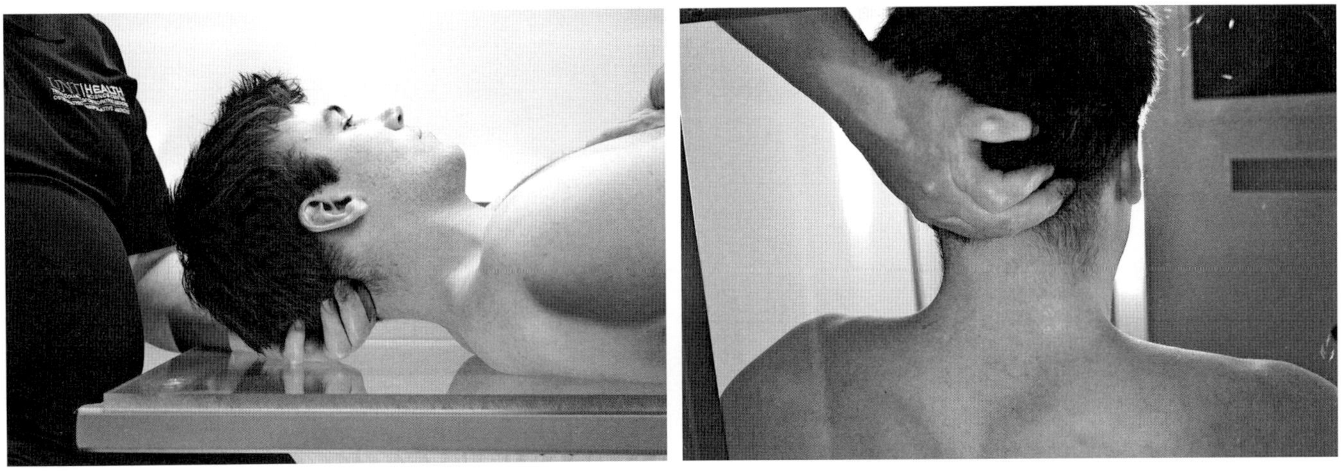

STEP 1

1. Place your left hand under their OA and turn the patient's head to the left side while flexing it, so as to gap open the right side. Then bring the arch of the atlas into prominence on that side

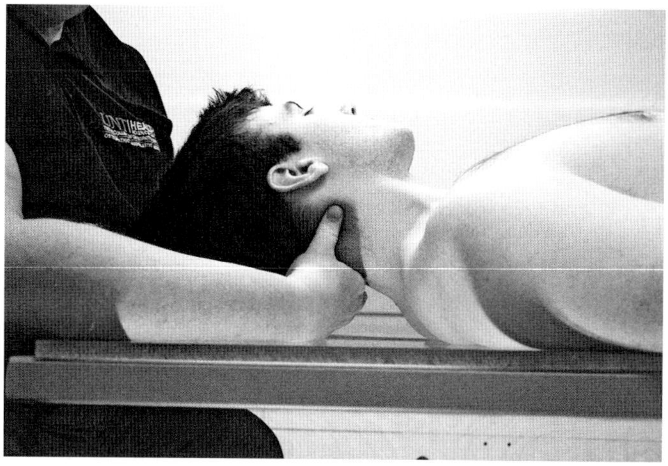

STEP 2

2. Insert your fingers or thumb of your right hand between the arch of their atlas and their occiput until your finger or thumb come into contact with the arch

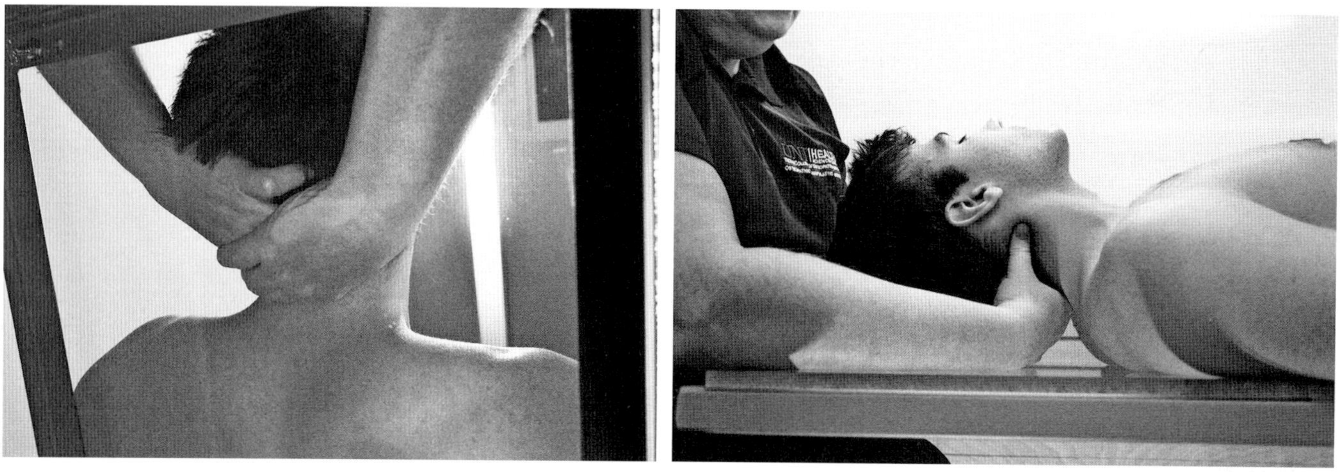

STEPS 3 – 4

3. Maintain pressure on their atlas with your right fingers or thumb and draw their neck back to the limit of motion to the right, until all articulations on the left are tensed
4. With a slight but quick further turning of their head in SLIGHT extension, the bone is lifted into place

Tucker's Posterior OA (Anterior Atlas) Technique

PHYSICIAN: Standing behind the patient
PATIENT: Supine

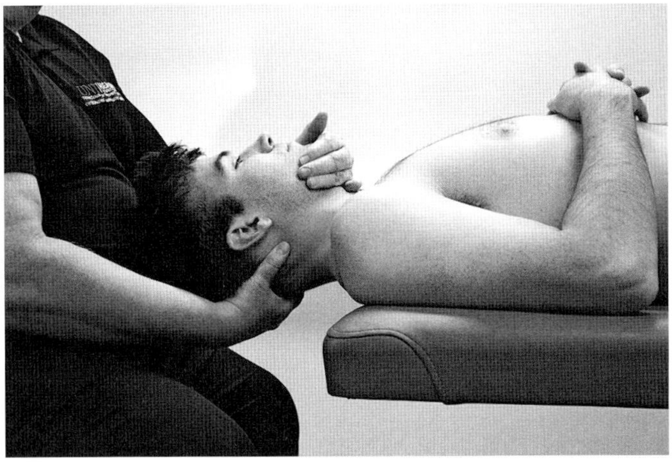

STEPS 1 – 2

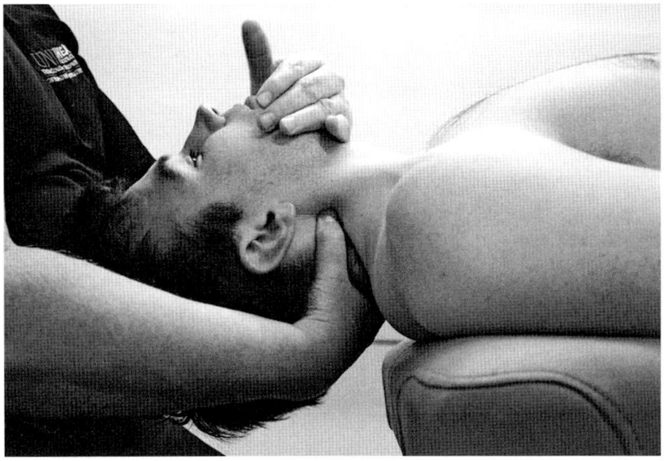

STEP 3

1. Bring their head slightly beyond the top of the table
2. Place your hand under the patient's chin and your other hand under the occiput
3. Lift their head, holding their face upward until the occipito-atlantal articulation is in full extension and the weight of the body of the occiput is dragged downward on the atlas

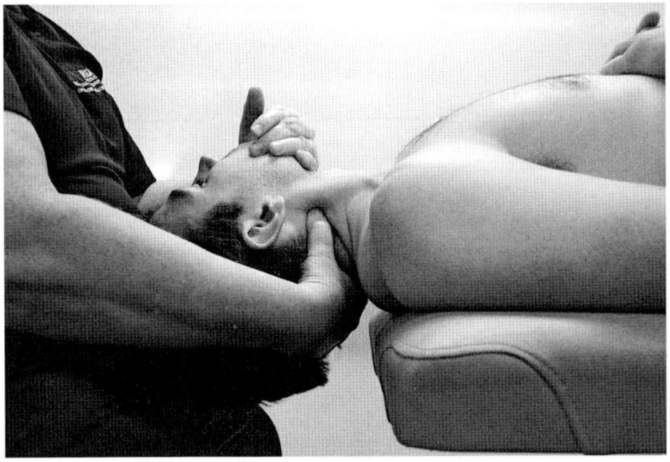

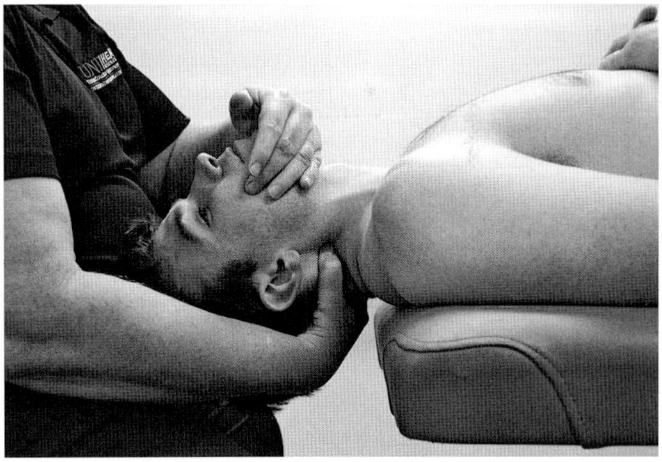

STEP 4

4. Carry the patient's head from side to side, focusing motion at their atlas, gapping open first one side and then the other side, until their atlas moves back to its normal position

OA Release Technique (1938 Yearbook)

"You can also normalize the nerve supply to the pituitary and often the vagus nerve with another technique which I will show you for adjusting the occiput. Most of these cases are curled up in the dorsal area and have the head back. That in itself narrows the chest and the occiput is anterior on their atlas."

PHYSICIAN: Standing beside the patient
PATIENT: Seated

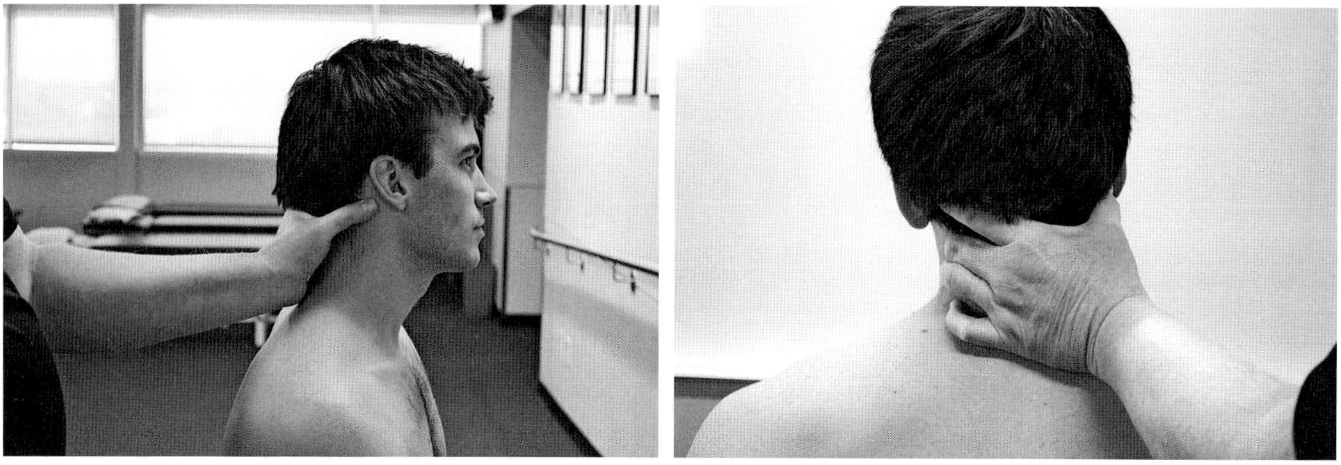

STEP 1

1. Place your left index and long fingers parallel along the articular pillar of their atlas with slight pressure while placing your left thumb in front of their ear. Your fingers should be up under their occiput so you feel the OA joint

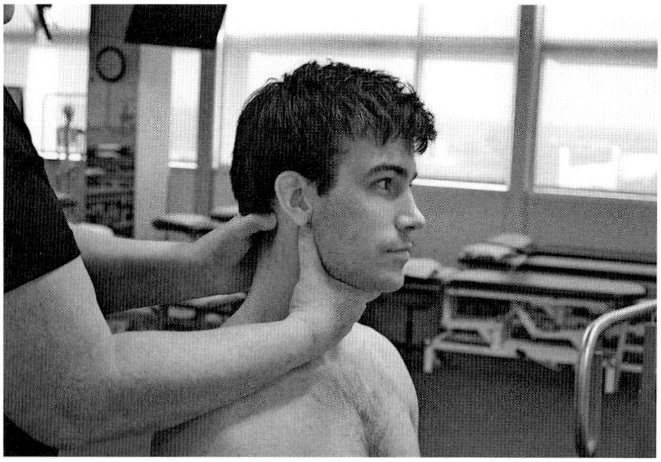

STEP 2

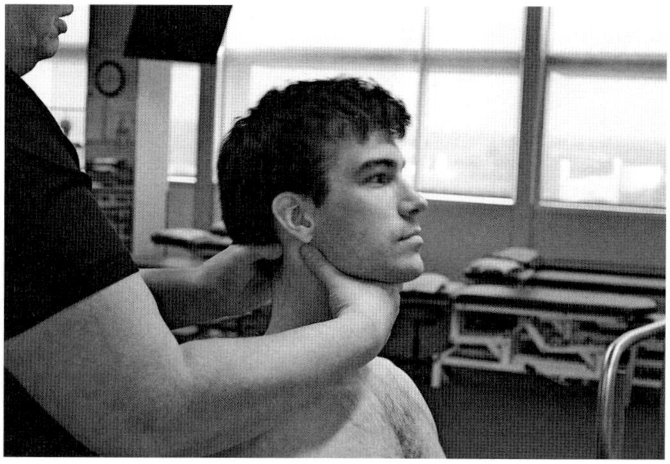

STEP 3

2. Reinforce your left ring and long fingers with your right index and long finger, so the fingers of your right hand are under their occiput and your right thumb is in front of their right ear. You have the joint between the occiput and their atlas so fixed that it alone moves
3. Lift their head cephalad (upward) and rotate their occiput back at the same time

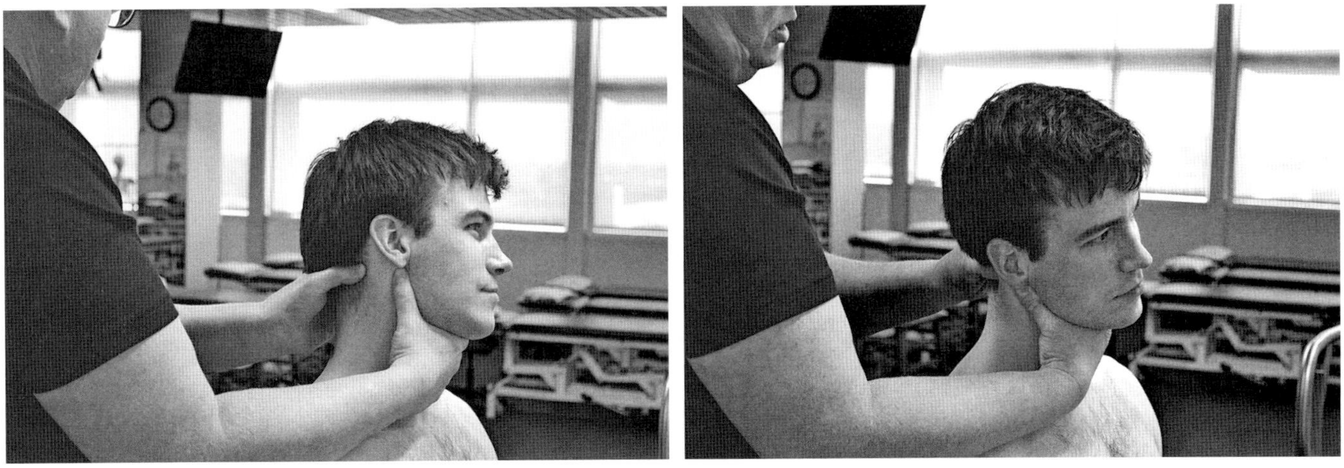

STEP 4

4. You then side-bend left and then right—freeing their sub-occipital musculature

1938 Yearbook: "The physician can feel definite movement directly between the occiput and atlas. You are turning the occiput back. If the occiput slides forward it also extends a little and laterally flexes to the other side. This technique will accomplish three motions—pushes the occiput back, laterally flexes it to the same side, and flexes the head anteriorly by the lift on the occiput."

Wales' Occiput Technique

PHYSICIAN: Seated behind the patient
PATIENT: Supine

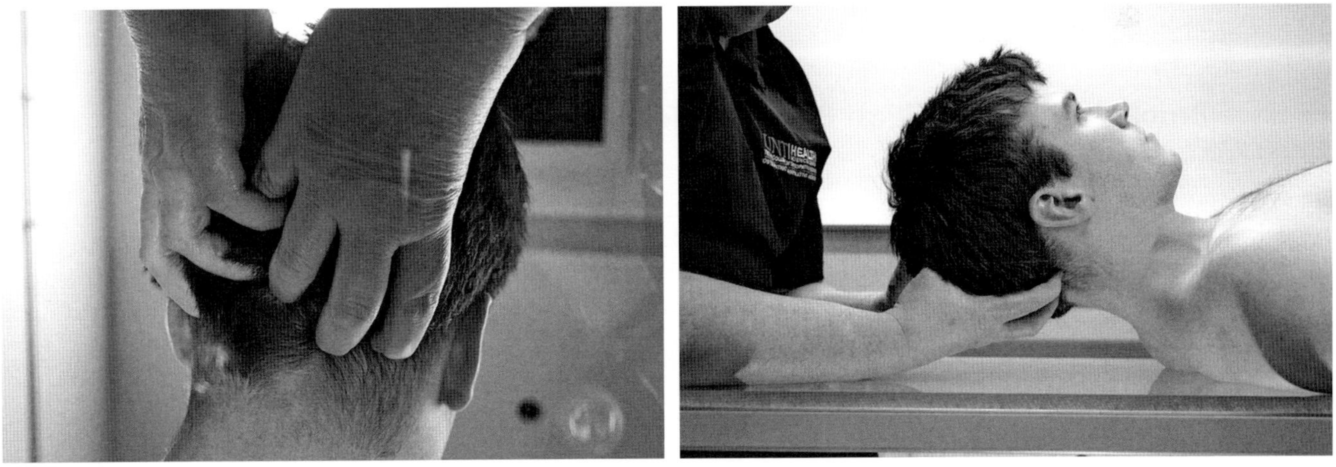

STEP 1

1. Place your thumbs on the patient's opisthion with your fingers cupped around the occiput and the tips of your long fingers on each side in contact with their atlas

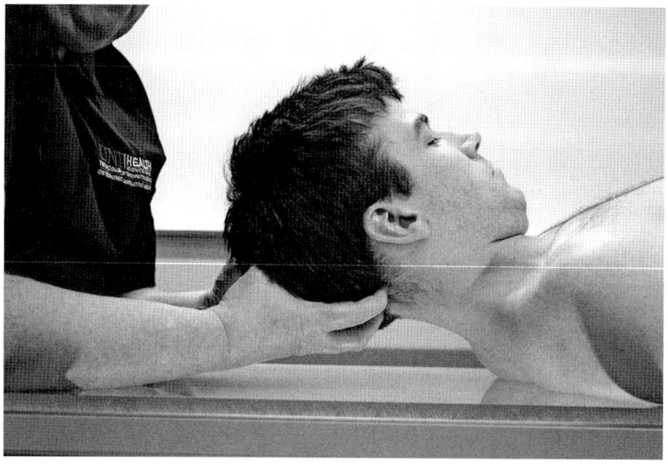

STEPS 2 – 4

2. Ask the patient to nod their head or nod the patient's head while keeping their atlas from moving with their occiput – your fingertips remain in contact with their atlas throughout
3. Their atlas meets your finger, then goes away because the occiput continues to move under the physician's pressure
4. Spread your fingers apart and wait for the release

Wales: All you want to do with the occiput is to have it nod, and to have it flex on the atlas so that the condyles go into the divergences. I find it convenient to have their head in my two hands with the occipital squamous in my hands. Then my two long fingers are at the posterior rim of the foramen magnum ready to meet the atlas. With either hand, I can turn the head to each side. It's a very small nodding motion. This is just what is convenient for me.

Brooks Walker and Elliott Blackman Technique for the Occiput

PHYSICIAN: Seated at the head of the table
PATIENT: Supine

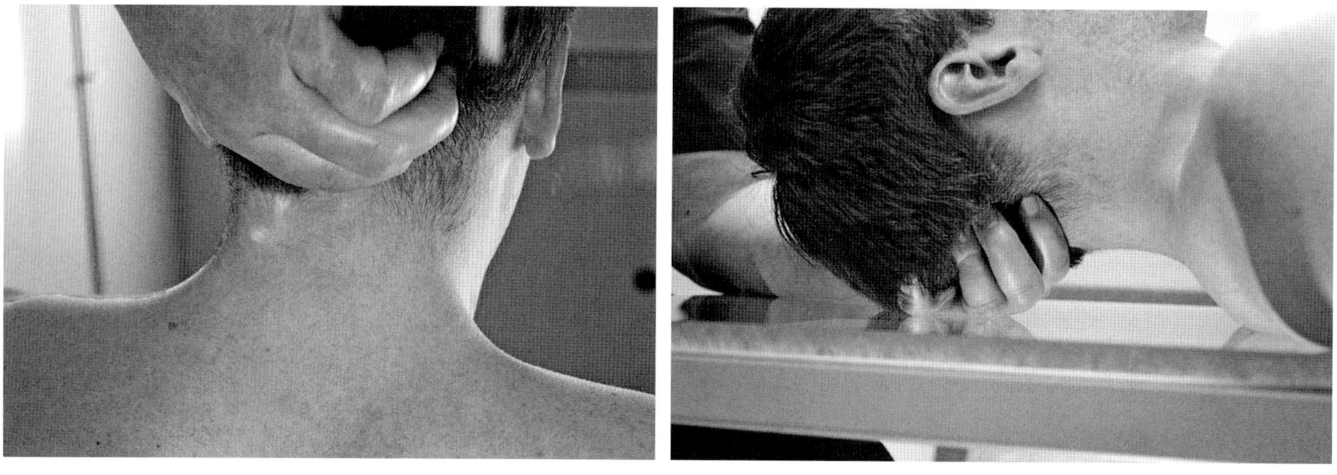

STEP 1

1. With your left hand take hold of the transverse processes of the patient's atlas between the tips of the mastoid processes and the angle of the jaw. Use your thumb on one side of their atlas and your index finger on the other side

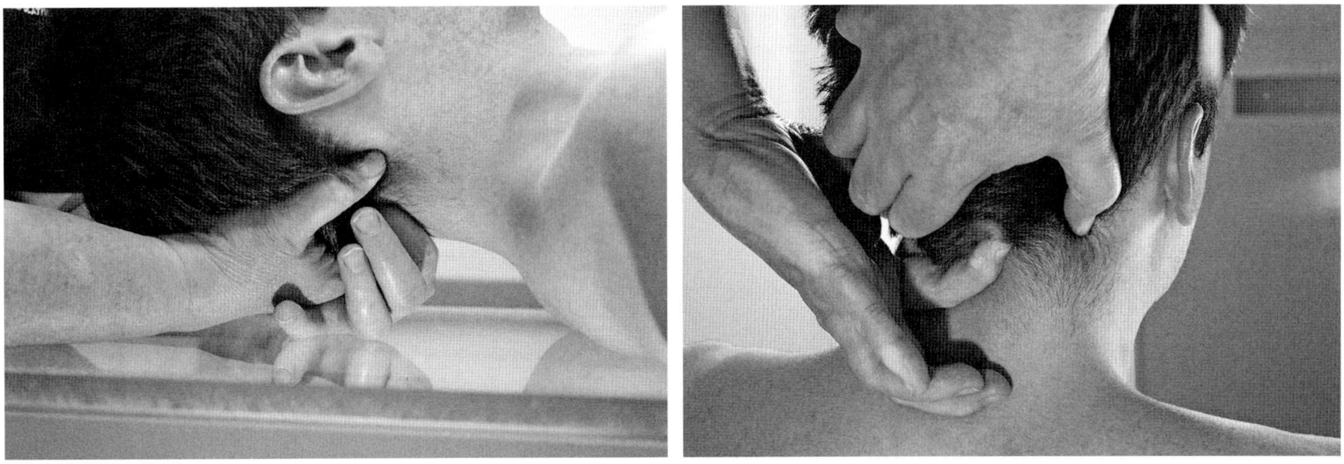

STEP 2

2. Take your right hand and place your thumb and forefinger on the base of their occiput near the foramen magnum

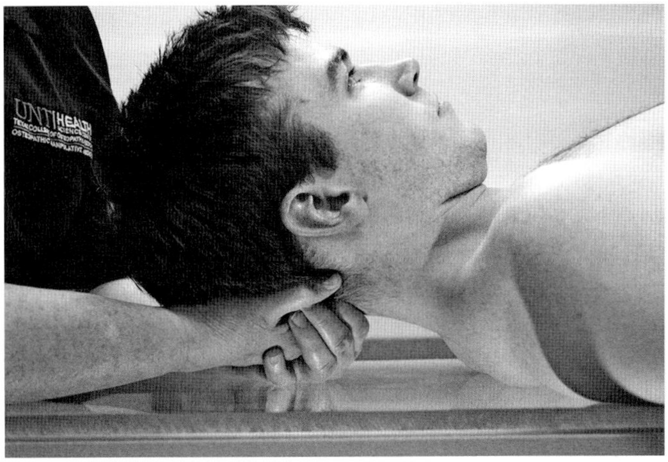

STEP 3

3. Ask the patient to bring their chin onto their chest and then balance the atlas against their occiput

Wales' Technique – the Base Spread

PHYSICIAN: Seated at the head of the table
PATIENT: Supine

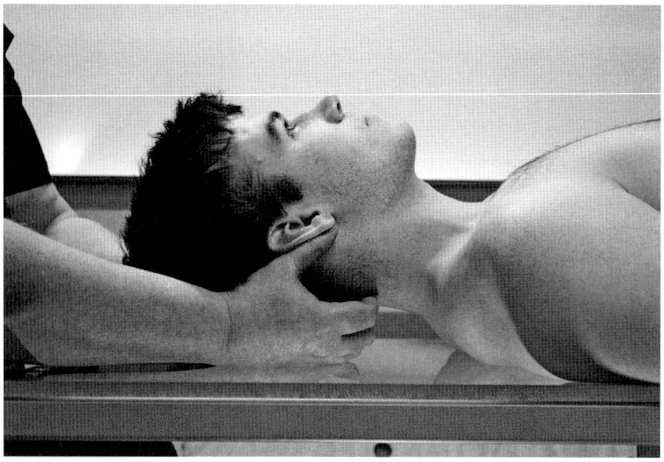

STEP 1

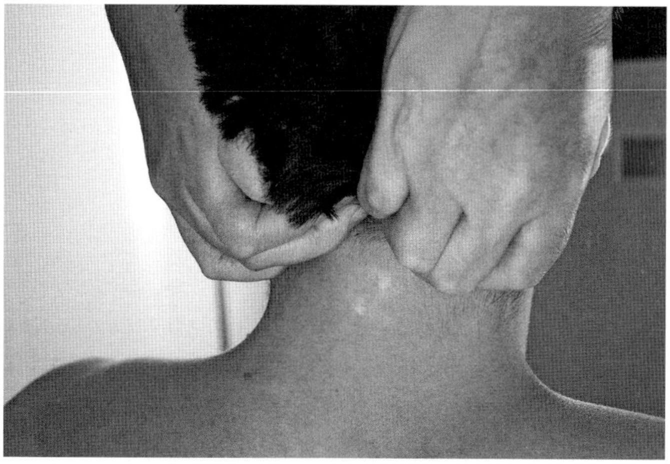

STEPS 2 – 3

1. Place your thenar eminences under the mastoid portion of the patient's temporal bone
2. Lean backwards, which will firm up your contact. Then take your thenar contacts laterally with both hands at the same time
3. Place your fingertips upon the articular processes of their axis so you can balance their axis with its relations to their atlas
4. After their axis moves freely, move your fingers to their 3rd cervical vertebrae and repeat

Wales: The base spread is one of the things which you do with the forepart of the occiput, as they may be compressed in infants. I do it with everybody at some time, because this recognition of the anterior and posterior divergence of the whole architecture of the skeletal system was emphasized by Dr. Sutherland. So much so that it keeps re-occurring as a mechanical principle in understanding the problem of compression. This is particularly in relation to the facets of the atlas and their relationship to the condyles of the occiput. The transverse atlanto ligaments of the facets of the atlas cannot move laterally as the condyles of the occiput come into the convergence. Consequently, at the anterior part of the foramen magnum the anterior part of the condylar parts are held in compression. That is something which happens with varying degrees of intensity.

The first thing you want to do is get the condyles of the occiput and the divergence of the atlas coming together and converging. So if you can hold the atlas and turn the occiput, the condyles will be in the divergence, and all this area will be released. You can do this any number of times if the atlas tightens up while you're treating the head.

I have said that you can't control the atlas. So Dr. Sutherland taught that you can go down the midline from the inion to the opisthion, and to the midpoint in the posterior rim of the foramen magnum, and hold your finger right there. When the patient nods their head the posterior tubercle on the posterior arch of the atlas will come up to your fingertip. That stabilizes the atlas. Then the condyles can move in the facets and the wider part of the occipital base. Otherwise the atlas and the occiput move together except in flexion and extension. I have modified my language because I said at a meeting that one couldn't control the atlas. Brooks Walker then tapped me on the shoulder and said "I control the atlas with one hand and the occiput with the other." Elliott Blackman, who practices in San Francisco, was sitting by him and he said he did too. So you see I should say "I can", and I made a point of this. But I had fallen into my own trap by saying you can't stabilize the atlas. I can't control the atlas by one hand on the transverse process, as I just don't have a big enough hand span, but they did. So they contact the transverse process on each side with one hand, and move the occiput with the other, and release this compression of the condyle parts of the occiput. That addresses this narrowing of the front part of the foramen magnum and the squeeze on the back part of the basal process. This may flip down or up or even turn. In which event what's going to happen to the other end of the sphenobasilar synchondrosis?

This is why this is so important not only in infants while the occiput is in four parts, but all through life. This is an important area to consider. The lateral ties of the occiput on which the condyles are placed may be turned so that you have a deformation of the foramen magnum. This is very important. Dr. Willard made a point of this, and he confirmed what I thought. I knew that the dysfunction was right there at the medulla and just inside the foramen magnum and the spinal cord. Just outside of it are the parietal tracks, the nuclei of the 12th cranial nerve and the 1st cervical nerve. What happens right there is of considerable importance from the osteopathic point of view. In the extreme situation the parietal tracks get entrapped around it, and that is one of the fundamental places where the roots of cerebral palsy begin. It is also a place where these lateral parts are compressed on the side, and where the canal through which the 12th cranial nerve exits.

3

Techniques for the Cervical Region

Crow: According to Dr. John Fox, my mentor, and one of the founding members of the Cranial Academy, Dr. Sutherland became upset with some of his students, who he said were "decapitating the body" by doing only cranial manipulation. He emphasized that what he was teaching was "OSTEOPATHY in the cranial field." In his 1947 course he taught what he learned from Dr. Still, while he was in attendance at the American School of Osteopathy. These techniques have been variously called BLT (balanced ligamentous tension techniques) or LAS (Ligamentous Articular Strain techniques). The techniques use balanced ligamentous tension to treat ligamentous articular strains.

West's Lateral Cervical Technique

EXAMPLE: C3 dysfunction
PHYSICIAN: Standing behind the patient
PATIENT: Seated

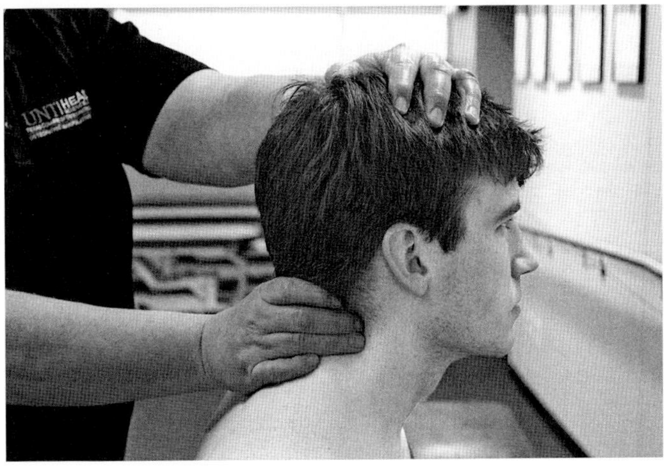

STEP 1

1. Place your right hand on the patient's C3. Your thumb and fingers are on the opposite articular pillars

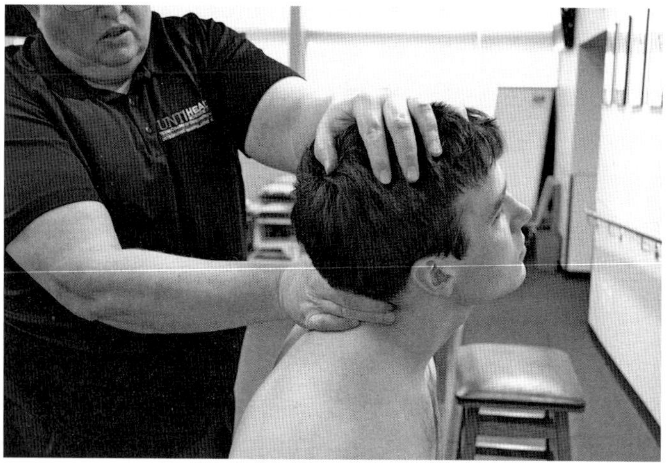

STEP 2

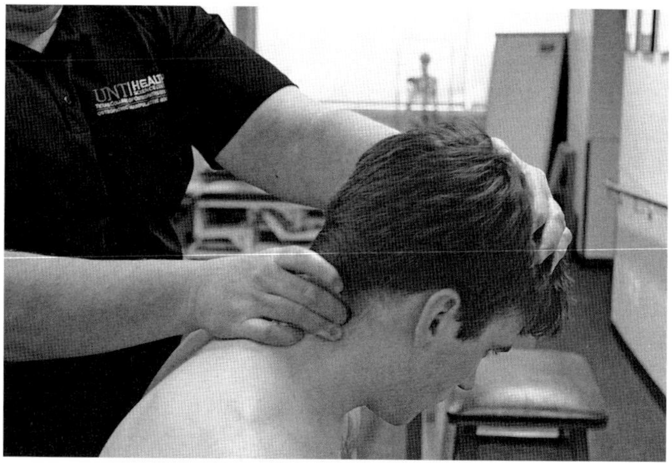

STEP 3

2. Take your left hand and place on the top of their head
3. Add mild compression and rotate their head in circles

West's Scalene Technique

EXAMPLE: Left scalenes in spasm
PHYSICIAN: Standing facing the patient
PATIENT: Seated

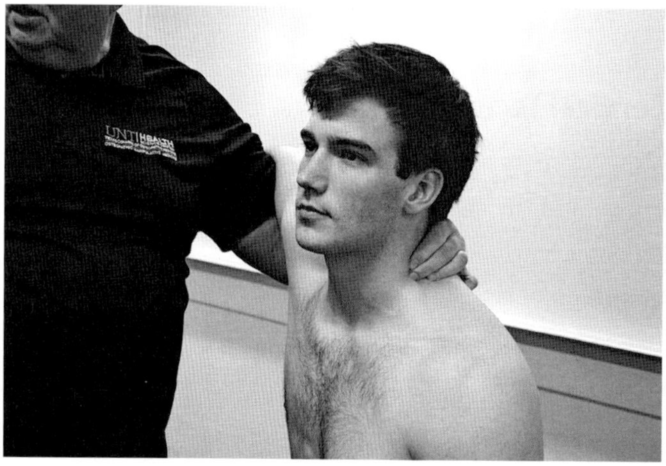

STEP 1

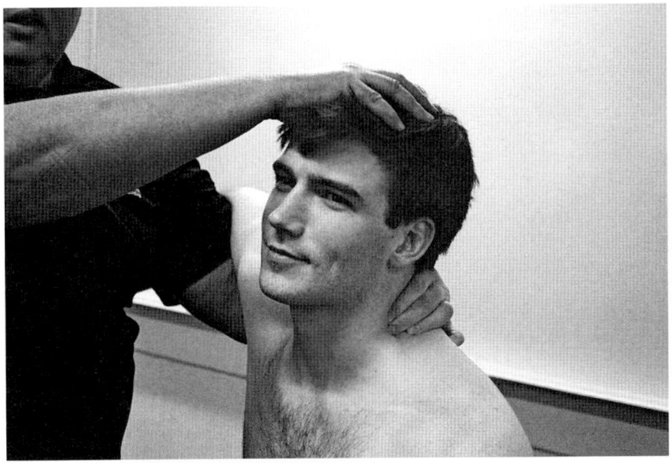

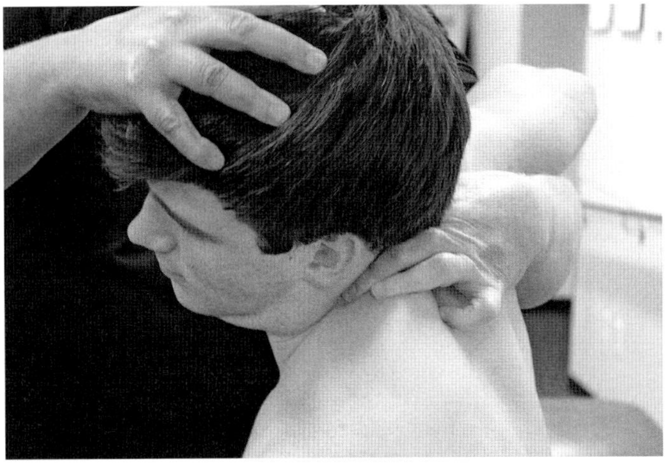

STEP 2

1. Reach under the patient's right arm and place your left hand upon the tubercle of their left first rib, close to their neck, with your fingers directed anteriorly
2. With your right hand on top of their head, stretch their head back upon your knuckle. Rotate their head forward while moving their head slowly

West's Anterior Cervical Technique

EXAMPLE: C3 dysfunction
PHYSICIAN: Standing behind the patient
PATIENT: Seated

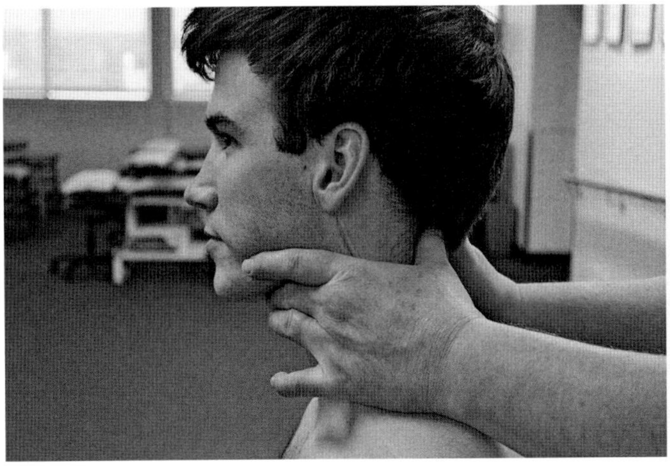

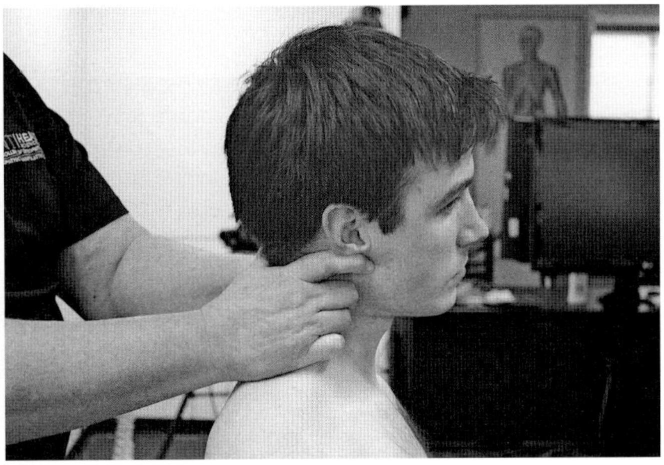

STEP 1

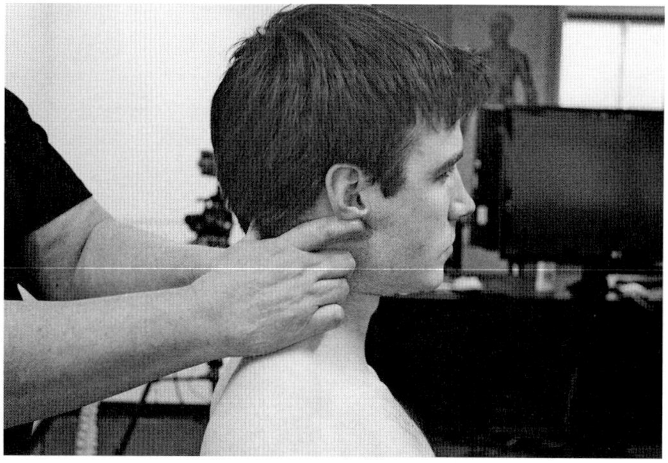

STEP 2

1. Place your right thenar eminence on their occipital protuberance and your long finger on the articular pillar of C3
2. Place your left fingers under their chin and your left thumb on the opposite articular pillar
3. Lift their head and add gentle pressure to the articular pillars with your fingers and thumb
4. Ask the patient to take a deep breath in and hold it until the cervical vertebrae release

Hazzard's Cervical Technique

PHYSICIAN: Standing in front of the patient
PATIENT: Seated

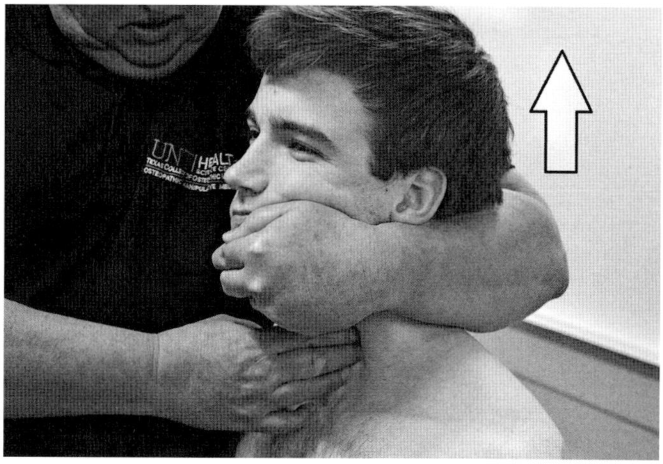

STEPS 1 – 2

1. Place your arm around the patient's neck so your elbow is just below their occipital protuberance posteriorly and with your hand beneath their chin
2. Their head is raised slightly
3. Palpate the cervical spine to find the area that is dysfunctional and then move their head to free the dysfunction

Hazzard's Technique for the Atlas #1

PHYSICIAN: Standing at the head of the table
PATIENT: Supine

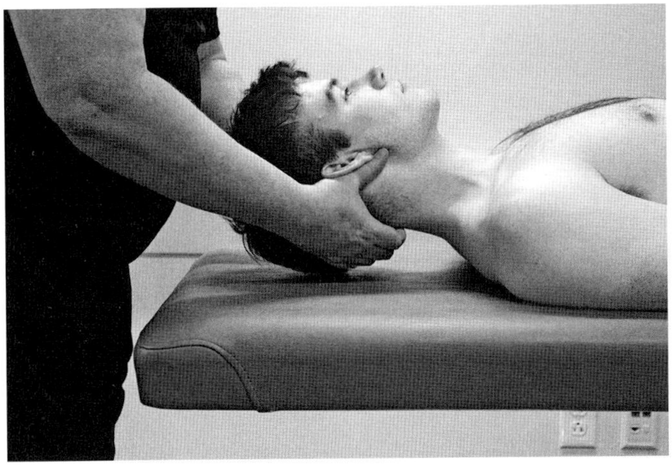

STEP 1

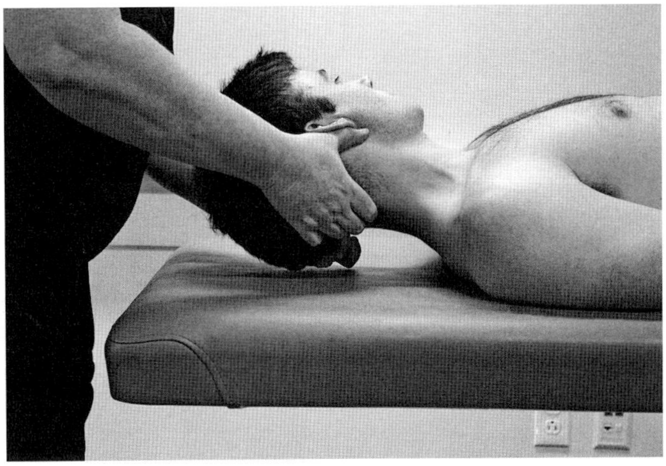

STEP 2

1. Hold their head between your hands, with your thumb or finger upon each transverse process of their atlas
2. Their head is now moved in a direction to exaggerate the lesion

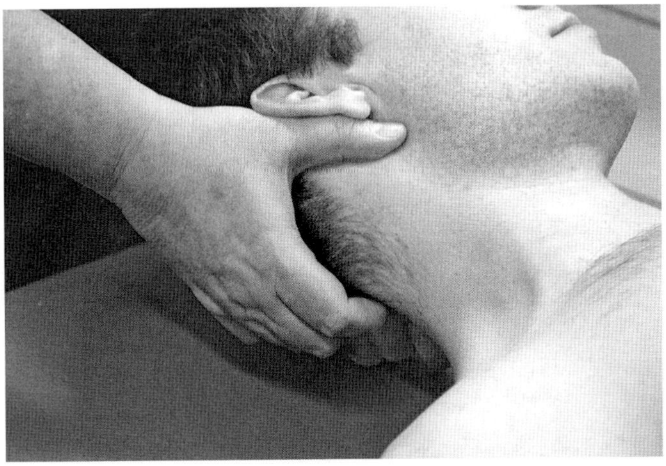

STEP 3

3. Add traction and rotate their head until the atlas begins to move into place. Then add pressure upon the articular processes until their atlas is forced toward its correct position

Hazzard's Technique for the Atlas #2

PHYSICIAN: Stands with one foot on the table
PATIENT: Seated facing you

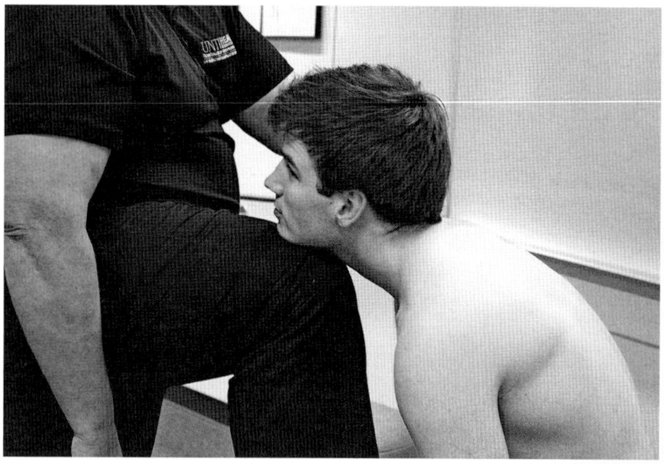

STEP 1

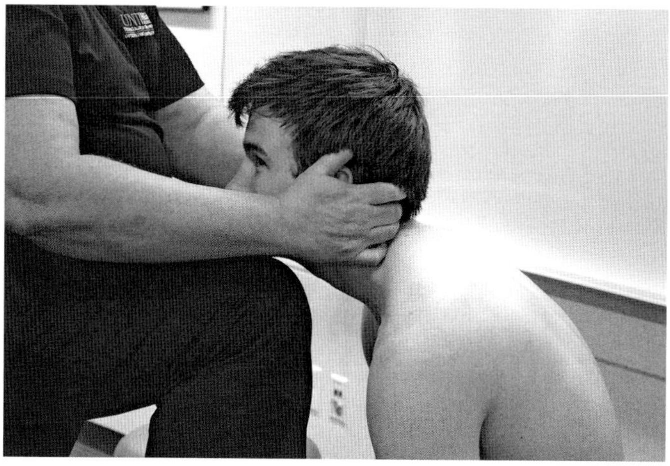

STEP 2

1. Place one knee beneath the patient's chin
2. Grasp the sides and back of the patient's head with your fingers firmly pressed upon the lateral arch of their atlas on each side

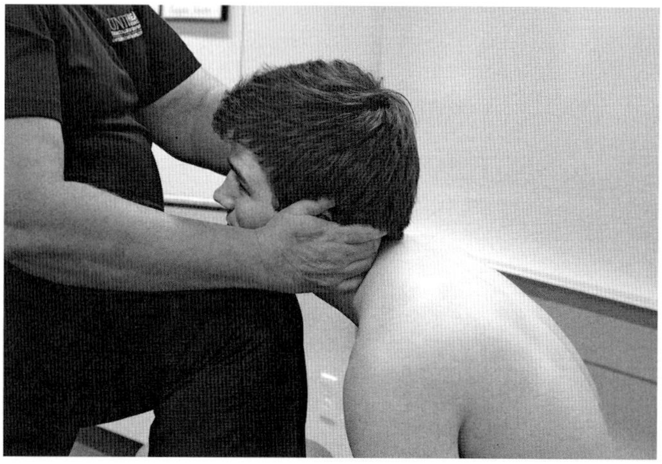

STEP 3

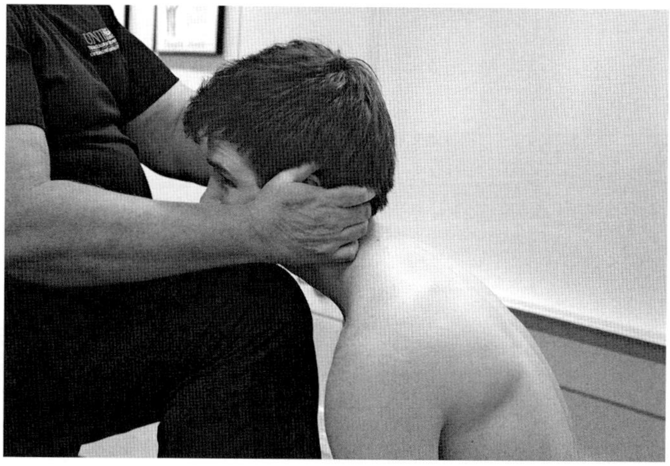

STEP 4

1. Their head is now moved in a direction to exaggerate the lesion
2. Add traction and rotate their head until the atlas begins to move into place. Add pressure upon the articular processes of their atlas

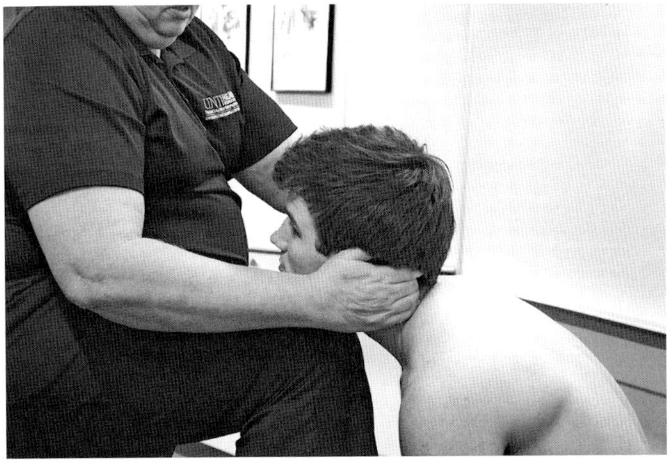

STEP 5

1. Their chin is slightly raised and drawn forward by the motion of your knee beneath their chin
2. The head is rocked upon the atlas gently, the requisite pressure being made upon the lateral arches to press the bone back to its position

Hazzard's Technique for the Atlas #3

Hazzard: Dr. Still uses the following movement in setting the atlas.

PHYSICIAN: Standing in front of the patient
PATIENT: Seated

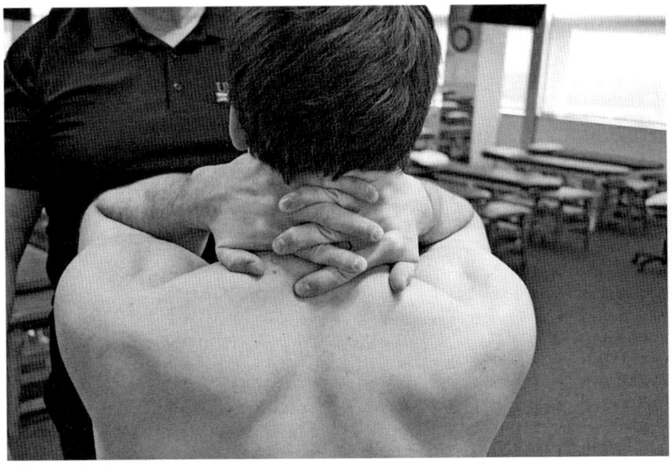

STEP 1

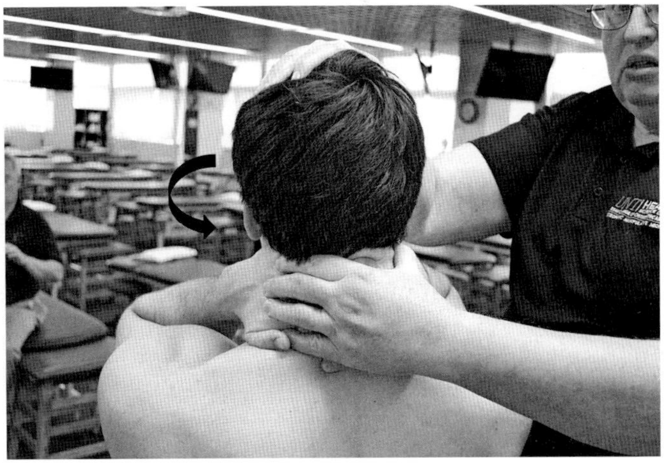

STEP 2

1. Ask the patient to clasp their hands behind their neck, just below the skull. Press their pisiform bones firmly against the lateral arches of their atlas
2. Rotate their head to the affected (lesioned) side

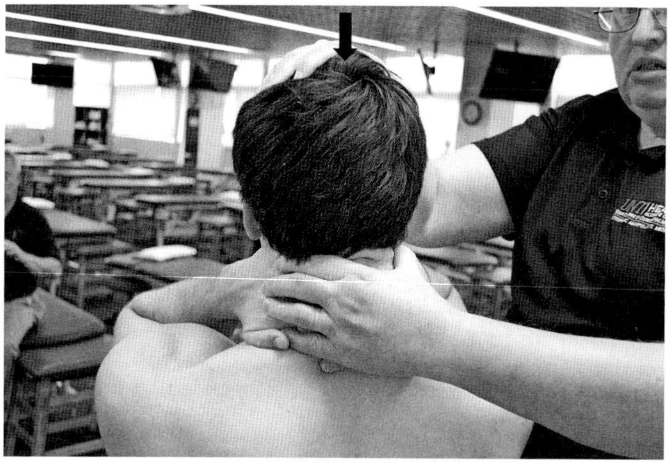

3. "Sink it down" upon their spine (press their head downward) and press their atlas into place

Ernest Eckford Tucker on Cervicals

Lesions of the cervical vertebrae are found to be in all directions. These are bilaterally posterior, unilaterally posterior, directly lateral, unilaterally anterior, and rarely bilaterally anterior. In the bilaterally posterior position it is evident that both articular surfaces have become separated from those below. This is a primary lesion of one side leading to a secondary gapping of the opposite side. This is also found in sacral lesions.

Unilaterally posterior lesions are the most frequent. There is not found to be necessarily a corresponding anterior displacement of the opposite side. More often it is the reverse. The point of engagement is some point of bony contact, of the lateral lip on that displaced side with the lip of the corresponding vertebra. A flexion lesion on the opposite side may bring about a separation posteriorly on the affected side, with the engagement of the transverse process against the superior edge of the articular process below. The mechanics of these very frequent lesions are not perfectly clear. It may be necessary to abandon the bony contact theory, and to adopt a view of the mechanics of these lesions based on passing the dead-center of the ligaments. Consider also the much slighter restraining power of simple friction, effective only because the tension of the ligament moves away from the load of the vertebra above.

Unilaterally anterior lesions, if maintained by points of bony contact, must be maintained by a catch of the superior border of the articular process of that side against the surface above. This causes a subsequent flexion of the vertebral column. There are no other points of bony contact in anterior lesions.

Directly lateral lesions, the least frequent of these, are maintained evidently by a catch of the lateral lip against the tissues at the base of the bone.

Tucker's Posterior Cervicals

EXAMPLE: C3 posterior right
PHYSICIAN: Standing at the head of the table
PATIENT: Supine

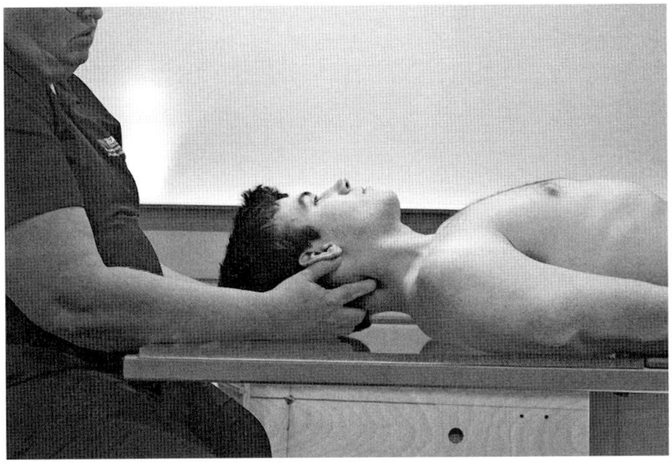

STEP 1

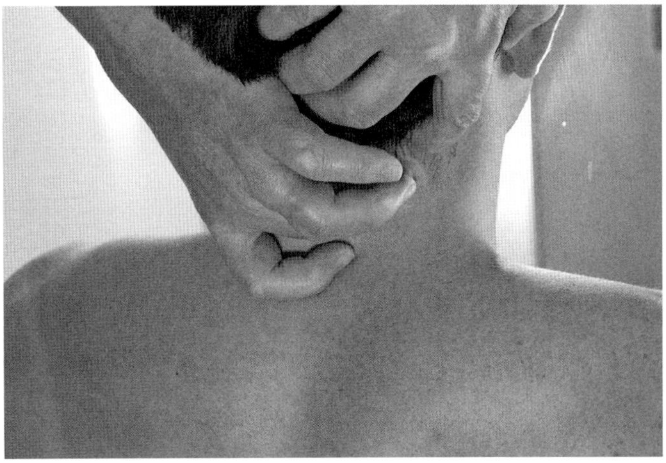

STEP 2

1. Place the proximal joint of your right index finger behind and below the prominent portion of the patient's C3. With your other fingers support their neck, with the patient facing straight ahead in the midline
2. Hold the patient's articular pillars of C4 with your left hand

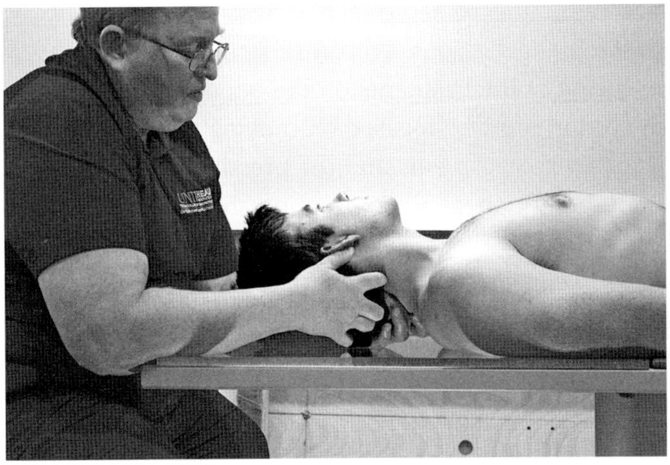

STEP 3

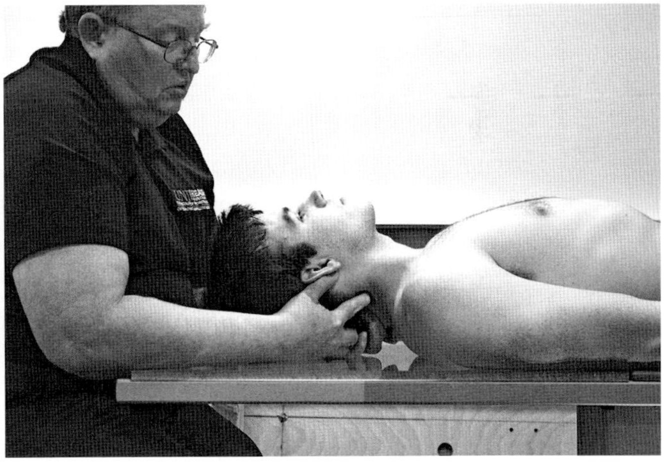

STEP 4

3. Side-bend their neck to the right without raising their head. Do not rotate their head until all of the tissues of the left side are on tension

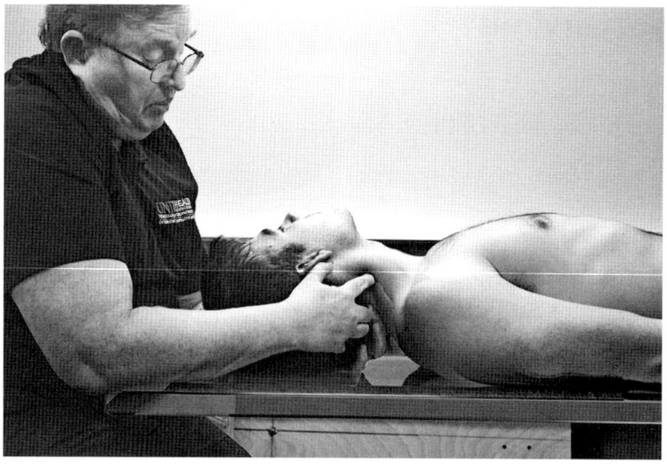

STEP 4

4. Turn their face to a forty five degree angle and at the same time draw their head back slightly. Press with your finger across their C3 in the direction of their nose—parallel to the plane of the articulation. In the average patient a very slight pressure is sufficient to reduce the lesion
5. At the moment of reduction the arches of their C3 and C4 are drawn by the pressure of your finger into two straight columns. The cervical vertebrae below are drawn taut and straight while still holding the patient's C4
6. The complete extension of the left side makes this side serve as a fulcrum

Tucker: Caution: The reduction of cervical lesions is always attended by a conscious shock for the patient. This is sometimes unpleasant and often unexpected by the patient. The word 'care' was invented to apply to techniques for cervical lesions. Preparatory stretching is especially advisable here. Aside from the tensing of the ligaments on the opposite side, which must be maintained throughout, all motion must be focused on moving the bone in the lesion. By means of the leverage of the tensed ligaments and the pressing finger, which limits motion in the plane of its natural motion, all your attention should be focused on the reaction of the patient to avoid unnecessary shock. The force used must be so graduated as to go no further than the point of correction. Indiscriminate 'cracking' of the neck without a definite plan for the correction of a lesion is a danger and often damaging to the patient. This should be regarded as little short of criminal.

Tucker's Anterior Cervical Techniques

EXAMPLE: C3 right anterior
PHYSICIAN: Standing at the head of the table on the patient's right
PATIENT: Supine

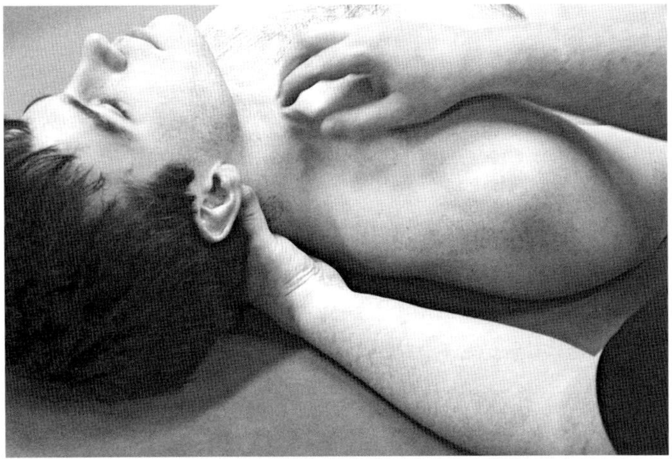

STEP 1

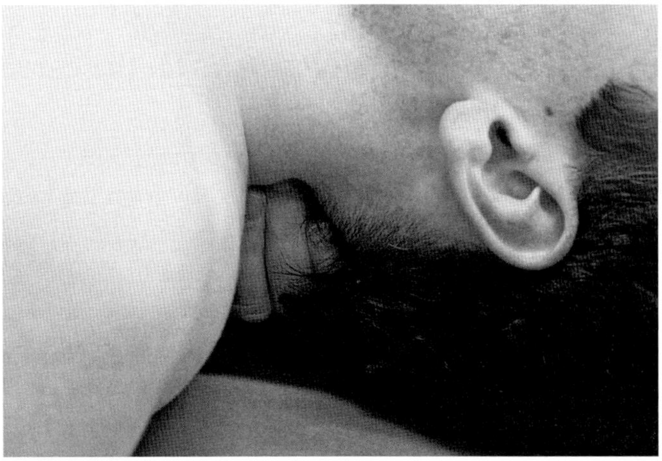

STEP 2

1. Place the palm of your left hand beneath their occiput, holding the patient's head in as low a position as possible
2. With your right hand move their sternocleidomastoid muscle out of the way and gently press down on their prominent right C3

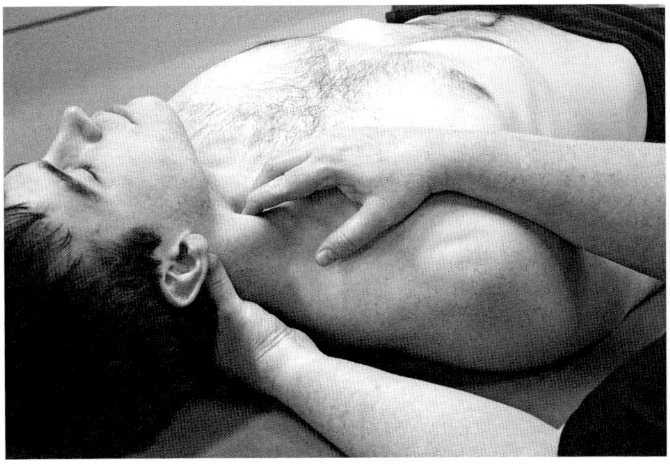

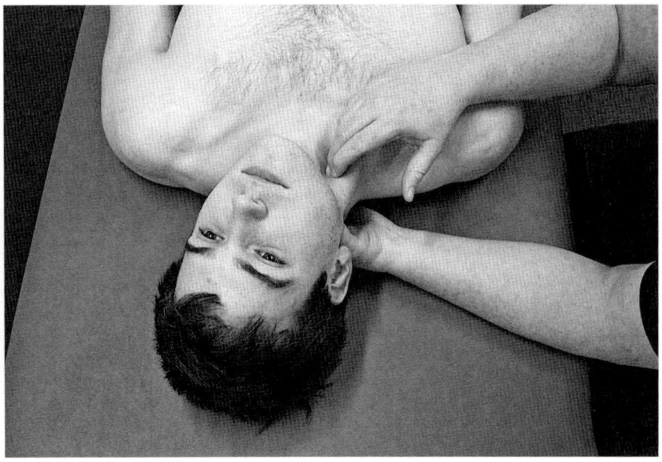

STEP 3

3. Side-bend their head to the left and to the physiological limit of motion. Without turning their head rotate their face slightly to their left. With your left thumb press down gently on the most prominent portion of the lesion
4. With a quick motion of your left hand turn their occiput to the left and their face to the right

Tucker: The effect of this technique is as follows, carrying the head to the limit of motion to the left locks all of the bony processes on that side against further motion. This makes that side of the cervical column the fulcrum for any further motion. At the same time the ligaments of the right side are all tense, tending to separate the bones in the lesion. Allowing the patient's face to turn back to the right as the neck is sharply carried to its limit of motion draws back on the right transverse processes of all cervical vertebrae. The fulcrum is on the opposite side, but especially with a lesion, as this is the farthest position of the vertebra anteriorly from normal. Since all vertebrae are separated already by the neck tension, a quick motion usually suffices to release the catch and carry the vertebra back to normal.

Sutherland's Technique for the Cervicals

Lippincott: From the axis to the seventh cervical vertebra, the articular surfaces lie in a plane that is tipped anteriorly from the coronal, so that in flexion the articular processes of one vertebra move upward and forward in relation to the one below. In rotation side-bending this movement is in that direction on the side that is anterior and convex. In extension the articular processes move relatively downward and posteriorly, as does the process on the posterior and concave side in rotation side-bending.

The anterior convexity of the cervical curve is reduced or straightened when the neck is bent forward in flexion, increasing the distance from the occiput to the shoulders. That distance is also increased on the anterior side in rotation side-bending. The distance from the occiput to the shoulder is reduced in extension, as well as on the posterior side on rotation side-bending.

The technique for correction of cervical ligamentous articular strains makes use of these principles. The articular processes that are relatively anterior, or that move anterior and superiorly more easily, are held anterior and superiorly to balance the tension of the capsular ligaments. The shoulders of the patient are placed so that the dysfunction position is exaggerated. The manner in which the patient holds their neck, especially in acute dysfunctions, and the altered bony relationships and soft tissue pathology noted under palpation, give evidence of the location and type of dysfunction.

The determining factor, however, is the freedom or restriction of motion. The articulation moves more freely and usually with less discomfort to the patient in the direction of the dysfunction than in the opposite direction. The technique is best applied with the patient supine and relaxed, but when circumstances do not permit this the physician can use his ingenuity in adapting the technique to the position that can be best assumed. It is said that Dr. Still, meeting a patient on the street, would even stand him against a tree to reduce a sacroiliac dysfunction. There is considerable latitude in applying Dr. Sutherland's technique providing the underlying principles are not violated.

The position of the shoulders is determined by no appreciable strain or tension of the muscles, the purpose being only to affect the ligamentous tension by altering the relative position of the attachments of the ligaments.

Sutherland's Cervical Flexion Dysfunction Techniques

PHYSICIAN: Standing behind the patient
PATIENT: Supine

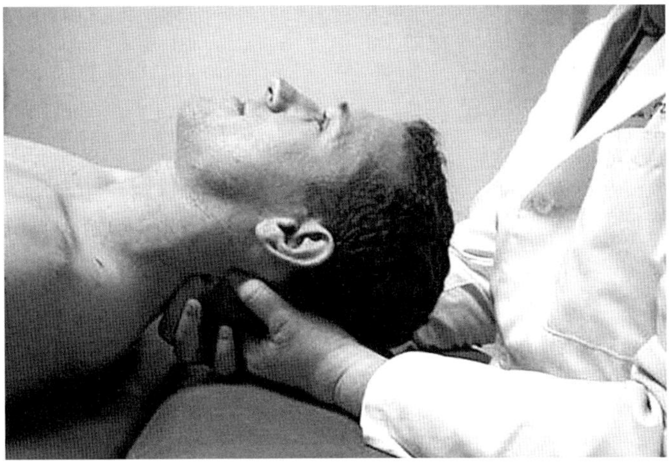
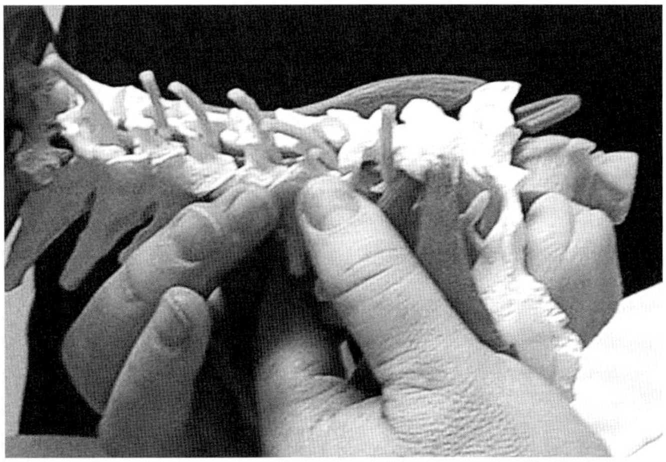

STEPS 1 – 2

1. The articular processes of the upper of the two vertebrae involved are held anterior and superiorly by the tips of your fingers (the direction being in the plane of the articular surfaces)
2. Ask the patient to lower both shoulders toward their hips and inhale and hold their breath. (Don't let the patient rotate their shoulder inwardly)

The point of balanced tension is found and held during respiratory co-operation in inhalation, which also tends to reduce the anterior convexity of the cervical spine.

Sutherland's Cervical Extension Dysfunction Techniques

PHYSICIAN: Standing behind the patient
PATIENT: Supine

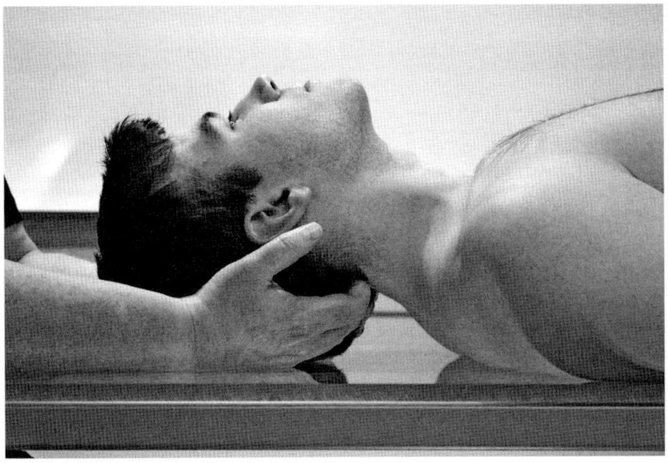
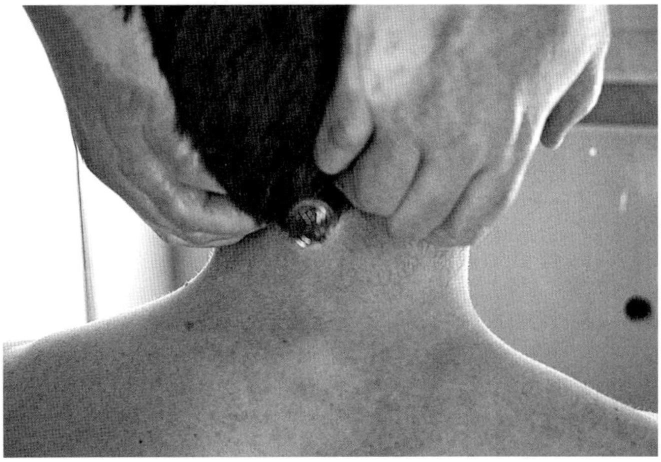

STEP 1

1. Place your fingertips on the lower of the patient's two dysfunctional vertebrae and hold it anterior and superiorly

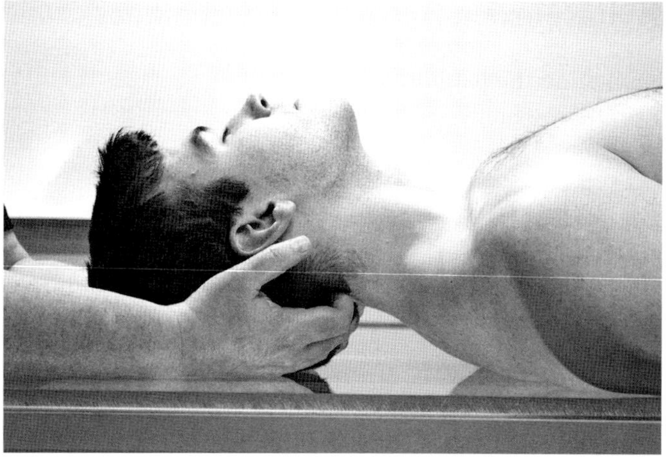

STEP 2

2. Ask the patient to bring their shoulders towards their head. Ask the patient to exhale and hold their breath out

Sutherland's Cervical Rotation Side-Bending Dysfunction Techniques

PHYSICIAN: Standing behind the patient
PATIENT: Supine

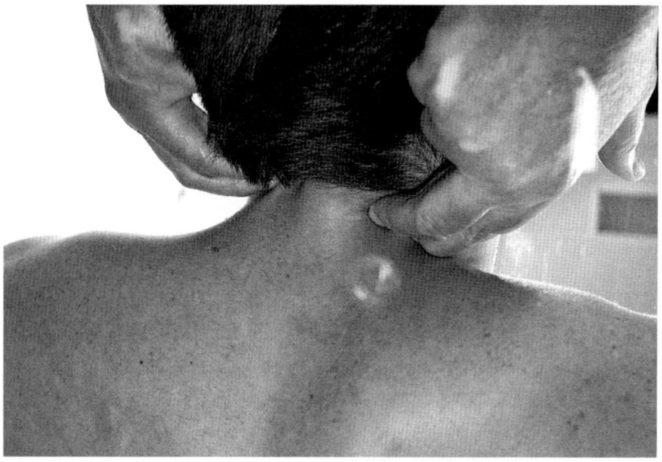

STEP 1

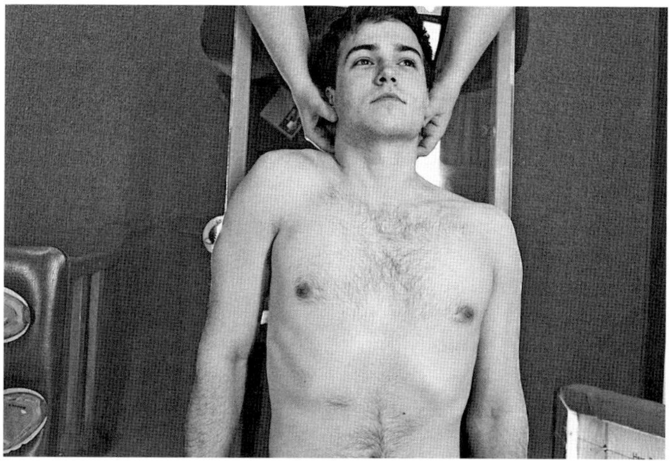

STEP 2

1. Hold the articular process of the patient's upper vertebra on the side of the convexity anteriorly and superiorly with the thumb and fingertips of one of your hands
2. Hold with your other hand the articular process of the lower vertebra anteriorly and superiorly under the inferior facet of the upper vertebra. This is relatively posterior and downward. In other words you rotate the dysfunction into ease. For example, the C5 is rotated right and the C6 is rotated left. Separate the two vertebrae and rotate one away from the other
3. Ask the patient to lower their shoulder on the side of the convexity to increase the separation of the facets, and to elevate the opposite shoulder to carry the superior process of the lower vertebra anteriorly and upward

4. Ask the patient to inhale or exhale until a balance point is felt

Lippincott: The patient holds their breath either in or out, sometimes depending on whether the strain is greater whether the articular processes are separated or approximated. Respiratory co-operation follows the general rule that inhalation is associated with flexion and external rotation, and exhalation with extension and internal rotation. The point of balanced ligamentous tension may be rather elusive, making it necessary to slightly alter the degree of pressure on the articular processes or the height of the shoulders. The greater strain may be in the ligaments on either one side or the other, so the tension may have to be varied to obtain balance.

Sutherland's Condylo-Atlantal Dysfunctions

Lippincott: The articular pits of the atlas converge anteriorly and inferiorly and they curve cranialward to a position anterior to the occipital condyles. The motion permitted is a nodding of the head as the condyles rock forward and back in the cup-shaped bits of the atlas.

PHYSICIAN: Standing behind the patient
PATIENT: Supine

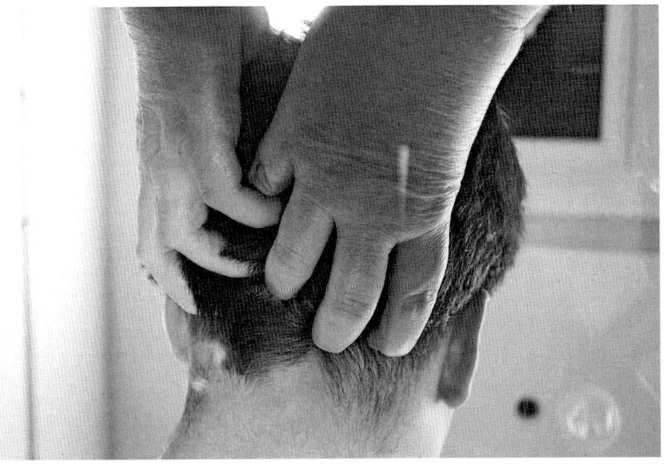

STEP 1

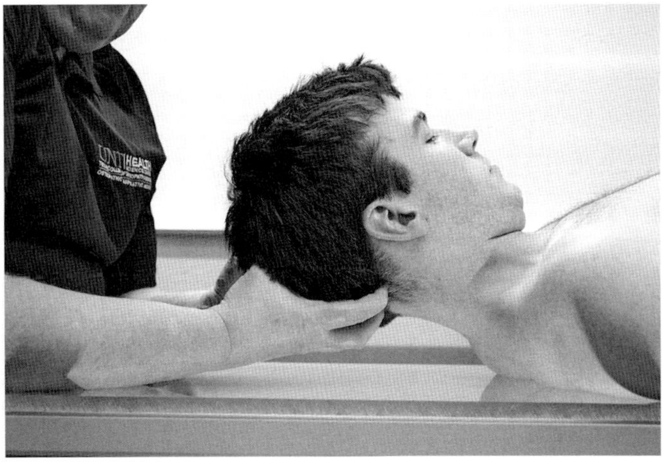

STEP 2

1. Place the tips of two of your fingers against the posterior tubercle of their atlas – one on each side
2. Hold the atlas anteriorly to prevent it from moving with the condyles, as the patient nods or tips their head forward. Avoid flexing their cervical spine. This rocks the occiput posteriorly in the pits, releasing the condyles from the atlas, and tenses the ligaments

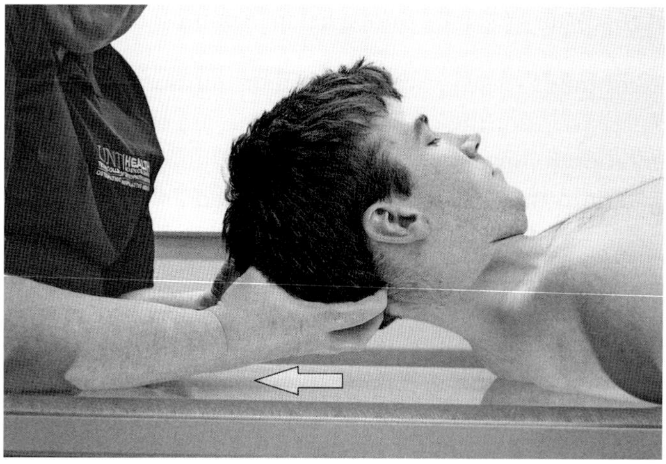

STEP 3

3. Gently draw your fingertips toward you. (This is a distraction technique using your hand on their forehead)
4. The right and left articulations will find a point of balance between them. This is perceived as a slight springing or elastic resistance of the ligaments
5. Ask the patient to hold their breath in either inhalation or exhalation. Ask the patient to take an inhalation first. If the tissue softens, then hold it. If it becomes tighter, then ask the patient to exhale slowly. When you feel the tissue releasing, ask the patient to hold their breath at that point

Lippincott: Release of the fixation is frequently perceptible to both the patient and you, usually during the respiratory efforts just before the patient must resume breathing. This technique is effective whether the dysfunction be unilateral or bilateral, or the condyles be held in the anterior, posterior or lateral position.

Wales' Cervical Vertebrae Technique

EXAMPLE: C3 rotation left and side-bent left
PHYSICIAN: Seated behind the patient
PATIENT: Supine

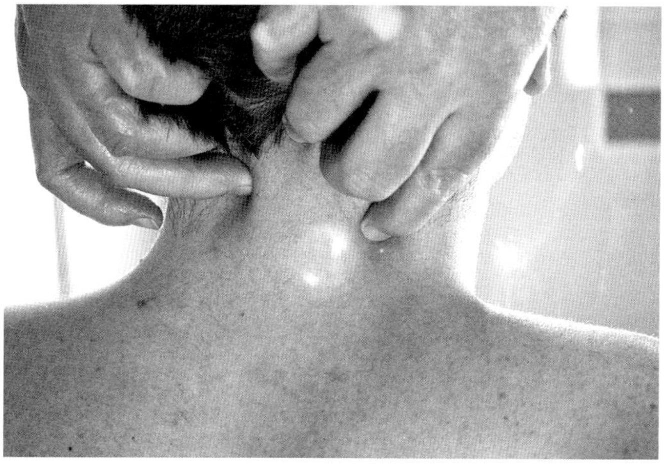

1. Place your thenar eminences on the patient's occiput
2. Place the fingertip of your left long finger on the articular process of their 2nd vertebra on the left
3. Place the fingertip of your right long finger on the articular process under their 3rd vertebra on the right
4. Bring your fingertips up toward the ceiling and turn the vertebrae in relation to each other.

Wales: I'm making an adjustment of the cervical spine between the 2nd cervical and the 3rd cervical, and the anterior spinal ligament is doing the work. I just turned the 2nd cervical through my palmar surface. I was on the articular process between the posterior and lateral cervical musculature. I think if you can just get right in there you are right on the back of the articular processes. I turn these processes on the right on the axis toward the ceiling, and the processes on the left toward the ceiling. Between the two of them the ligaments and the bodies move to a point of ligamentous articular tension. The patient's breathing and the anterior longitudinal ligament provides rebalancing.

But there are some situations where there are anomalies in the neck. I may as well speak of that now. Normally the occipital condyles move in the facets of the atlas for the nodding motion. Otherwise the atlas goes with the occiput. The cranial vertebral junction, the atlas, axis and associated ligaments and structure have their own anatomy and mechanics. I might as well add what Dr. Sutherland said about the cranial vertebral junction. Its function is as a ligamentous articular mechanism to function in relation to the reciprocal tension membrane in the head. This is much like the tension spring which regulates the balance wheel of a watch. The balance wheel is the falx and the tentorium. The cranio-cervical junction works like a tension spring to regulate that mechanism in relation to the cranial base.

How does a tension spring on a watch work anyhow? I don't usually pay any attention to one. I thought I finally understood it when I was sitting in Grand Central Station in New York. There is a huge cube which is a clock with four faces on it. Each side has hands on it, so you can watch the inside machinery work. I watched the tension spring in that mechanism regulating the balance wheel in that mechanism, and I finally got the point. This has a great deal to do with the situation at the cranial vertebral junction, because here there is the superior cervical ganglion which is the sympathetic nervous system. This resembles all the other ganglia, which is vasomotor and secretory to everything inside the head.

Crow's OA Technique and Upper Cervical Technique

PHYSICIAN: Seated behind the patient
PATIENT: Supine

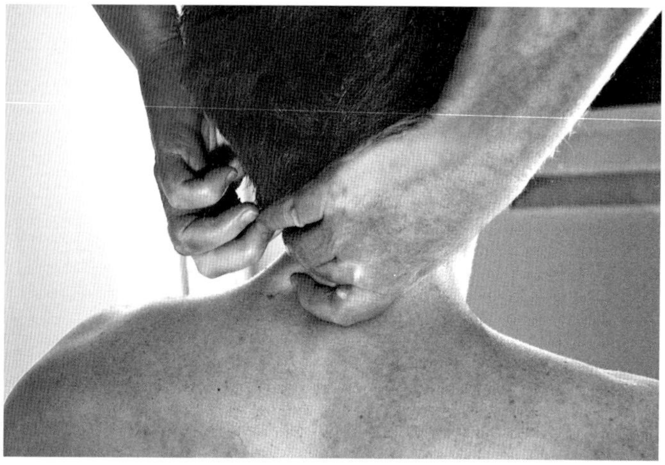

STEPS 1 – 2

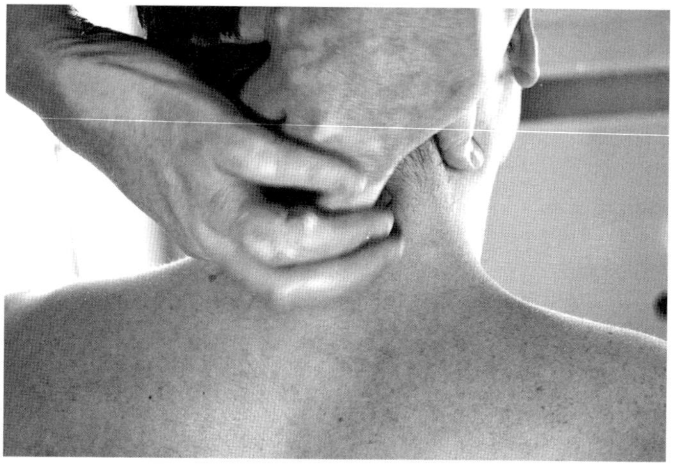

STEPS 3 – 4

1. Place your right thumb on the right side of the patient's articular pillar of their C1
2. Place your right index finger on the left side of the articular pillar of the patient's C1
3. Place your right long finger on their OA
4. Place your left thumb on the left side of their C2 articular pillar
5. Place your left index finger on the right side of their C2 articular pillar
6. Separate the OA from the C1 by pushing your right long finger and pulling your index finger to the right
7. While you're separating the OA and C1, take their C2 in the opposite direction of their C1. This should free the upper cervicals

Crow's Lower Cervicals Technique

EXAMPLE: C4 on C5
PHYSICIAN: Seated behind the patient
PATIENT: Supine

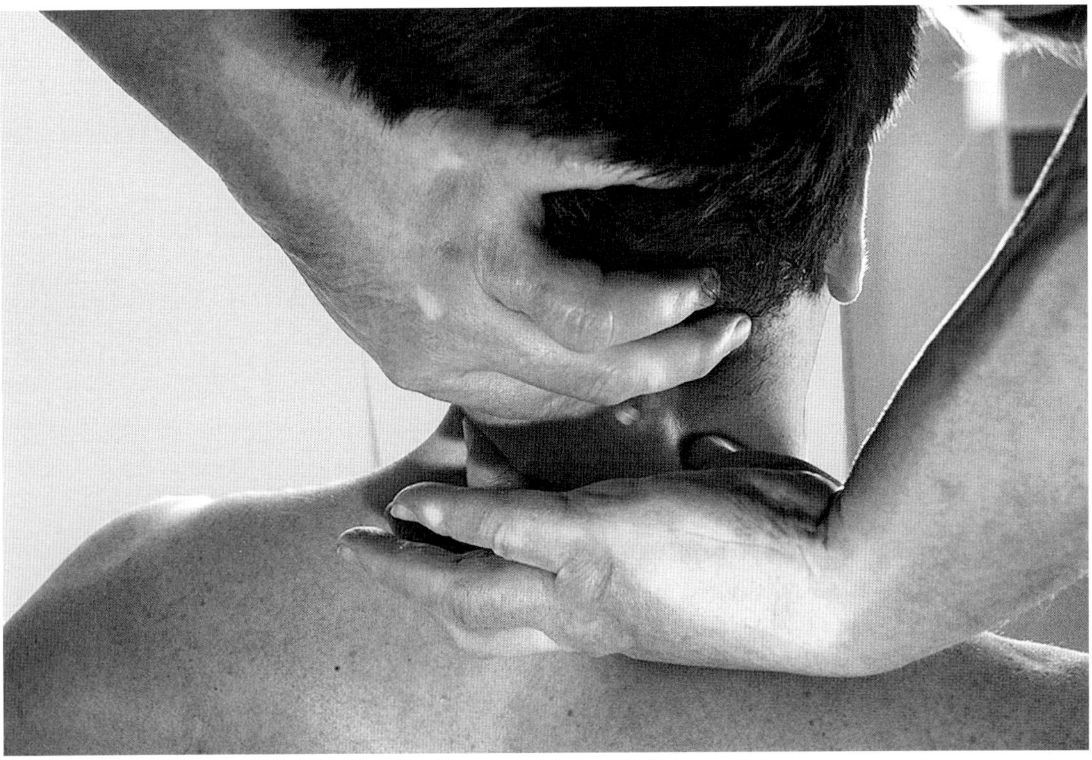

1. Place your right thumb on the right side of the patient's C4 articular pillar
2. Place your right index finger on the left side of the articular pillar of their C4
3. Place your left thumb on the left side of their C5 articular pillar
4. Place your left index finger on the right side of their C5 articular pillar
5. Take the C4 in the opposite direction of their C5. This should free the lower cervicals

4

Techniques for the Thoracics

Tucker on Thoracics

The chief limitation to motion in the dorsal [thoracic] region is perfectly obvious—it is the flatness of the top and bottom surfaces of the bodies, and the thinness of the intervertebral discs. These do not prevent motion of pure rotation, but they do all but prevent any other kind of motion—except to slight degrees. Motion to slight degrees is consequently all that we find in the other directions. But it matters not how slight is that degree, the shape of the articular surfaces has adjusted to this motion, and when it is exceeded, the danger of a 'lesion' is just as great as though it were highly mobile.

Limitation of motion of extension is from the tension on the discs and bony contact of the articular processes with the bone below. Exaggeration of this motion and lesion is very rare.

Limitation to flexion is first the flatness of the bodies and the thinness of the intervertebral discs. Second it is the interspinous and other ligaments posteriorly. This is the yellow elastic cartilage where they are in line with the motion, and white fibrous cartilage where they lie radially to it. When the limitation to motion has been reached in flexion, the anterior edge of the body acts as a fulcrum, and any other motion tends to gap open the spinal and costal articulations behind. But under the forward pressing weight, which causes flexion, these may slide forward over the anterior edge of the one below, bringing the surface of the inferior articular processes (upper of the two in each joint) against the top edge of the surface below. This has the possibility of indentation and lesion. The ligaments, all tensed by this exaggeration of motion, serve to drive it with greater force against this edge and to hold it there. A lesion in the midline is not so frequent as lesions in other positions. This is merely because in the midline the ligaments are at maximum resistance strength. Yet pure flexion lesions are by no means infrequent in the dorsal region. However, in a position of extreme flexion, when other exaggerated motion is added, then there is the greatest danger of lesion. This is because the ligaments of only one side are bearing the strain, are more stretched and allow greater exaggeration of motion for any given force. This causes engagement against a corner instead of a side, with greater indentation and more power to hold.

In pure rotation the first limitation to motion is the costal articular surface on the inferior border, which allows rotation around a center not far from the center of the body for a short distance. But this deflects it upward, transforming it into a rotation/side-bending lesion. The spines rotate to the right, with the side-bending, carrying the transverse processes up on the right. In the lumbar region the axis of rotation is behind, the bodies rotate while the spine is open, and stationary. Rotation means rotation of the bodies to the right and side-bending down on the right. In the dorsal region this is reversed. The axis of rotation is in front, the spines rotate, with the body being often stationary at its front edge. Side-bending is up on the same side.

The limitation of motion in rotation/side-bending in the dorsal region is wholly ligamentous, unless the head of the rib may be regarded as such a limitation. Probably all of these ligaments are so adjusted that they reach the point of limitation at about the same time. Pure rotation/side-bending is added to the flexion movement and such lesions do occur. The strongest of the retaining ligaments is beyond doubt the intervertebral disc, whose action is to throw the axis of rotation nearer the center of the body. This causes jamming of the upper articular surface against the upper and outer corner of the articular process below on the convex side, with indentation and lesion. On the concave side, the joint is gapped open. This is doubtless only a momentary state. When to this motion flexion is added without recovery from the rotation, it simply strains the point of contact to a point farther down on the articular surface. More distortion, greater ligamentous pressure, deeper indentation and more likelihood of lesion occurs.

Dorsal Region: Movements

Tucker: There is a slight movement of flexion and extension in the dorsal region, but except at the lower two or three dorsals and the upper two dorsals it is very slight. With the spine in an erect position and the practitioner's hand on the head, causing passive flexion and extension, this is felt more as an elastic yielding than as a motion. It should be remembered that the spinous process, twice as long as the distance from the axis of flexion (articulation of rib) to the articular surface, moves twice as much as the articulation itself.

The axis of flexion and extension is the head of the rib where it articulates with the lower facet of the vertebra. The narrowness of the disc itself shows how slight is this flexion and extension. Additionally, the articulation at the head of the rib is not shaped for such motion at all, providing only a slight elastic yielding at the axis of motion. Rotation of the spine as a whole occurs in the dorsal region. In an extended position it occurs almost wholly in the lower dorsal and upper lumbar vertebrae. In an erect position this occurs in the lower dorsal, and in a semi-flexed position in the mid dorsal. It is only present in a flexed position in the upper dorsals. The factor or at least one factor determining this may easily be shown. It is simply that when in the fully flexed position of any vertebra rotation occurs. It is accomplished by the extending of one side. That movement involves extension, and cannot occur if the flexion is fully maintained. Flexion occurs first in the lower vertebrae and last in the uppermost ones. Therefore, rotation is lost first in the lower dorsals and last in the upper dorsals.

Movements of rotation in single vertebrae are also very slight. This is indicated by the smallness of the articular surfaces and the way in which the inferior articular surface of the bone above overlaps at its edges the slightly smaller surface below (indicating motion is restricted to the larger surface). Also, the smallness of the articular facet of the rib (which is the axis of flexion and extension, but not of rotation) must also move in rotation. There is always limitation set by the tissues surrounding the ribs.

Nor is it probable that movements of rotation are pure, but are a combination of rotation and side-bending to most probably equal degrees, especially as we approach the limits of motion. This is indicated by the costal facets and by the shape of the upper articular surfaces. The costal facets are so placed that they could allow a slight degree of rotation in the horizontal plane around an axis near the center of the body, by pushing the rib down on its inferior facet, yet the position of the facets indicates motion at an angle of about forty-five degrees from the horizontal. Direction of motion is determined by the articular planes, and that of the dorsal vertebrae would be in the direction common to the two planes of the facets, and of the spinal articular surfaces themselves, which are about forty-five degrees up and forward.

Now if we examine the actual bones, we will observe that the facets on the lower borders of the vertebral bodies (those for the upper facets on the heads of the ribs), are the best formed and defined. They are the ones on which motion evidently occurs. The facets on the upper borders (those for the lower margin of the head of the rib) are evidently those by which the ribs adhere to the bones. The rib belongs with the lower of the two bones as it is a branch from the upper edge of each segment. This is proven by the eleventh and twelfth ribs, and by the joining to the transverse processes of those vertebrae. Motion occurs at both of these facets in respiration and other motions of the ribs, sometimes doubtless in the motion of the vertebrae themselves. But it is evidently the facets on the inferior border that determine the motions of the vertebrae. Placing a finger in such a position that it is flat against both of these articulations (costal and spinal), it will be found that the facets point up and forward and out. Up at an angle of about forty-five degrees in the lower dorsals, with the angle growing less until it is almost horizontal in the third or fourth dorsal, and is practically lost on the second. The costal surface there is not a plane, but often a cup-shaped surface, showing little or no motion. On the first dorsal the first dorsal articulation provides the predominant fixed facet surface for the movement of the seventh cervical. This angle determines the amount of side-bending, which is greatest in the lower dorsal and is lost in the upper dorsals.

The forward angle of the pointing of the practitioner's finger (indicating the angle of rotation) likewise changes. In the lumbar region, it is backward. In the twelfth dorsal it is also backward. In the eleventh dorsal the practitioner's finger usually points directly outward. In the tenth slightly forward. As we ascend the direction of the finger moves more forward until about the fifth, when it changes again. In the second or first it is directly out, or may even point backward as such vertebrae have no rotation at all, but only unilateral flexion and extension.

This again coincides with previous studies, where it was found by all students that the centers of rotation were in front of the articular surfaces in the dorsal region, and were farthest away in the lower and upper dorsals. This was determined as nearest in the mid dorsals, where rotation was greatest and sharpest. The center was at infinity in the eleventh or tenth, and in the second or first, and being for the most part near the front of the body of the vertebra in the average mid-dorsal vertebra. In many spines that were examined the centers of rotation of the upper dorsal vertebrae were extremely irregular, on account of the extremely slight degree of true rotation in that area. In those vertebrae whose centers of rotation are at infinity there is of course no rotation. Rotation of the trunk is nevertheless aided by unilateral flexion and extension as the articular surfaces are sloped forward. In such vertebrae it is to be noted that the rib does not articulate with the vertebra above, and has only the one facet on the body. A curve formed by continuing the line of the pointing fingers on the two sides inward until they meet would define the arc of movement of the vertebra. This arc points up, out and forward on both sides.

A further illustration of this side-bending/rotation is found in the shapes of the superior articular surfaces. Rotation up, out and forward would naturally cause the upper and outer corner of the superior articular surface to be bent forward. Examining the articular surfaces we find this to be the case, at least in the lower three or four vertebrae, where the articular surfaces are bent like propeller blades. This is apparent chiefly in these lower vertebrae because it is here that side-bending mainly occurs. All motions are less in the upper dorsals. Among other reasons, this is on account of the shortness of the ribs.

The best way to fix these facts in mind is to make practical use of them. Note that a strain beyond the normal is likely to affect different parts of the spine, according to the direction of the force. Strain of rotation in the erect position is likely to be felt in the lower dorsals. In the semi-flexed position it is felt in the mid dorsals. In the fully flexed position it is felt in the upper dorsals. Anyone may quickly and easily test this matter in his own body. The greatest danger of a lesion is where the limitation to motion is greatest. It is a mechanical law that there is a point of mechanical weakness where a large part joins a small part. As in a nail driven into a wall, the nail will bend just where it leaves the wall. The danger of a rotation lesion is therefore greatest just at the upper part and of the part that is locked against rotation by flexion. It is lower down in extension and higher up in flexion.

To focus the corrective force of a rotary nature on the lower dorsals, the upper dorsals should be kept straight, by means of an arm under the chest. To focus it in the mid-dorsals the lower dorsals should be flexed, the upper ones extended as in bowing of the spine, while the head rests on your folded arms. To focus force on the upper dorsals, the head and neck should be used as levers. They are protected against injury by the supporting hand on the patient's neck, while the spine below the point to be treated is flexed.

Lower dorsals are carried to the limit of their normal motion by flexion/side-bending/rotation. Mid dorsals by flexion/rotation and upper dorsals by rotation. Strains of a different character have a tendency to produce lesions, especially if they occur at the limit of motion.

In diagnosis, while exploring for limitation to motion, it must be borne in mind that individual skeletons vary. Much research and comparative study needs to be done on this point before safe generalizations can be made. So far as such work has been done, it points to the fact that the side-bending, or unilateral flexion and extension, is greatest in the lowest dorsals. True rotation does not occur here, but is greatest in the mid dorsals. Practically all motion beyond a mere elastic yielding is often lost in the upper dorsals.

It must then be borne in mind that one occasionally finds a single vertebra that has acquired such great freedom and width of motion that they are practically never in the median line. When apparently in lesion to one side, they move easily to the opposite side with the least effort on the part of the physician.

These occur usually when there is an abnormal limitation to motion above and below. They are found with greater frequency in the eleventh dorsal, on account of the limitation to rotation in the lumbar spine, which arises from the civilized habit of sitting or standing with the lumbar spine fully flexed. Rotation does not occur in the fully flexed spine, so long as flexion is maintained.

Side-bending is greatest in the lower dorsals and least in the upper dorsals, where it is practically lost. A side-bending strain involving the whole spine will take effect chiefly in the lower dorsals. If it involves the upper dorsals, however, it is much more likely to produce an exaggeration of motion and so a 'lesion'. Such a lesion is pretty sure to show itself as a unilateral flexion lesion, with rotation of the spine to the side of the lesion. Measurement with a tape line reveals that whenever there is lateral deviation there is almost certain to be separation, with compensatory approximation above and below. Examination for limitation to motion is of very little value in the upper dorsals.

Side-bending corrective force is focused on different parts of the spine chiefly by pressure with the thumb. Also by different use of the muscles of the patient's shoulder. Keeping the shoulders well up tenses the long muscles down to the lower dorsals. Drawing the shoulders forward in mid position tenses the muscles down to the mid dorsals. Drawing them down tenses the muscles to the upper dorsals. Side-bending of the upper dorsals is best accomplished through the head and neck.

Taking up to the point of movement as determined by the muscles, we discover the astonishingly simple fact that the costal facets on the inferior borders of the vertebrae always point toward the shoulders. They are in line with the muscles that cause their motion. Can further simplification be discovered by this characteristic? We find, of course, that the spinal articular surfaces are in line with the pull of the erector spinae muscles. We find that they are concave toward the line of the center of gravity. We note that they are directly behind the base of the bodies of the vertebrae, and perpendicular thereto.

Tucker's Thoracic Technique

PHYSICIAN: Standing in front of the patient
PATIENT: Seated

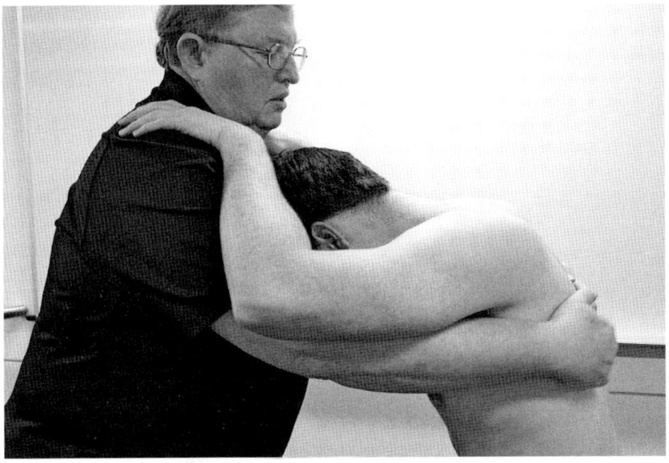
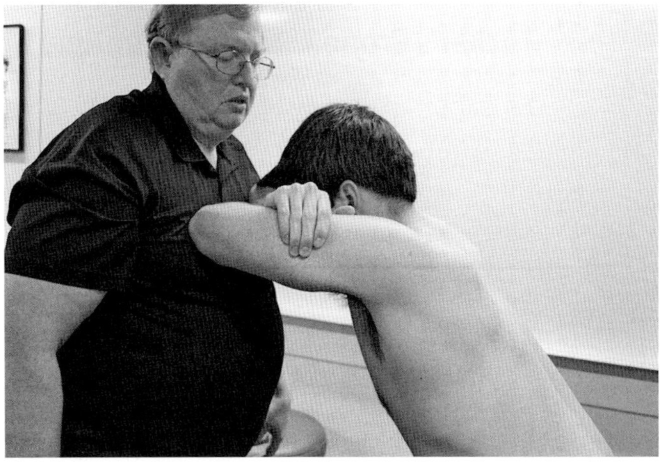

STEP 1

1. The patient places their hands on the physician's shoulders, and their head against the physician's manubrium. (Alternately, ask the patient to cross their arms and lay their crossed arms on the physician's manubrium, and then ask the patient to lay their head against their crossed arms)

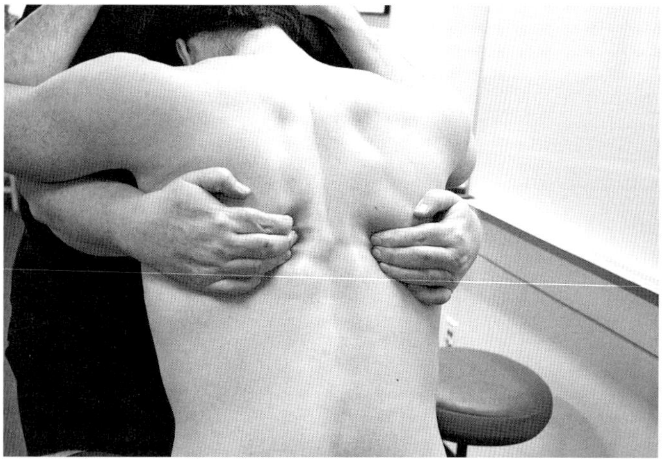

STEP 2

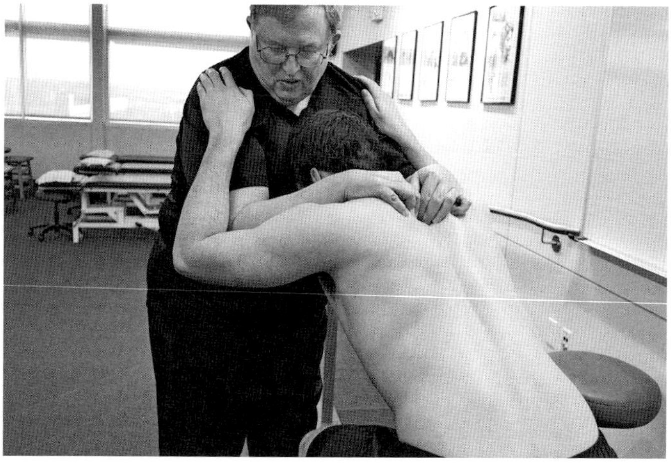

STEP 3

2. The physician reaches their hands around the patient and places fingers on either side of the spines of the upper thoracic vertebrae
3. The physician leans back carrying the patient's spine into full extension. At the same time lift the patient's arms and elevate their ribs

Tucker: In the lesion, the upper edge of the lower articular process is engaged against the surface of the one above. This throws the latter into flexion, or separation. In this technique the fingers pressing against the patient's articular processes below tend to carry them away from the point where they are engaged. Pressing against the spine above tends to flatten it out, making the lower edge of the upper articulation the fulcrum for releasing the surface from its midway catch against the edge of the lower vertebrae. Note that the articular process is opposite the base of the bone (opposite the cartilaginous joint). In the fifth to the tenth dorsals, the tip of the spinous process is directly opposite the articular process of the next one below. The practitioner's finger may press on both spinous processes of the bone above, and also on articular process of bone below, at the same time.

Tucker's Prone Thoracic Technique

PHYSICIAN: Standing beside the patient
PATIENT: Prone

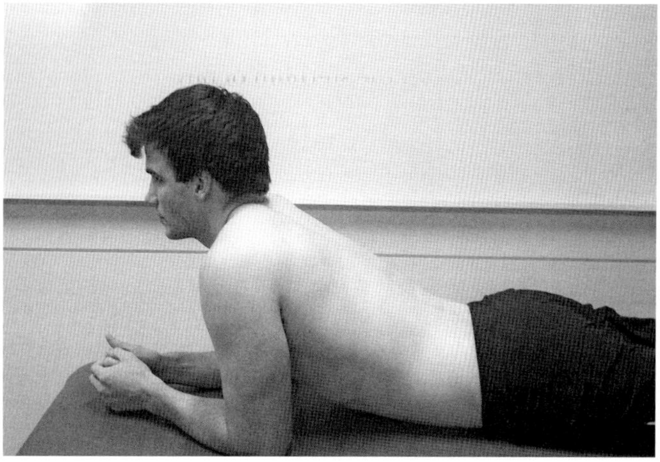

STEPS 1 – 3

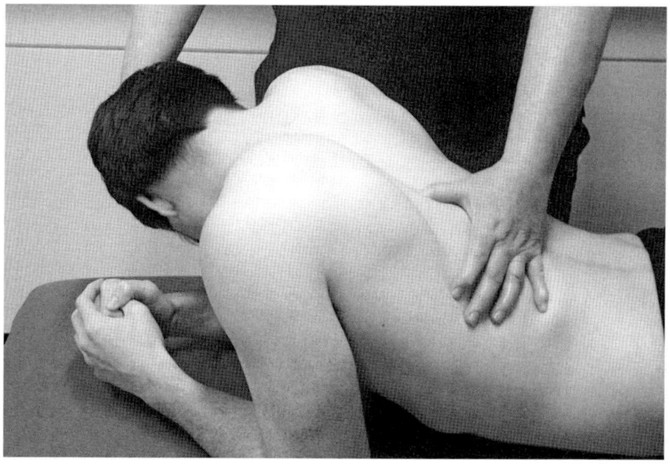

STEP 4

1. Ask the patient to rise up on their elbows, so that their upper arms are vertical, with their forearms lying along the table
2. Stand at the side of the table; place your thumb on the articular process of the lower of the two dysfunctional vertebrae, pressing down (tending to directly release). Alternately, on the upper of the two bones, press down and out on the spinous process, thus making a fulcrum of the lower vertebrae
3. The patient is asked to let their head hang down
4. With your other hand rotate their head (with their face slightly turned to the side) from side to side to the limit of motion in each direction
5. If extra leverage with their head is necessary, the physician may brace the patient's shoulder on either side against their abdomen to prevent pulling the patient and so that the upper arms are not vertical. It is an important point to keep their arms vertical

Tucker: The rib on the side of the dysfunction belonging to the dysfunctional vertebra is thrust forward, and so bears a relatively heavier tension than the rest. This technique tends to press the vertebra backward and so release the dysfunction.

Tucker's Supine Thoracic Technique

PHYSICIAN: Standing beside the patient
PATIENT: Supine

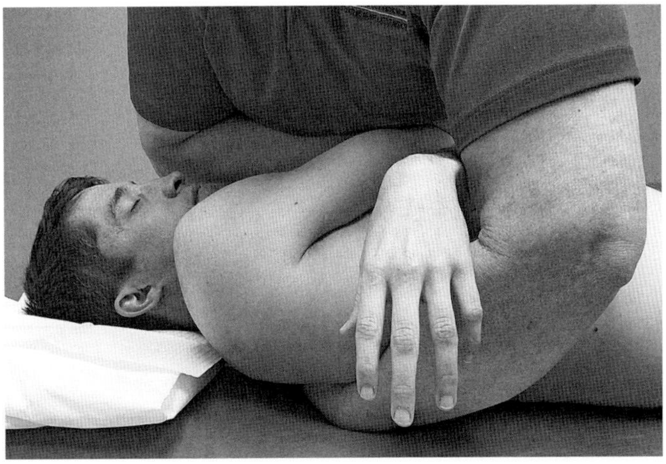

1. Ask the patient to cross their arms over their chest, the arm nearest the physician being the arm below. Otherwise the patient's elbows will be in line with the sternum of physician, with the near arm below the other arm. The arms are on opposite sides of the manubrium as the physician presses their chest against them. The patient's elbows in this position present a broad surface for pressure on the physician's chest, and reduce the risk of injury to the physician
2. The physician draws the patient's arms down against the patient's chest so as to bring pressure against their ribs, and to tense their pectoral muscles
3. Wrap your arms around the patient and place your knuckles underneath with your fingers at the level of the thoracic dysfunction
4. The physician lightly but firmly presses against the patient's elbows with their chest while exerting firm pressure upwards against their dysfunction with their knuckles

Tucker: Some practice is necessary to use this technique to the best advantage. Properly used, it is one of the most effective. It is effective in some patients as low as the eleventh dorsal and as high as the third. In adjusting the patient's lower lesions the elbows should be carried farther down on the patient's chest and the direction of pressure of the physician's chest is lower. In adjusting the upper vertebrae the patient's arms and the pressure of the physician's chest are more nearly vertical. This technique is especially valuable in mid and anterior upper dorsal warps.

CAUTION: In some patients the coracoid processes are long and the patient's arms in this position exert uncomfortable pressure against the physician. This technique should not be painful nor require undue force. In patients this technique should be used with proper skill. Physicians should take into consideration sensitive or degenerative shoulders and slightly built patients with this technique. In patients with valvular (heart) lesions it is contra-indicated.

Tucker's Upper Thoracic (T1-T3) Technique #1

The technique for the upper three dorsals is more difficult than that for the rest. Here motion is slight, and lesions frequent. Here the shoulder muscles have little value. Recourse is usually made to leverage of the patient's neck.

EXAMPLE: T3 rotation right and side-bent left
PHYSICIAN: Standing beside the patient
PATIENT: Supine

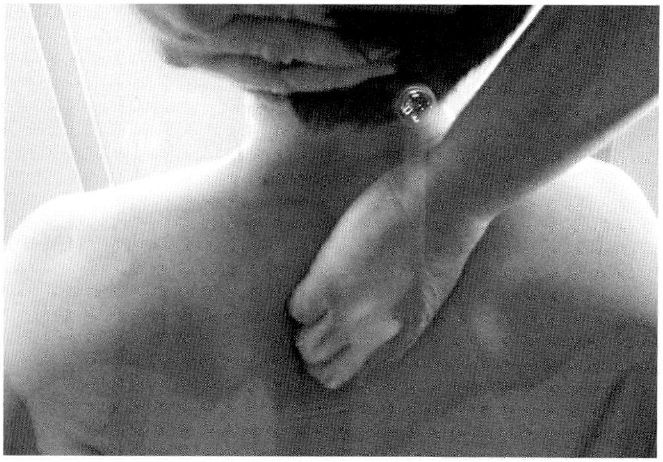

STEP 1

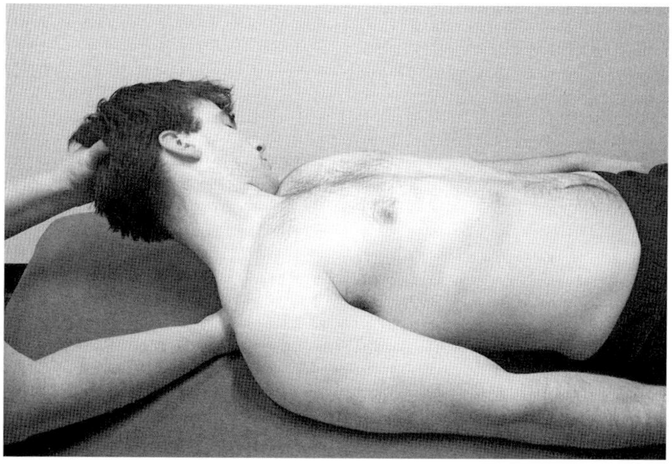

STEP 2

1. Place your right thumb against the prominent side of the spinous process of the patient's T3 vertebra, and the MIP (middle joint of your index finger) on the opposite side stabilizing the joint
2. The patient's head is drawn forward to full flexion and to the left, which is opposite to the side of the dysfunction, stretching the ligaments on the right side

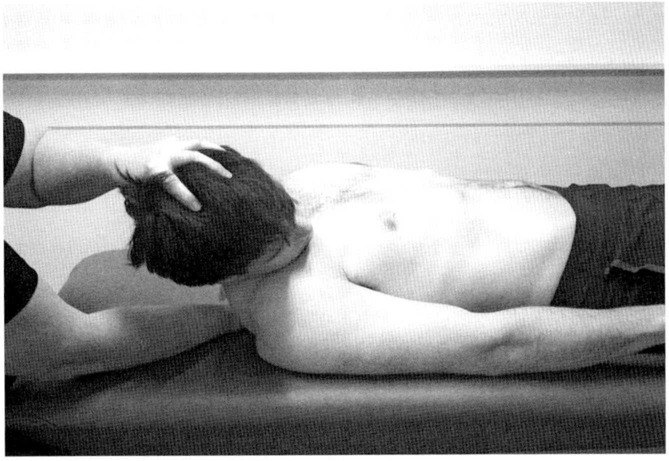

STEP 3

3. Swing the patient's head to the right without releasing the flexion to the limit of motion, while holding their T3 in place

Tucker's Upper Thoracic (T1-T7) Technique #2 (Side-Bending Technique)

EXAMPLE: T3 rotation right side-bent left
PHYSICIAN: Standing behind the patient
PATIENT: Lying on their left side.

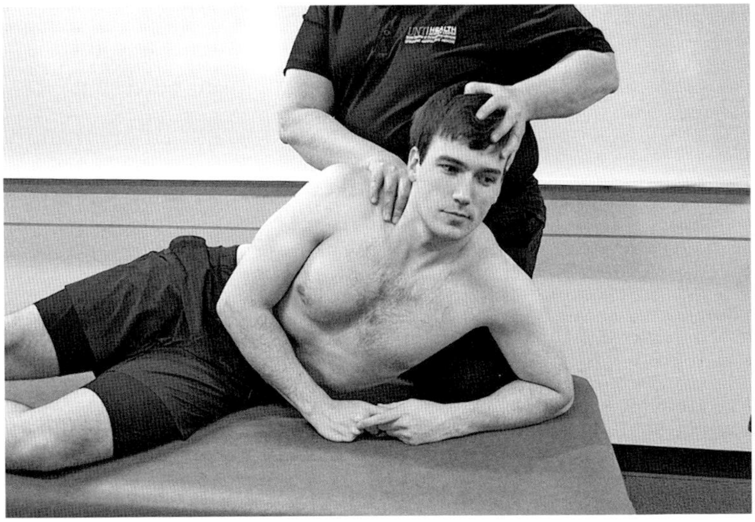

STEPS 1 – 2

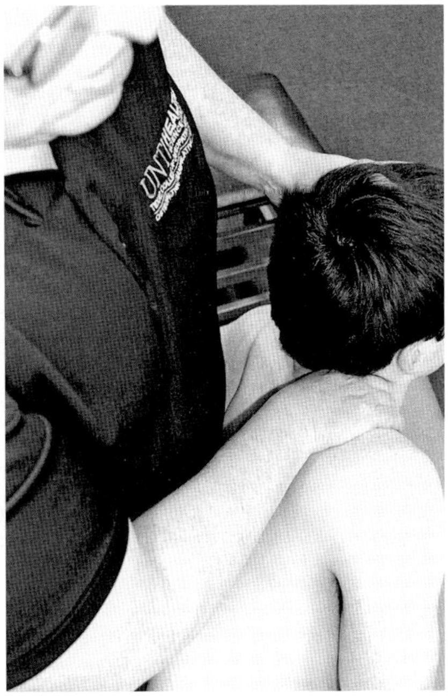

STEPS 3 – 4

1. Lift the patient's shoulders off the table, and place your left leg on thc table
2. Lower the patient across your thigh so that your leg fits into their axilla, the patient's arms being up and forward, out of the way
3. Place your right thumb against the prominent side of the spinous process of their T3 vertebra and the MIP (middle joint of your index finger) on the opposite side stabilizing the joint

4. Press the patient's head down to the limit of motion, stretching the ligaments on the dysfunctional side. Then lift their head up to their limit of motion (always remembering to keep their face towards the side-bending)
5. Repeat by going back and forth until the vertebra frees

Tucker: In this technique the rib braced against the thigh aids in fixing the vertebra below and in focusing the corrective force. This technique is available from about the seventh dorsal to the first dorsal. With traction upward instead of downward it is effective, for lesions of the opposite side (to the left). It is useful for many rib lesions.

Sutherland's Thoracic Vertebrae Principles of Technique

Lippincott: The facets of the superior articular processes face dorsally, cranially and laterally. Those of the inferior processes face ventrally, caudally and medially. Consequently, in flexion the transverse processes of one vertebra move anteriorly and superiorly in relation to those of the one below. In extension, the processes move postero-inferiorly. In side-bending/rotation the transverse process on the side of the convexity moves cranially, anteriorly and slightly medially away from the one below. On the side of concavity the two processes approximate and the upper one moves dorsally.

Elevation of the patient's shoulders tends to separate the transverse processes and move the inferior articular facets antero-superiorly on the superior articular surfaces of the vertebra below. This approximates the relationship which exists during flexion. When the shoulders are lowered the articular processes assume the relationship present in extension. Elevating one shoulder separates the transverse processes on that side and the upper one moves anteriorly, on the side of convexity in side-bending/rotation. Lowering the shoulder produces the relationship which is present on the side of the concavity.

Sutherland's Thoracic Diagnosis – Palpation for Motion

PHYSICIAN: Standing behind the patient (if the patient is seated); seated at the head of the table (if the patient is supine)
PATIENT: Seated or supine

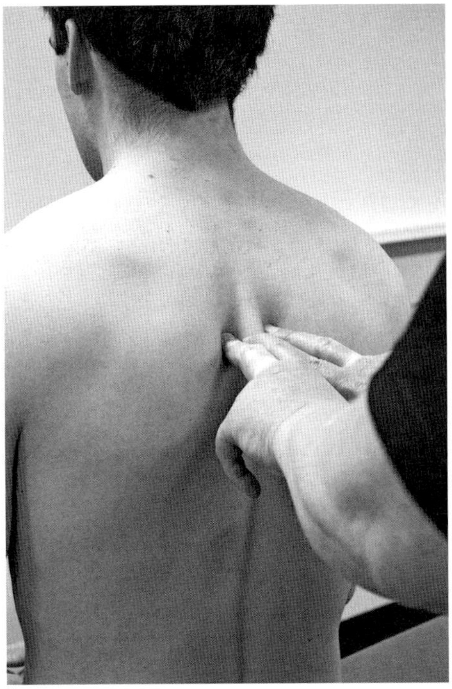

STEP 1

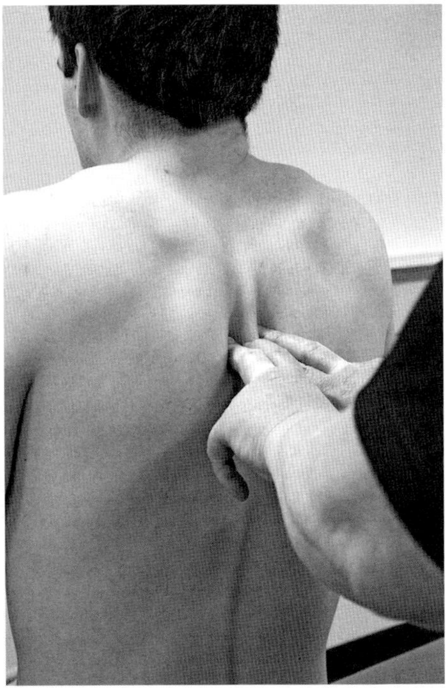

STEP 2

1. The physician places a finger on each transverse process of the patient's thoracic vertebrae
2. Ask the patient to elevate both shoulders slowly, and then lower their shoulders towards their hips

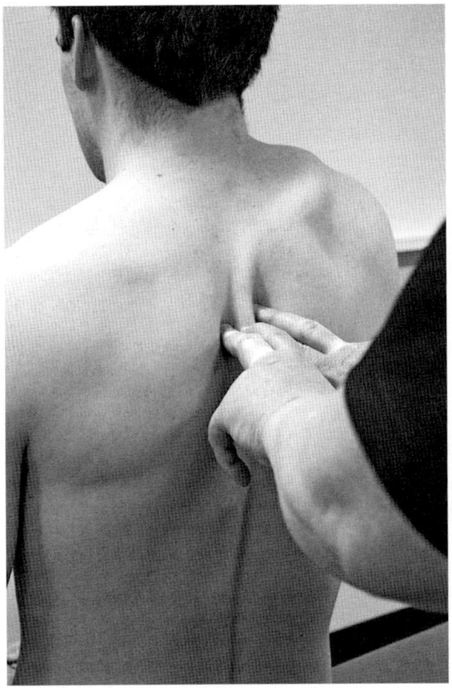

STEP 3

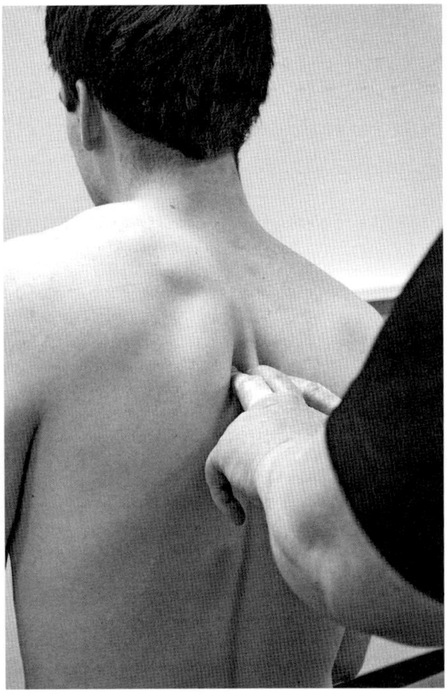

STEP 4

3. Ask the patient to raise one shoulder and lower the other shoulder alternately while you palpate for freedom of motion

4. The transverse processes of their involved vertebrae are in a relatively anterior position
5. These vertebrae are held anteriorly in the plane of their articular facets to exaggerate the dysfunction position

Sutherland's Technique for Thoracic Flexion Dysfunctions

PHYSICIAN: Standing (if the patient is seated); seated (if the patient is supine)
PATIENT: Supine or seated

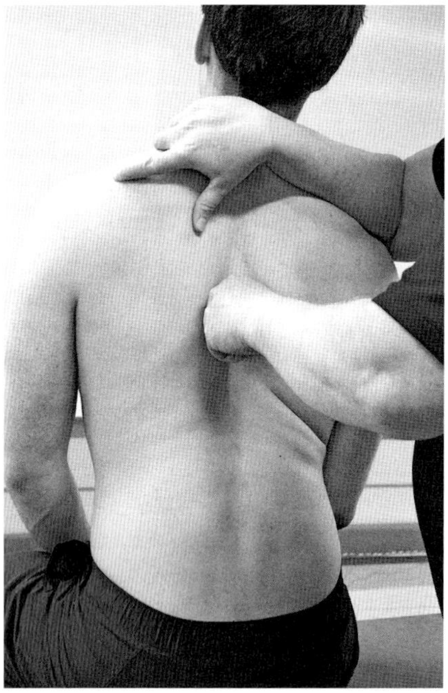

STEP 1

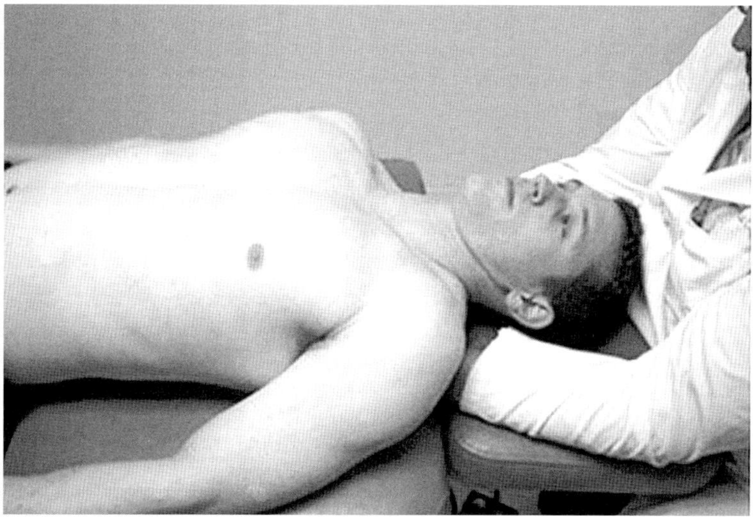

STEP 2

1. The physician holds the processes of the upper of the patient's two vertebrae while pushing anteriorly and superiorly with their thumb and index finger. If seated, your other hand is on the patient's shoulder
2. If the patient is supine, use your finger tips on each of the upper of their two vertebrae while pushing anteriorly and superiorly
3. Ask the patient to elevate both shoulders to balance the ligamentous tension. This position is held while the patient inhales and holds their breath in

Sutherland's Technique for Thoracic Extension Dysfunctions

PHYSICIAN: Standing (if the patient is seated); seated (if the patient is supine)
PATIENT: Supine or seated

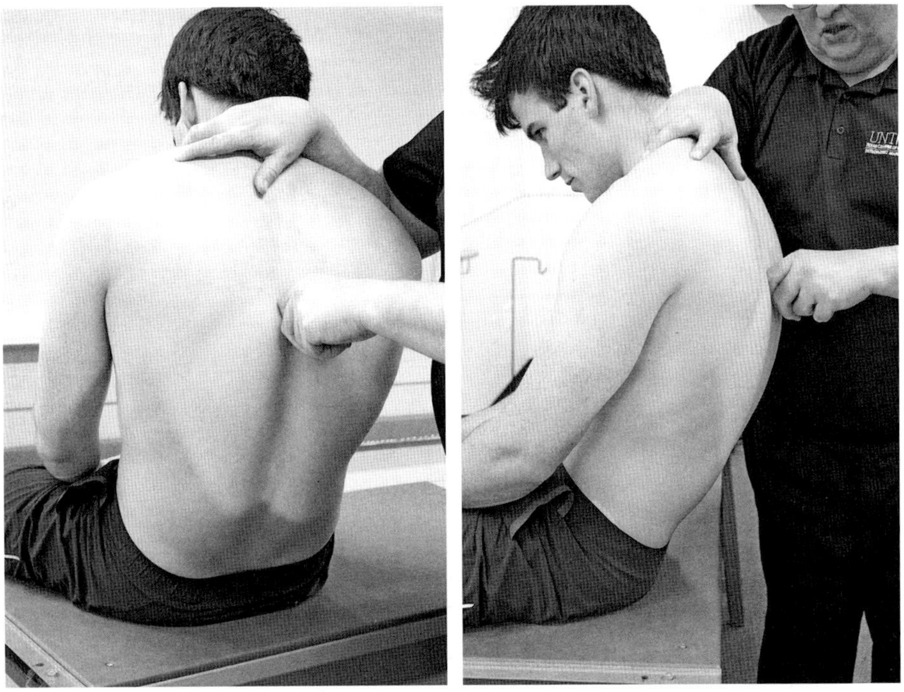

STEP 1

1. The physician holds the transverse processes of the lower of the patient's two vertebrae anteriorly and superiorly between the physician's thumb and finger; if seated, with the physician's other hand on the patient's shoulder

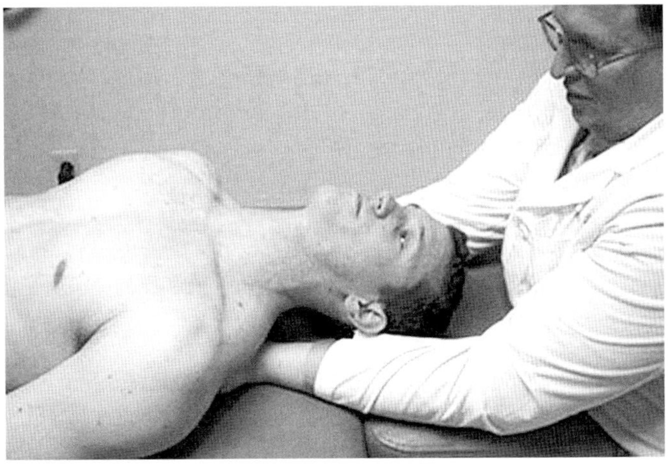

STEP 2

2. If the patient is supine, use your finger tips on each of the transverse processes of the lower of the two vertebrae anteriorly and superiorly
3. Ask the patient to bring their shoulders towards their feet. Ask the patient to exhale and hold their breath

Sutherland's Technique for Thoracic Side-Bending Rotation Dysfunctions

PHYSICIAN: Standing (if the patient is seated); seated (if the patient is supine)
PATIENT: Seated or supine

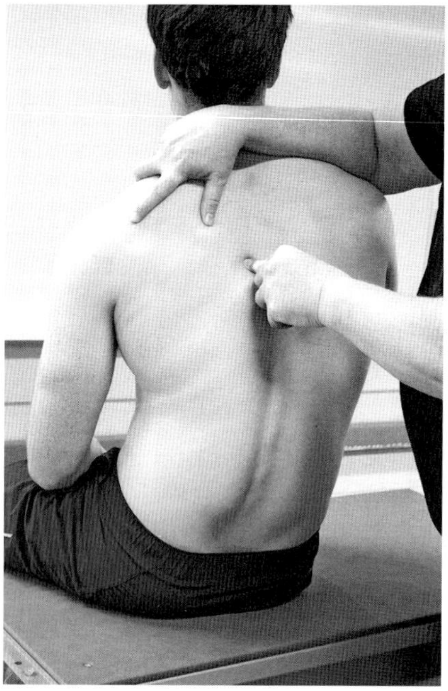

STEP 1

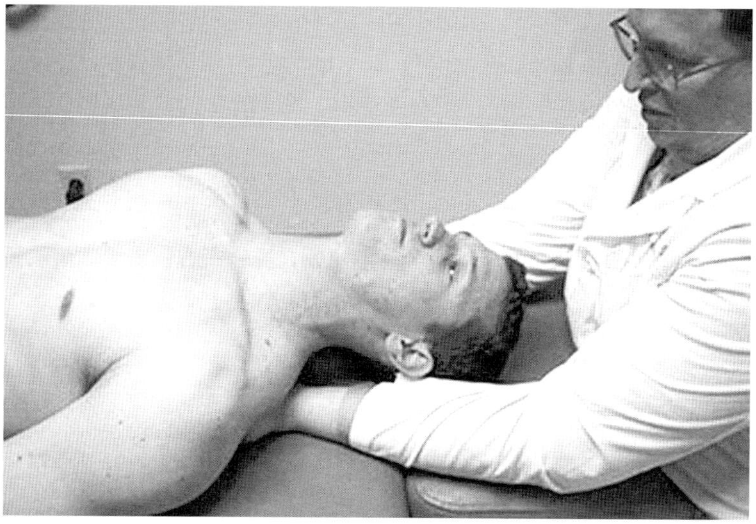

STEP 2

1. On the side of the convexity you will be moving the transverse process of the patient's upper vertebrae with your thumb or fingers by pushing anteriorly and superiorly. On the concavity the transverse processes of the lower vertebrae is held by the physician. You are rotating the vertebrae in opposite directions. In other words you 'over-rotate' the dysfunction. For example, if T5 is rotated right take it more right, and if T6 is rotated left take it more left. Then you separate the two vertebrae and rotate one away from the other
2. Ask the patient to elevate their shoulder on the side of convexity, and carry it slightly anteriorly or forward. Then ask them to lower the opposite shoulder and carry it slightly posteriorly or backward
3. Ask the patient to inhale and exhale until the point of balanced ligamentous tension is reached and ask them to hold their breath. Usually inhalation is used if the ligamentous imbalance is mainly on the side of the convexity. Exhalation is used if the imbalance is on the concave side.

Wales on the Thorax and Ribs

The ribs are the making of the thoracic cavity. The shape of the thoracic cavity which contains these viscera is determined by the excursion of the diaphragm. The point is that it not only changes its shape, it has to change its size. If you breathe in air there has to be more room for it to go into. I didn't know that Dr. Sutherland made it clear that the thoracic cavity changes its size at the back of the cavity in front and then posteriorly via the ribs. The ribs come around and have a gliding articulation with the transverse process of their respective vertebrae. They converge anteriorly to the articulation at the head of the rib with the body of the vertebra. The three radial ligaments at the head of the ribs are merged into the anterior longitudinal spinal ligament.

The next ribs are all in line and they create the space at the back of the thoracic cavity. You don't normally think of that. You think of rib cage movement where it moves most, and where you can see it. But posteriorly at the back, in order for it to do that, the neck of the rib has to go into rotation.

Dr. Sutherland said that the necks of the ribs rotate in the plane so that they function like venetian blinds. When they all line up they make the wall flat, and it makes more room for inhalation. Then, with exhalation they move the other way. It has helped me a great deal to have a picture, because you don't realize how many people breathe inadequately until you watch them, and analyze what they are doing. Singing teachers and others, especially Dr. Sutherland, have said that the correct way to breathe is to have both lower ribs move laterally with inhalation, and medially with exhalation. If we do this properly, everything else works right.

There is a joint between the manubrium of the sternum and the body of the sternum. With inhalation of the whole chest, the manubrium goes backwards. He had a great deal to say about the disadvantage to the body of this military posture on parade. You're standing there sticking your chest out and staying like a stick. It isn't good for effective respirations as you don't breathe completely even though the upper lobes of the lungs go up almost into the back of the clavicles. They just simply have alveoli that fill. Your bronchial tree gets the air to them, and the blood has to be there in this delicate distribution involving the alveoli in order for there to be an interchange across that interface between the blood and the air. The carbon dioxide can go out and the oxygen can come in.

This is another place in the body which in osteopathy we aim to enhance. Breathing is done by the diaphragm, but you watch the posture of a lot of people and you will see that they aren't breathing with their diaphragm. They are puffing away with the upper part of their rib cage.

Release Technique for the Erector Spinae Muscles and Longitudinal Ligaments of the Spine

Crow: This technique works on the erector spinae muscles. Either in a small group complex of two vertebrae, or a large group if a long muscle is involved like the longissimus coli.

PHYSICIAN: Standing beside the patient
PATIENT: Prone

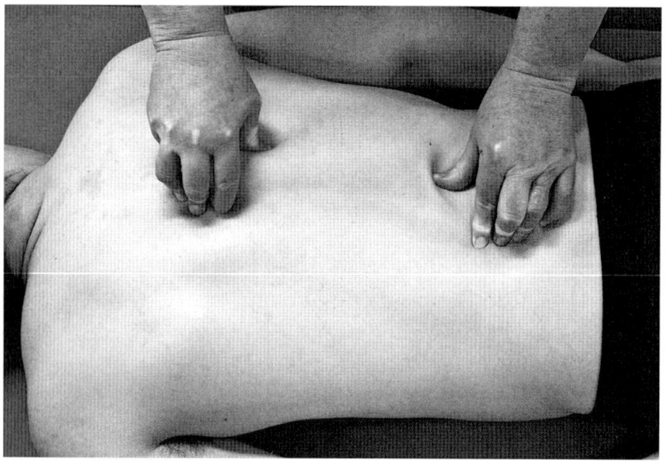

LONG LEVER

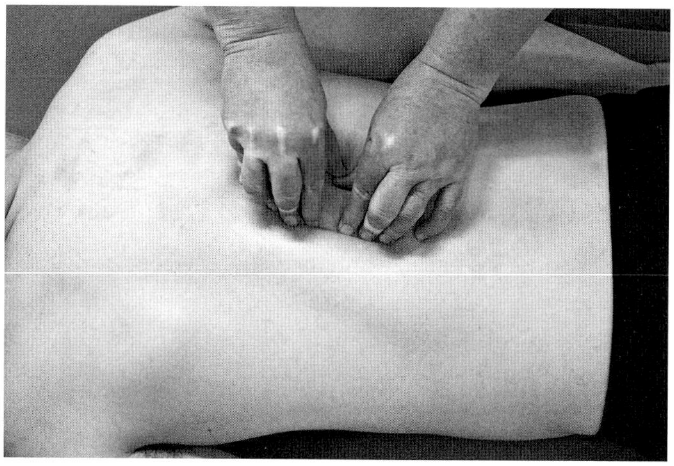

SHORT LEVER

1. Locate a lesioned vertebral complex, type 1 or type 2, or an area of the spine which does not appear to give anteriorly when pressure is added. Apply your fingertips or your fingers at their interphalangeal (IP) joints to the spinous processes of the patient's vertebra
2. Try to ascertain the general position of the vertebra (XYZ axes), as you will try to guide against these barriers once they are determined. This is not absolutely necessary to the success of the treatment, but may assist in a more complete release
3. Apply a very firm anterior force, as firmly as you can without creating pain in the patient. This is often an uncomfortable technique for the patient, so care is required to keep the pressure within the bounds of patient tolerance
4. Maintenance of the pressure is continued until softening occurs. This will often be in segments, rather than the whole area that has been placed under ligamentous strain
5. Maintain pressure on the points that fail to yield until the overt return of the CRI or generalized softening occurs. This is also accompanied by a greater sense of pulmonary respiratory motion
6. Apply pressure again as part of re-checking for improvement. If a release has occurred, the sense of anterior translation will be greater than when first assessed

5
Techniques for the Ribs

Wales' Sternal Release Technique

PHYSICIAN: Standing beside the patient
PATIENT: Supine

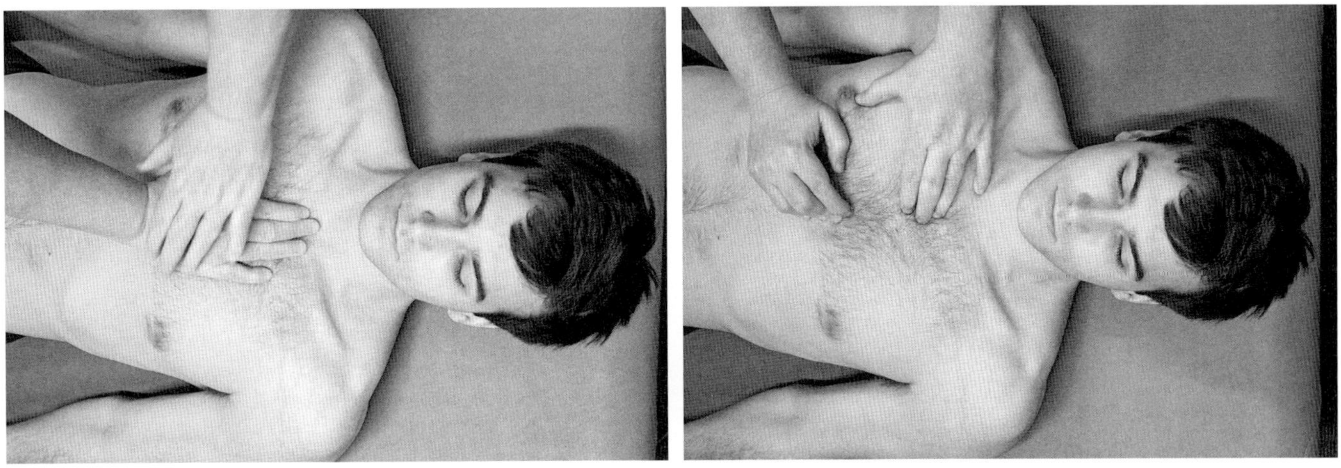

STEP 1

1. Place only your hand on the manubrium with your fingers pointing towards the patient's head

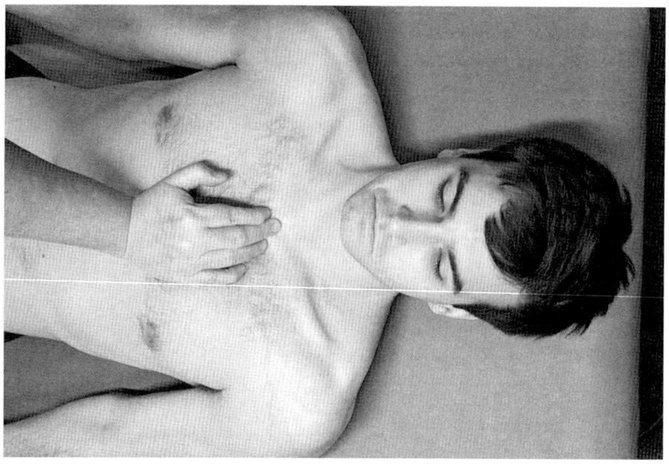

STEPS 2 – 3

2. Gently compress the patient's manubrium and find a point of balanced tension
3. Ask the patient to take deep breaths—in and out

Wales: This will shift all the fascia around the thoracic outlet, and all you do is hold the manubrium. When you're doing it you will have a good opportunity to note if the manubrium goes in when the patient breathes in. When they breathe out, if it goes forward and out, this is not the way the body of the sternum normally moves. The manubrium does move.

I can do the same thing with the upper ribs and the upper thorax, or I can make a regional adjustment. I'm thinking of the sternum as a whole in relation to the mediastinal fascia. I use both hands to shift the whole rib cage around this fascia. I can move the sternum to the right, to the left, and then I can come back to neutral. I can move it down. I can move it up. I want to leave it up.

West's First Rib Technique #1

EXAMPLE: Left 1st rib
PHYSICIAN: Standing beside the patient
PATIENT: Seated

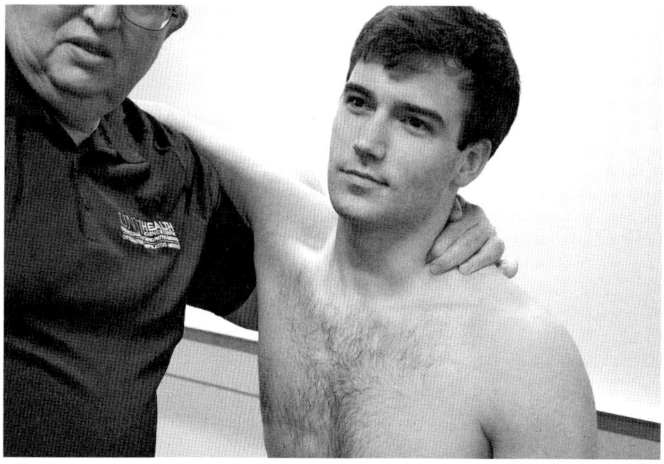

STEP 1

1. Reach under the patient's right arm and place your left hand upon the tubercle of their left 1st rib, close to the patient's neck with your fingers facing downwards

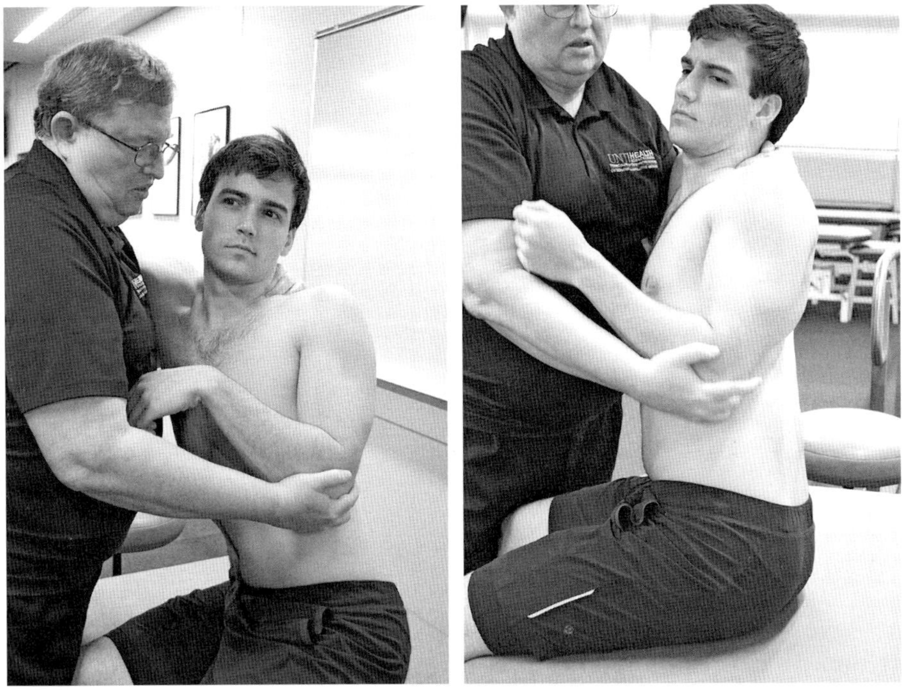

STEP 2

2. Place your right hand under their left elbow. Raise their elbow and their shoulder strongly, straight up in the mid-axillary line

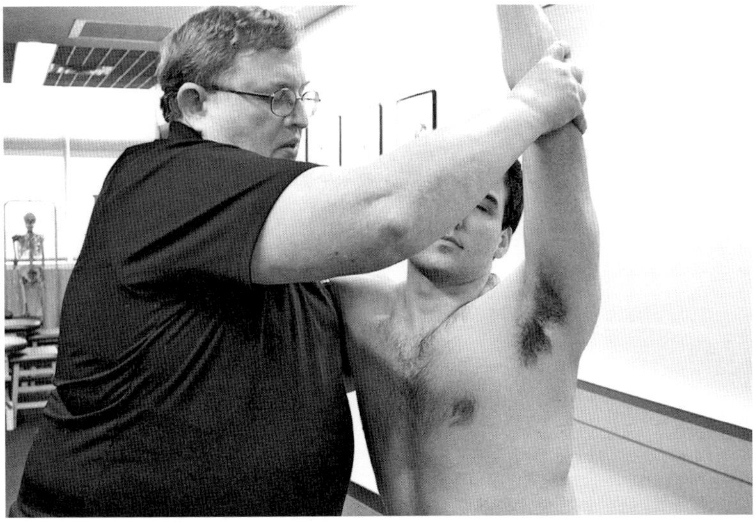

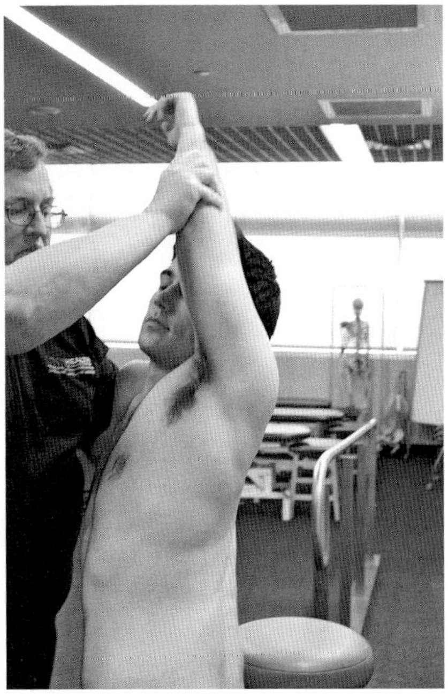

STEP 3

3. Bring their elbow back up and swing their upper arm in a backward rotation of their shoulder while maintaining strong pressure on their rib at the tubercle

West's First Rib Technique #2

EXAMPLE: Left 1st rib
PHYSICIAN: Standing beside the patient
PATIENT: Seated

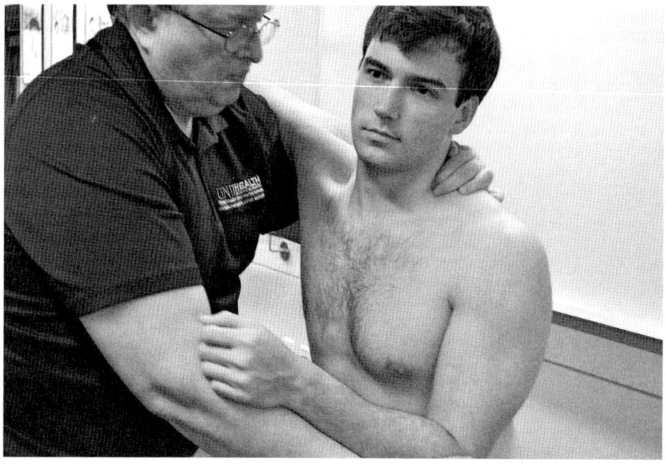

STEP 1

1. Reach under the patient's right arm and place your left hand upon the tubercle of their left 1st rib, close to their neck with your fingers facing downwards

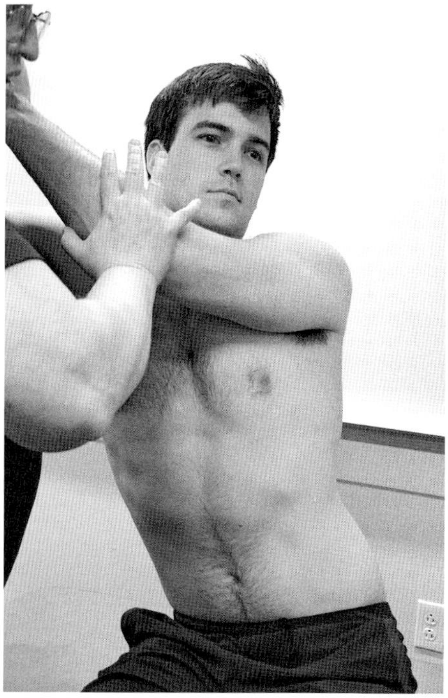

STEP 2

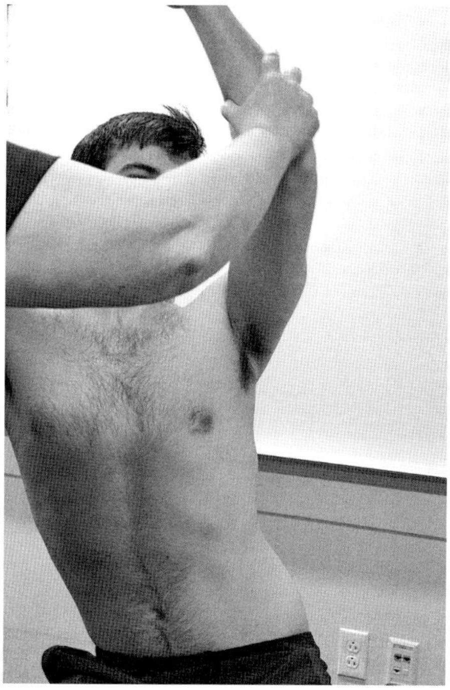

STEP 3

2. Draw their forearm down sweepingly over their abdomen and across their mid-line, up close to their body
3. Then, with an outward rotation of their arm, throw their shoulder strongly back to stretch their subclavius muscle

West's First Rib Supine Technique

EXAMPLE: Left 1st rib
PHYSICIAN: Standing at the head of the table
PATIENT: Supine

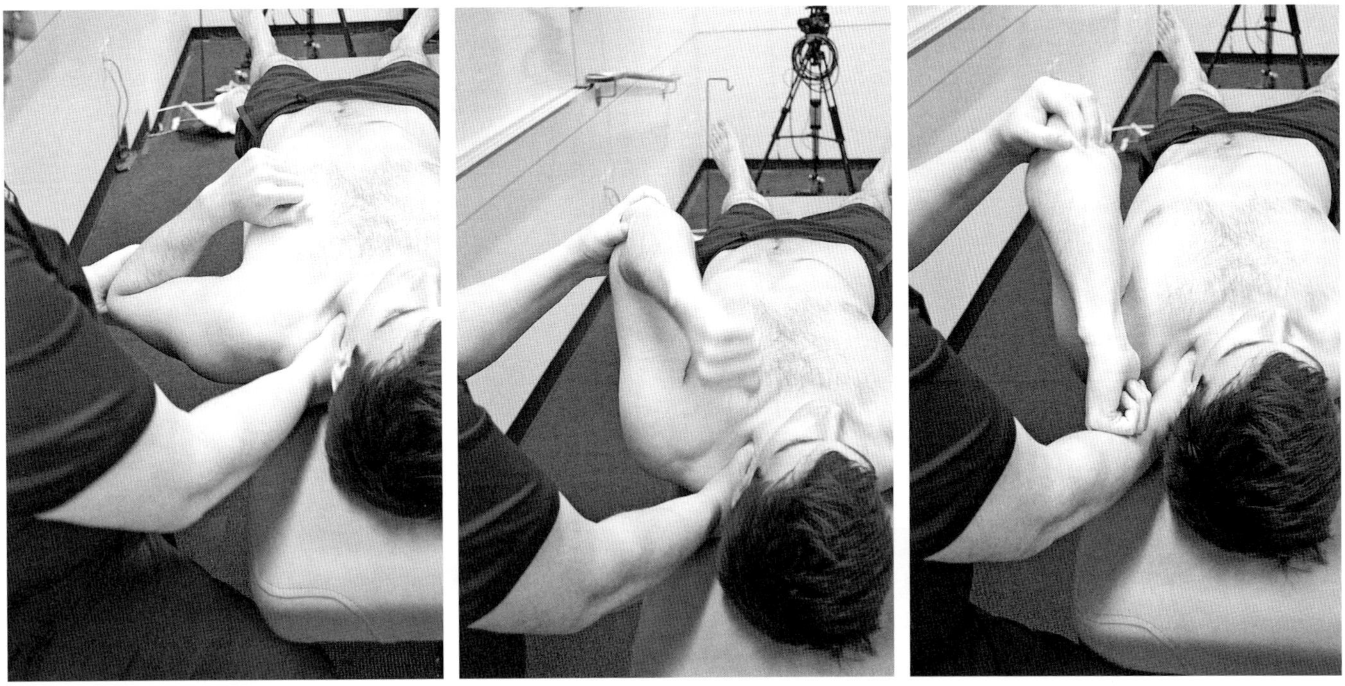

STEP 1 STEP 2 STEP 3

1. Place the thumb or fingers of your right (inner) hand between the patient's neck and clavicle
2. Take your left (outer) hand and elevate their left arm by means of their elbow
3. As "one" press down on their 1st rib to make a complete rotation of their arm at the shoulder

Tucker on First and Second Ribs

The motion of these two ribs is much slighter than that of the others. The motion of the sternum is forward and up. The excursion of the lower part of the sternum is much greater than that of the upper part, leaving very little movement for these first two ribs. Beside this they have a slight wing motion, under the traction of the scalene muscles, opposed by the intercostals. This is little more than a ligamentous yielding.

DIAGNOSIS

Tucker: On account of the thickness of the over-lying muscles, it is very difficult, as a rule, to examine effectively these two ribs except at the sternal ends. Unevenness on the two sides in front argues the probability of a lesion. But to know which side is in lesion, one must rely upon relative sensitiveness. Lesions upward at the transverse process draw the sternal end backward, making it seem smaller than its fellow, and making it also sensitive. If the lesion is downward, it is the reverse. About one inch of the first rib may be felt beneath the collarbone. By drawing the shoulder blade away and slightly lifting it in thin subjects the spinal ends may sometimes be felt. But usually they bend almost directly forward from the transverse process, leaving little surface for examination and little certainty therein. With the patient lying on their side and shoulder blade lifted, the thumbs may find and examine one side at a time.

DYSFUNCTIONS

Tucker: As in the other ribs, lesions at the transverse processes cannot be distinguished (if slight) from those at the head, up and forward or down and back. The curve can be diagnosed if the latter exists. Lesions at the transverse process are up and forward or down and back. They seem more prominent if up, on account of the spacing. Less prominent if they are down.

Tucker's First Rib Technique #1

EXAMPLE: Right 1st rib to be downward on transverse process
PHYSICIAN: Standing behind the patient
PATIENT: Seated on the table

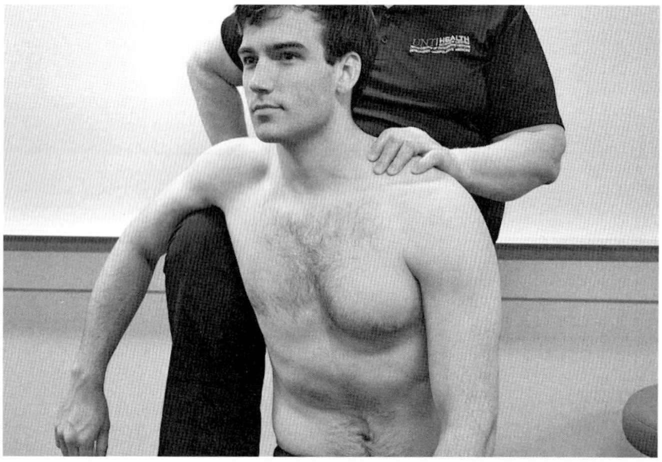

STEP 1

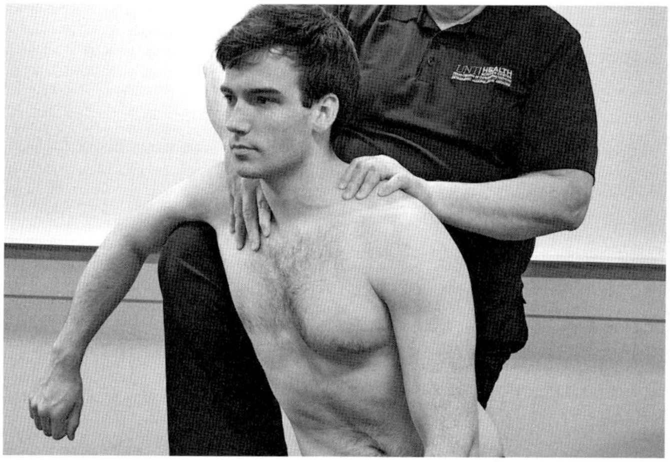

STEP 2

1. Place your right foot on the table and place your right knee under the patient's right axilla with the patient's right arm hanging down
2. Press down on the patient's right arm to carry their shoulder blade away from their spine and to put upward tension on their subclavius and pectoralis minor muscles

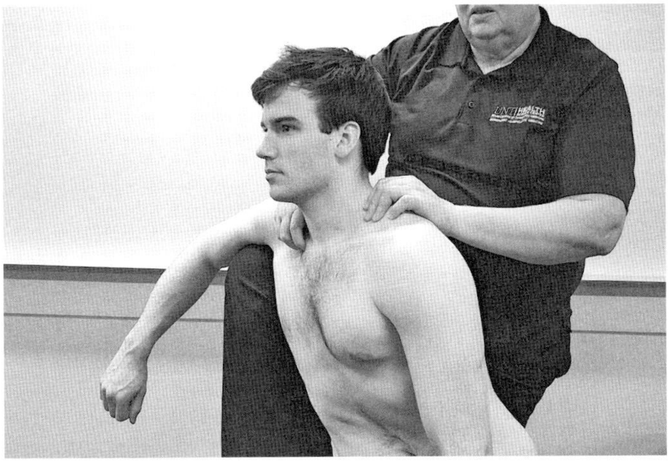

STEP 3

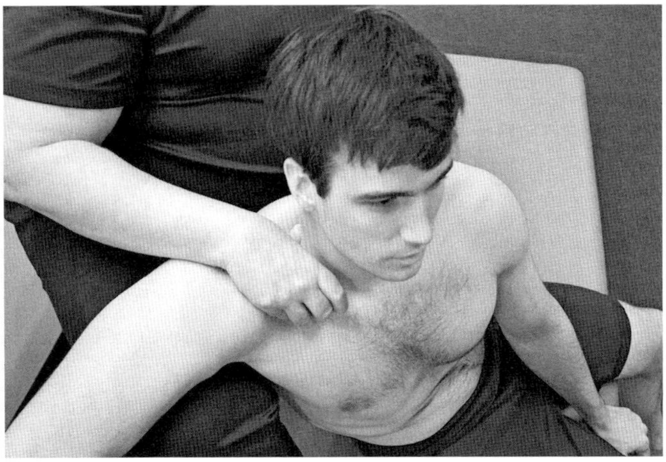

STEP 4

3. Swing your right knee with the patient's body slightly to the right to secure full extension of their ribs
4. Place your right thumb against the angle of the rib where it leaves the transverse process. Endeavor to get beneath the rib—between this rib and the second rib
5. Place your left hand on the patient's head and carry their head to the left to the limit of motion to produce tension on their scalene muscles
6. In this position you turn the patient's face first towards the left to lift the transverse process and produce an angle between it and the rib. Then you turn the patient's face to the right and backward to carry the transverse process backward away from the ribs, thus changing the angle
7. With gentle exaggerations of these tensions the rib may be brought back to normal
8. If necessary swing their head and neck into extreme side-bending from extreme left to the extreme right. Repeat until the lesion is reduced

Tucker's First Rib Technique #2

PHYSICIAN: Standing beside the patient
PATIENT: Supine

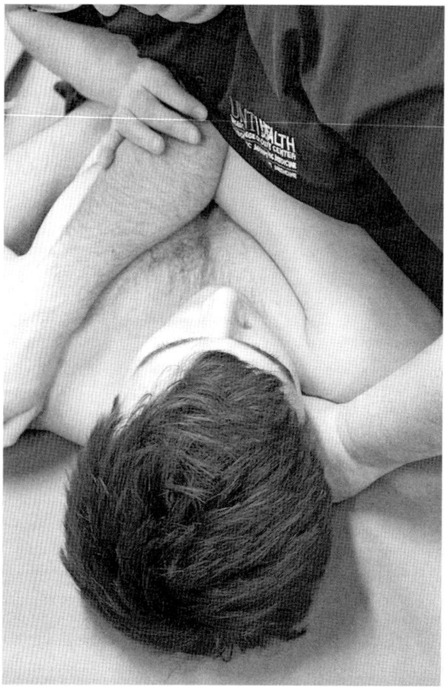

STEP 1

1. Draw the patient's right arm across their chest, with their arm high up and bent at the elbow

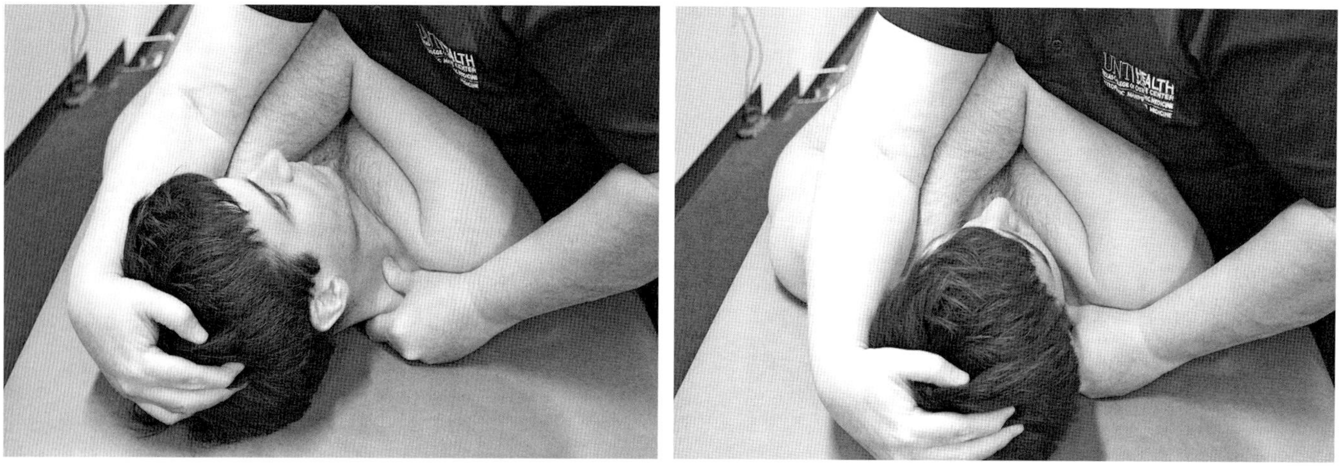

STEPS 2 – 4

2. Place their right elbow against your sternum
3. Place your left hand under their 1st rib, your knuckles against the table, and your fingers bearing up against their rib
4. With your right hand carry their head to the left side, and then to the right. Gentle exaggeration of all of these tensions will tend to bring the rib back to normal

Sutherland's Rib Dysfunctions and Technique

Lippincott: A rib dysfunction is considered as an articular strain of the capsular, radiate and intra-articular ligaments connecting the head of the rib to the bodies of the vertebrae. Diagnosis is made in the usual manner—considering history of trauma, pain and tenderness, tissue tenseness and induration, possible abnormality of position, and restricted motion. If the first and the last two diagnostic points indicate a rotation of the rib in a particular direction, that position may be held in exaggeration for the correction. Otherwise the simple disengagement of the costo-central articulation alone is used.

In this corrective technique the ligaments are tensed by using first degree leverage of the rib to lift its head anteriorly and laterally away from the facets on the vertebral bodies. The rib is shaped like a horseshoe with a long arm from the angle to the anterior end, and the short arm from the angle of the head of the rib. In other words, you hold the 'bolt' while the patient turns the 'nut' to release the dysfunction.

Sutherland's First Rib Technique

PHYSICIAN: Standing at the side of the patient
PATIENT: Seated

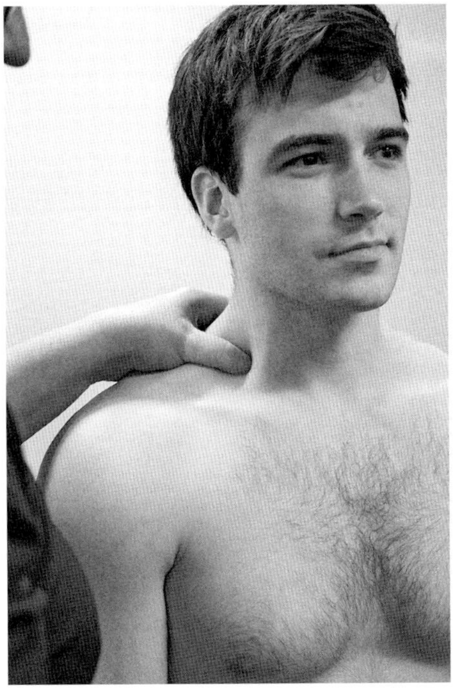

STEP 1

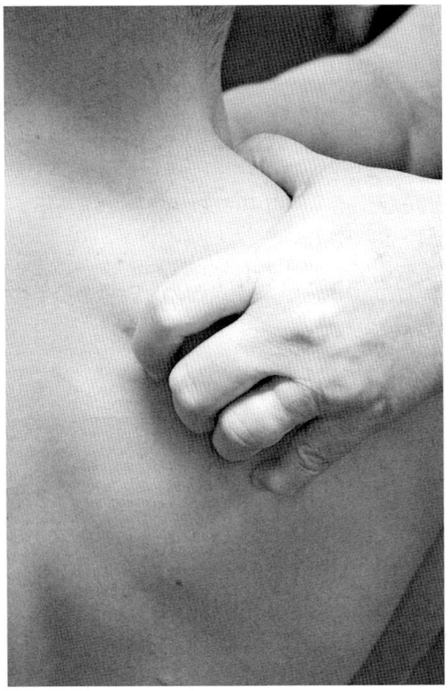

STEP 2

1. The thumb of your posterior hand is placed anteriorly to the patient's trapezius and follows their rib posteriorly and medially under that muscle
2. Advance your thumb posteriorly as the patient inhales and exhales, until you arrive at the posterior surface of the rib. If necessary the hold may be through the muscle itself

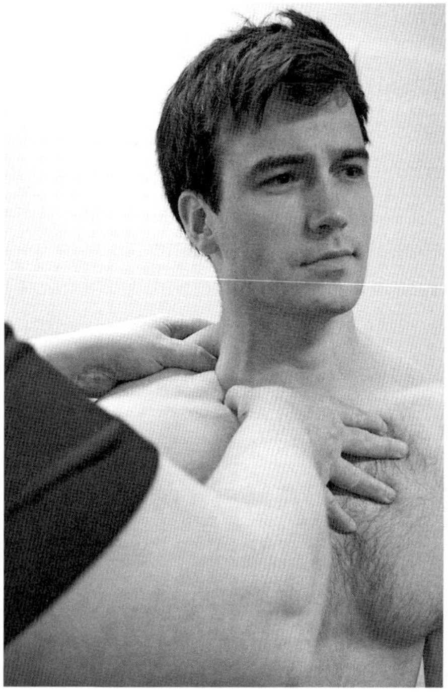

STEP 3

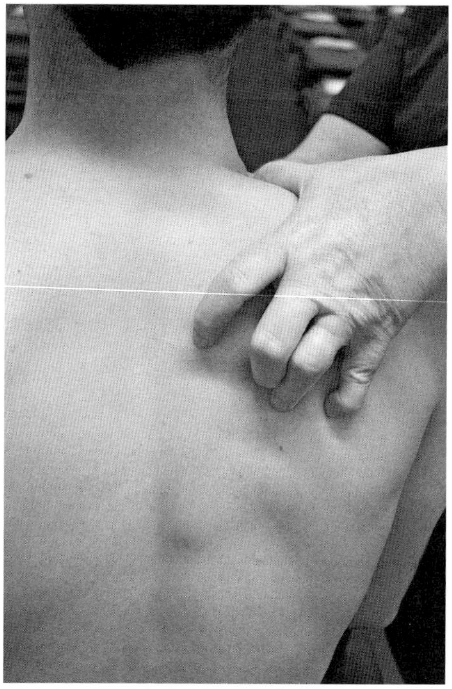

STEP 5

3. Place the thumb of your other hand on the anterior portion of their 1st rib
4. Maintain firm contact while the patient gently lowers their shoulder on the dysfunctional side
5. Place the fingers or the palm of your posterior hand at the inferior part of the lateral border of their scapula. Hold their scapula medially, posteriorly and upward away from your other thumb
6. Ask the patient to lean towards you
7. Ask the patient to keep their head erect and not turn their neck as they turn their body slowly away from you. Ask them to carry the opposite shoulder posteriorly to the point of balanced tension of their ligaments
8. Ask the patient to inhale and hold their breath in

Wales on Ribs

One of the things which we osteopaths have as a great advantage is our knowledge of the rib cage. What we can use it for is to influence the vasomotor blood supply and secretory nerve supply of this whole region of the sympathetic ganglion. This is located in front of the ribs on the back wall of the thoracic cage. You can't have a tight rib cage without having some sluggishness in the function of the sympathetic nervous system under those conditions. So the point is to move the heads of the ribs out of the demi-facets at the articulations with the body of the vertebrae.

So all I have to do is lift and hang on to the angle of the ribs and just lean back to change my position. I'm lifting the ribs by their angles laterally. The neck of the ribs that articulate with the transverse processes of the vertebrae and the heads of the ribs that articulate with the bodies of the vertebrae, will glide on both these articulations and hold them there. As the patients breathe, the heads of the ribs move much more widely than they had been able to previously. That gives the whole sympathetic chain of ganglia a treatment. This gives me better control of what I am doing. When the sympathetic ganglions are more functional the patient will feel better.

Therefore, you are seeing a mechanical function of the rib cage as a whole architectural unit. The patient is doing the work. The diaphragm is going up and down and their mediastinal fascia is thereby being moved. Each rib comes around the sternum on the costal arch and the patient's thorax is now 'breathing'. Which it was not doing very thoroughly beforehand. I don't have any words for what it was doing because it wasn't doing it. I can feel it loosening up with their breathing, so that all the ribs are moving toward their head and then toward their pelvis. This is the normal excursion of ribs on the transverse processes and I haven't moved my position at all.

There are times when these are called a rib lesion. This is what I call a tonic osteopathic treatment for the treatment of some systemic problems, such as the common cold, grippe, and the flu. The body has been through some compensatory process, and the body is still bogged down in some aspect of it. All I am doing is stirring up the patient's body machinery to do a little better work on its own. What I like about Will's techniques is that they don't hurt. If they hurt, it's actually inflammation from the patient's existing problem and I can use this inflammation to help them heal.

Wales' 1st and 2nd Ribs Technique

EXAMPLE: 2nd rib right
PHYSICIAN: Seated or standing beside the patient
PATIENT: Seated

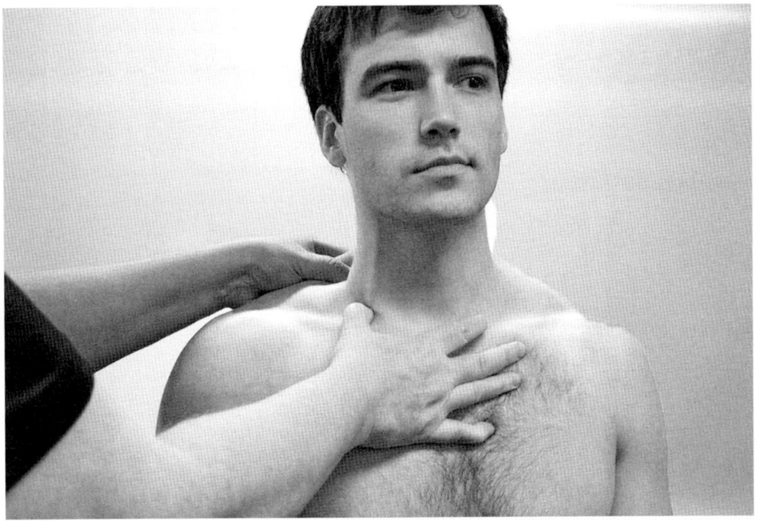

STEP 1

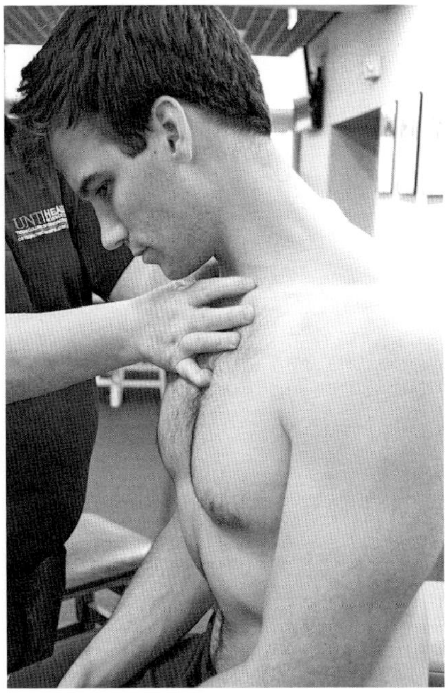

STEP 2

1. Ask the patient to raise their right arm above their head
2. Place your left thumb under their right scapula at the level of their second rib and your fingertips on the angle of their scapula

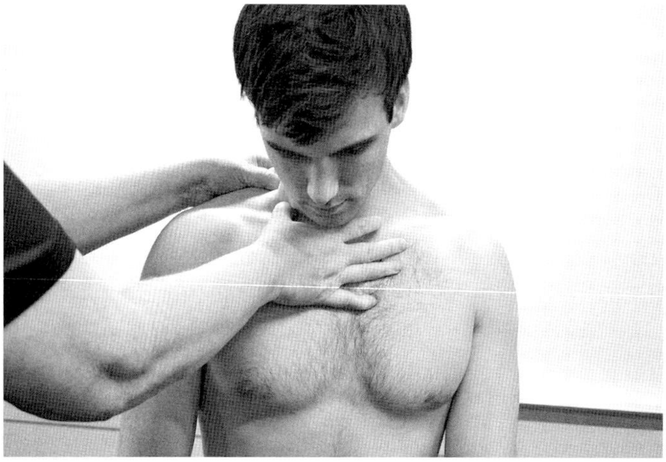

STEP 3

3. Ask the patient to lower their arm while you maintain contact with their second rib
4. Place your right thumb or fingers on their 2nd rib
5. Ask the patient to lower their weight onto your hands
6. Ask the patient to then take their left shoulder backwards and inhale

Sutherland's 2nd and 3rd Ribs Technique

PHYSICIAN: Standing beside the patient
PATIENT: Seated

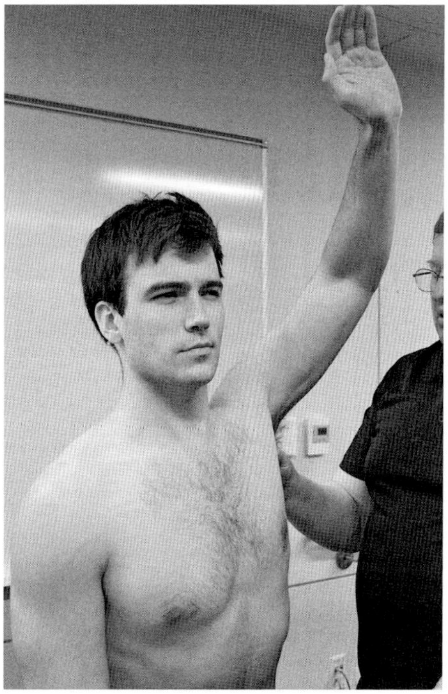

STEP 1

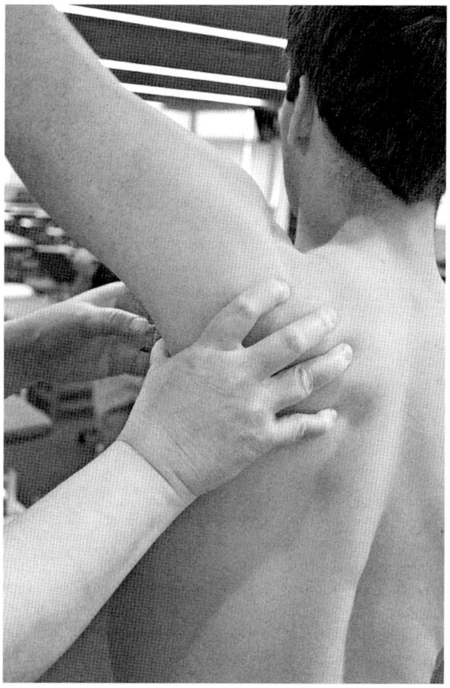

STEP 2

1. Ask the patient to raise their shoulder on the dysfunctional side
2. Place one hand on their anterior chest wall with your thumb in their axilla. Your thumb

travels upward and back toward their scapula while your contact on their second or third rib is as near to the rib angle as you can get

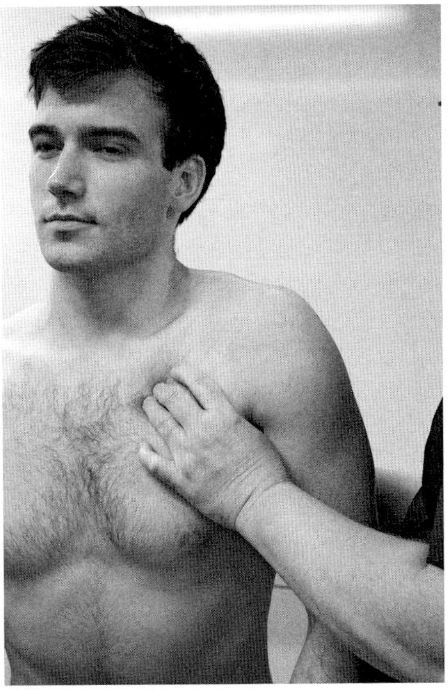

STEP 3

3. Ask the patient to lower their shoulder on the dysfunctional side
4. The thumb of your posterior hand is placed at the inferior part of the lateral border of their scapula and holds the scapula medially, posteriorly and upward away from your other thumb
5. Ask the patient to lean towards you
6. Ask the patient to keep their head erect and not turn their neck as they turn the body slowly away from you. Ask them to carry their opposite shoulder posteriorly to the point of balanced tension of the ligaments
7. Ask the patient to inhale and hold their breath in

Sutherland's Alternate Technique for Upper Ribs

PHYSICIAN: Standing in front of the patient
PATIENT: Seated

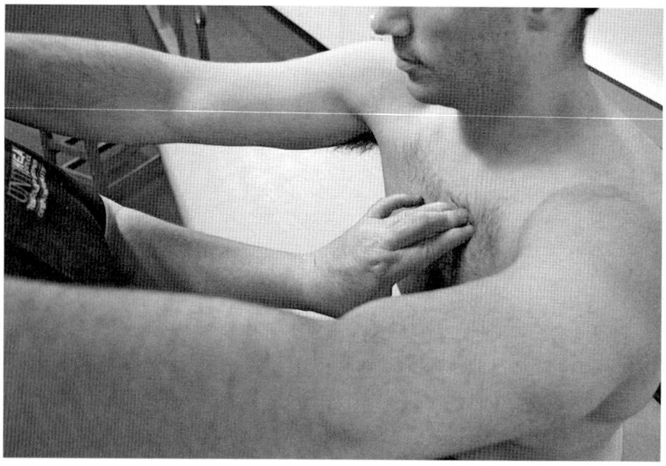

STEPS 2 – 3

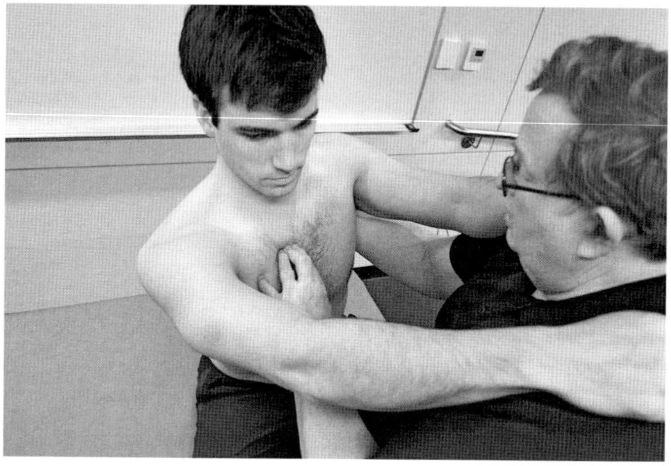

STEPS 4 – 5

1. Ask the patient to be seated with their hands resting on your shoulders
2. Hold the sternal end of their rib posteriorly with your fingers
3. Ask the patient to place his hands or forearms on your shoulders
4. Ask the patient to rotate their body, carrying their shoulder opposite the dysfunction in a posterior or backwards direction
5. Ask the patient to inhale and hold their breath in

Wales' Rib Technique

Wales: You can treat with the patient sitting up or standing up if you have to. I like to treat with the patient lying down—supine. I proceed to slide my hand underneath by the angle of the patient's rib yet medial to it. I reinforce my contact, and lean away so that I put lateral traction on the rib at the rib angle. That is putting tension into the ligamentous articular mechanism with the transverse process and the head of the rib. All I have to do is hold it, and all this time the patient is breathing. You can feel this principle, what Dr. Sutherland called the nut and bolt principle. The bolt is the rib. The nut is the vertebral column. We have to hold the bolt and have the patient turn the nut.

PHYSICIAN: Seated beside the patient
PATIENT: Supine

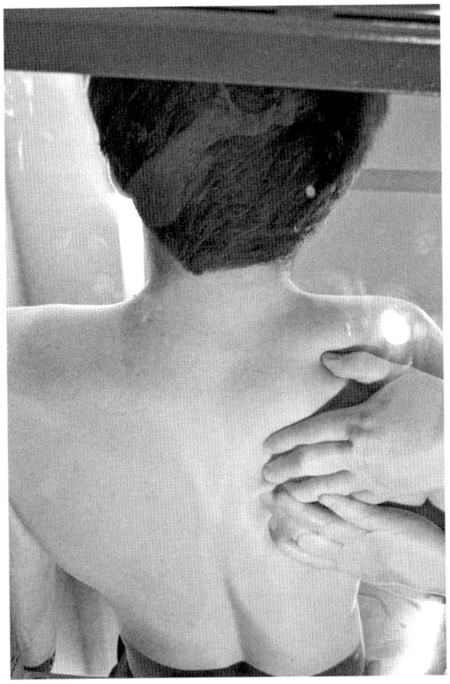

STEP 1

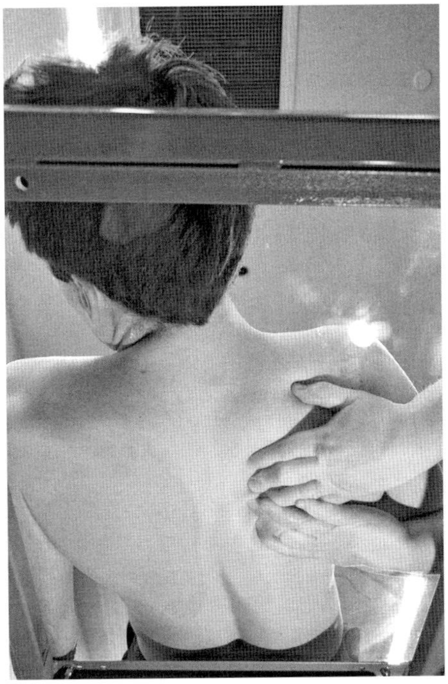

STEP 2

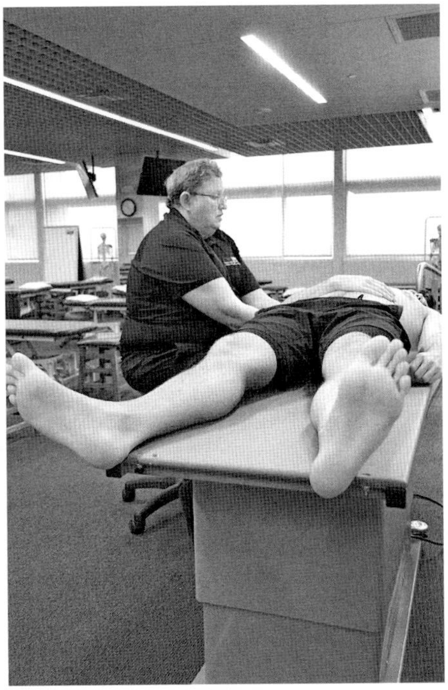

STEP 3

1. Place your fingers medial to the patient's rib angle
2. Ask the patient to turn their head toward their opposite shoulder
3. Ask the patient to dorsiflex their opposite foot
4. You should then lean backwards
5. Ask the patient to take a breath in and out
6. After that rib releases, then move down to the next rib

Wales: The flexion of the opposite foot, the diagonal from where you are, is to stabilize the whole fascial system of the body so as to amplify the actions of the ligaments and free up the subluxation. The weight of the patient lying supine is your counterforce, so you don't have to lean on the patient.

If it has happened that a group of thoracic vertebra have gone into hyper extension, these wedge shaped heads of the ribs may have gone with them sufficiently to jump out of their demi-facets and may be a subluxation or may have come back somewhat. In that case the heads of the ribs will prevent you from correcting the hyperextension of the vertebra. So you get the ribs out of the way first before you treat the thoracic spine.

This technique works beneficially for the postural mechanics of people with some degree of osteoporosis without any contraindication. There are some contraindications for some osteopathic procedures on a spine, which has osteoporosis or osteomalacia (adult rickets), or any pathology that you may know about.

Hazzard's Rib Technique

A most effective treatment is shown by Dr. Still.

EXAMPLE: Rib 3 right and stuck in inspiration
PHYSICIAN: Seated on the left side of the patient
PATIENT: Seated

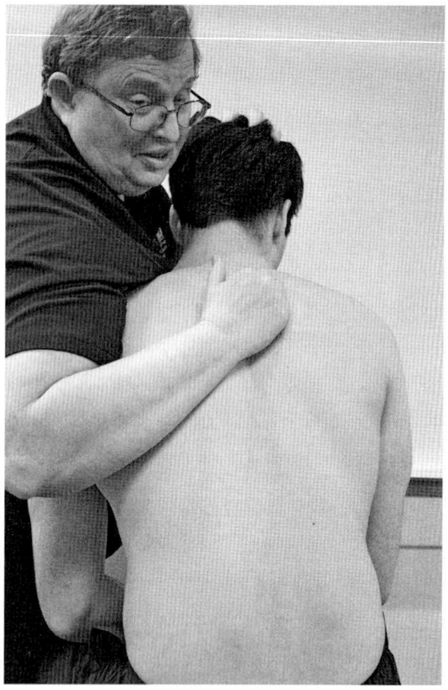

STEPS 1 – 2

STEP 3

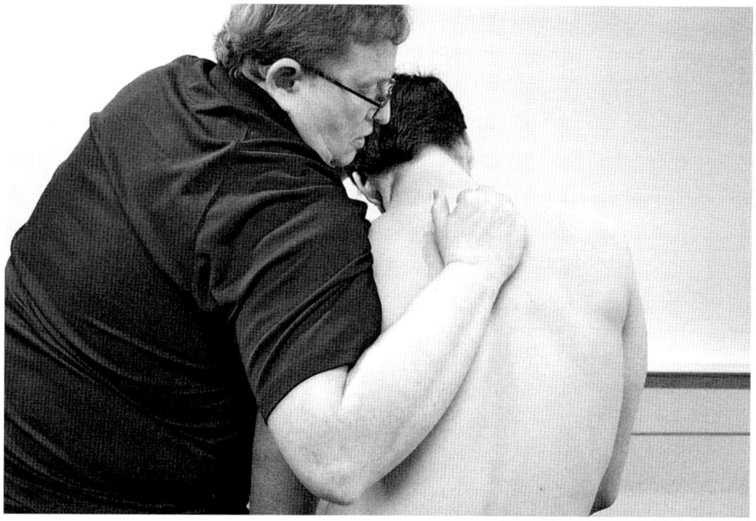

1. The operator's axilla should be over the patient's shoulder and place your fingers on the upper aspect of their 3rd rib
2. Place your left hand on the patient's head
3. First the patient's head is drawn toward you while their body is pushed slightly away

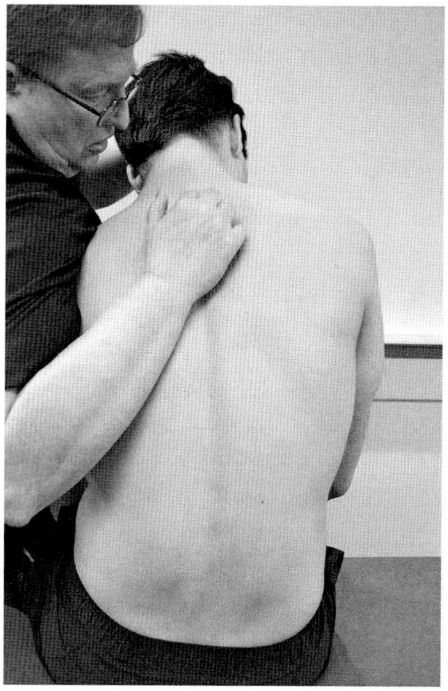

STEP 5

4. This 'swerves' the spinal column and throws the subluxated rib up higher, exaggerating the lesion
5. Now their head is pushed well away from you, while their body is drawn towards you. Accompany this movement with strong pressure of your right hand downward upon the shaft of their rib

West's 2nd to 6th Ribs Technique

EXAMPLE: Left 2nd rib dysfunction
PHYSICIAN: Standing at the head of the table
PATIENT: Supine

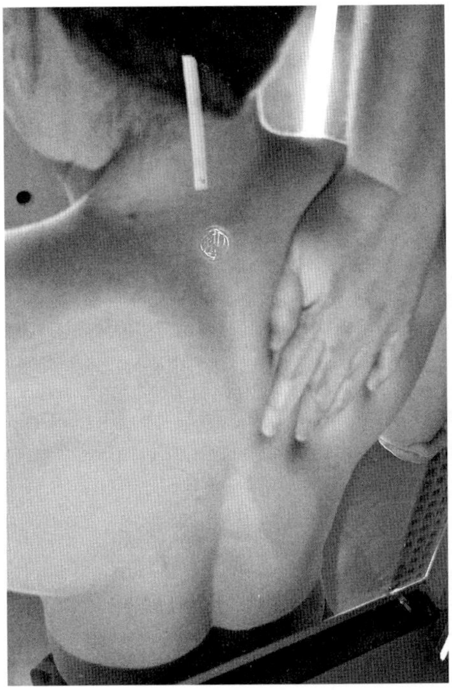

STEP 1

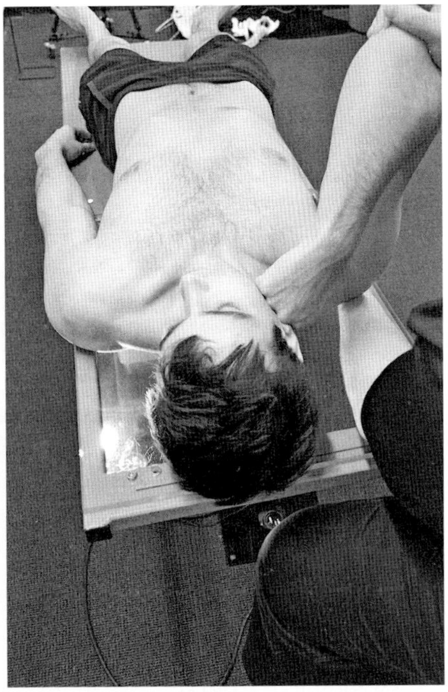

STEP 2

1. Place your left (inner) hand to use as a fulcrum under their 2nd rib between the angle of the rib and the rib head
2. With your right hand draw the patient's left arm up and back into full extension, so as to pull up the front of their 2nd rib by their pectoral muscles

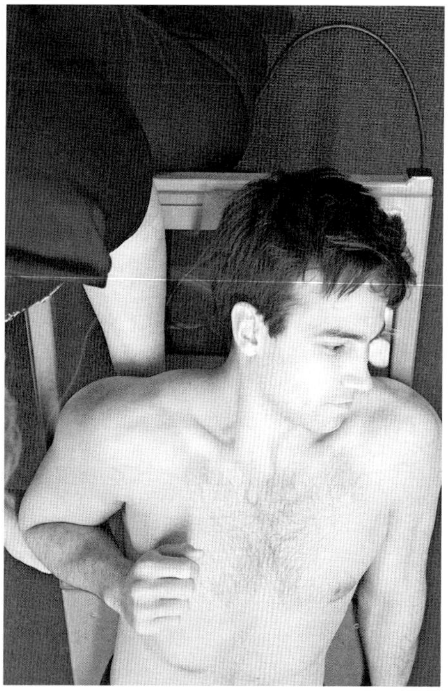

STEP 3

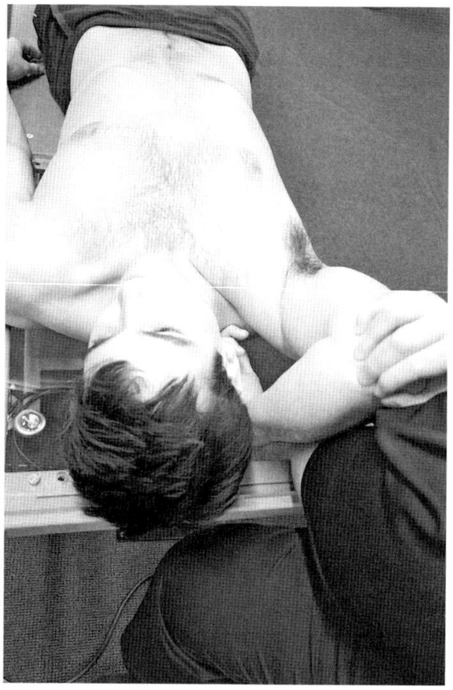

STEP 4

3. The patient is asked to bend their elbow and place the flat of their hand over the front end of their rib and inhale
4. Next the patient is asked to forcibly exhale. With slight pressure on their elbow, their upper arm is brought quickly down using the physician's posterior hand as a fulcrum to move the rib

Hazzard's Rib Technique for Ribs 3 to 10, Seated

EXAMPLE: 4th rib right
PHYSICIAN: Standing in front of the patient
PATIENT: Seated

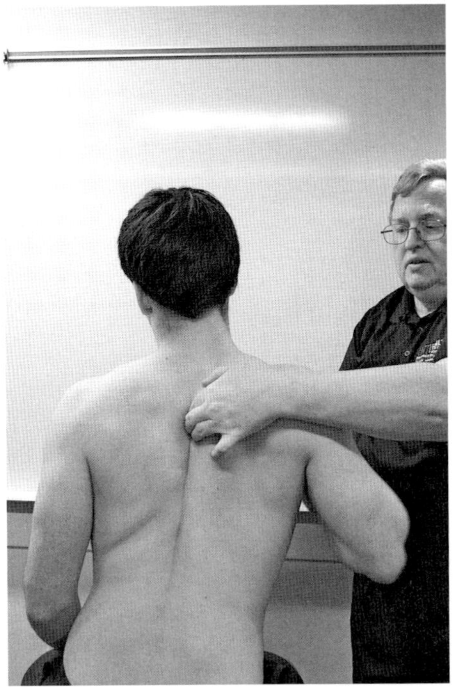

STEP 1

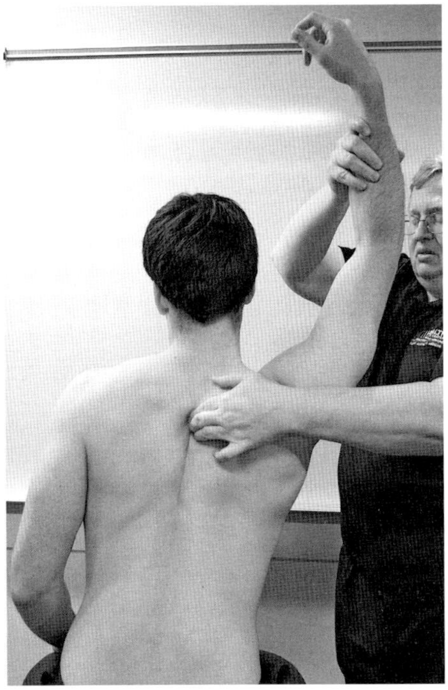

STEP 2–A

1. From the front reach to the patient's back and press your fingers upon the angle of their right 4th rib with your left hand
2. With your right hand raise the patient's right arm in front of their body and high over their head. Then rotate the arm downward and backward. This brings traction upon the pectoral muscles and soft tissues of the whole anterior aspect of the side of their chest. This elevates that entire side and effects particularly the ribs at the rib angles on which pressure is being made

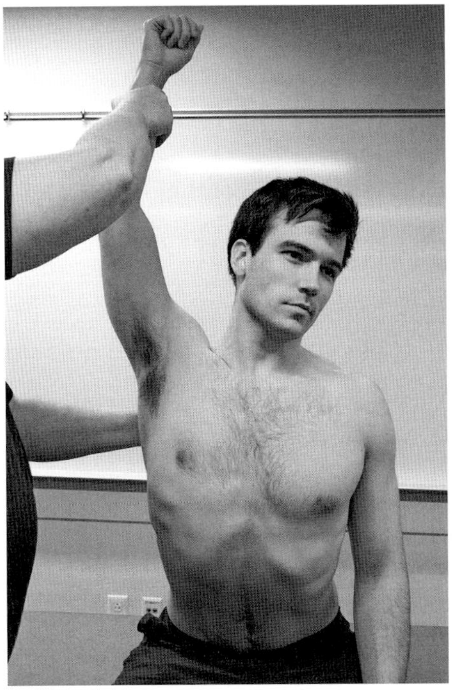

STEP 2–B

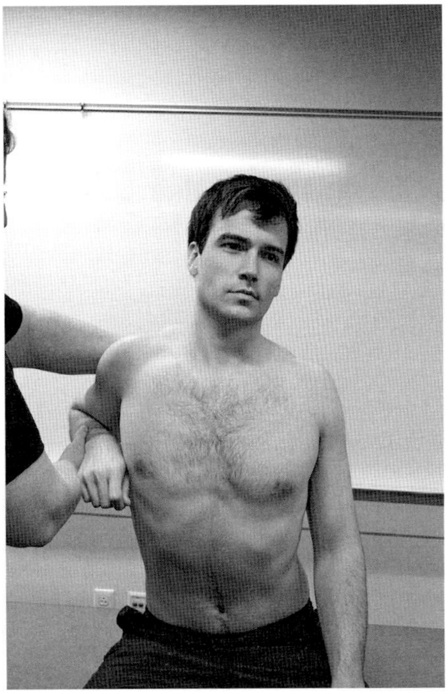

STEP 2–C

3. Care must be taken to maintain this pressure until the end of the movement of their arm
4. This motion may be repeated, your pressing hand traveling down their back to each successive rib in need of treatment

This treatment elevates all the ribs and tones all connected muscles, ligaments, vessels, nerves, etc.

Hazzard's Rib Technique for Ribs 3 to 10, Side Lying

EXAMPLE: 4th right rib
PHYSICIAN: Standing behind the patient
PATIENT: Lying right side up

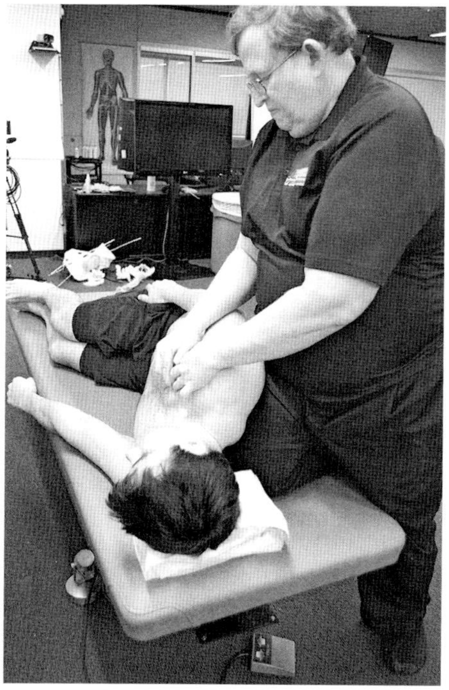

STEPS 1 – 2

1. Place your bent knee on the table against the posterior angle of their rib
2. With your left hand place pressure against the sternal attachment of the 4th rib
3. Ask the patient take a deep breath in
4. Their arm may be rotated either forward and up, or downward and back—quickly
5. Great caution must be exercised in any application of your knee to their chest. Use the knee only as a fixed point or fulcrum—not as an adjustive force

Tucker's 3rd through 10th Ribs Technique

In inspiration the ribs turn slightly on the transverse processes, slide forward on the lower, and backward on the upper facet, against the bodies of the vertebrae. From extreme expiration to extreme inspiration, the total motion is rarely more than two inches at the tips of the longest ribs. In some of this movement the vertebrae themselves share. A maximum of two inches at the tip of the rib means very slight motion indeed at the transverse processes and facets. Even the slightest apparent motion is diminished by the motion of the vertebra itself, and the yielding of the elastic cartilages and ligaments involved. In flexion and extension of the body the ribs move as in inspiration and expiration.

In side-bending of the body each rib moves with the vertebra to which it belongs. The vertebra above slides on the superior facet of the rib below. It may even press the rib down on the concave side, with the rib sliding down and out on its inferior facet, and out on the tubercle of the transverse process. Doubtless this motion is in all cases exceedingly slight, but it explains the discrepancy between the center of rotation of the articular processes and that of the costal facets. In this motion the tips of the ribs remain relatively stationary on both sides. They are fastened together in front, unless there is inspiration at the same time. On the convex side the extreme lateral part in the axillary line moves relatively down (unless there is inspiration at the same time). On the concave side the rib moves up, with corresponding turning at the transverse processes.

In rotation/side-bending each rib moves with its related vertebra. The transverse process of the vertebra moves up and out and forward on the convex side, carrying with it the rib. However, the ribs are all fastened together in front by the cartilages which attach them to the sternum. So the ribs on the convex side must separate in the axillary line. Since the spine turns relatively more than the ribs, these must slide upward on the transverse processes. On the concave side, it is the reverse, giving the downward motion to individual ribs as noted in the preceding paragraph. Any confusion of thought that arises here may be clarified by recalling that the tubercle-transverse process joint is concave on the transverse process and convex on the tubercle. Thus, as in the shoulder, motion down of the shaft means motion up in the socket. Since this is exactly the point where the 'lesions' occur, the picture should be clear.

LESIONS

Tucker: Limitations of motion are due to the ligaments of the joints, and the intercostal aponeurosis, drawing down and in, below and up, and out above, with a slightly greater distance from the spine on the lower side. The general tendency is to an upward location of the ribs. This is particularly true of the human subject, standing erect with the full weight of the ribs and muscles bearing downward on the ends of the ribs. This is the reverse of the general direction of pressure in an animal such as a horse. Here the pressure from the weight of viscera carries ribs down and forward, and from muscular effort toward the head. Lesions may, however, be either up or down at the tubercle. Lesions of the rib head, if they exist, are indistinguishable from those at the tubercle.

The intercostal muscles, along the full length of the rib, act in lesions so as to distribute the tension. Certain fibers will be over-strained and others relaxed. Those 'in-between' remain normal. The latter should be found at the juncture of the middle third of the rib with the anterior and posterior thirds. These are therefore apparent centers of rotation. The intercostal muscles so act, however, only when in tension. This is not the usual state in the erect trunk of the human subject. The position of a rib in lesion is therefore determined usually by the position of the tubercle and of the rib head and tip. When up at the tubercle its lower edge will be exposed behind, and its tip will be drawn back and depressed. When all of the intercostal muscles are in tension this tends to correct the lesion.

To become familiar with the motions of the ribs, have the patient seated with physician standing behind. Place the thumbs of both your hands on the corresponding ribs on two sides, with your thumbs as near to the spine as possible when still distinctly feeling the bone. Place your fingers on the margins of the same ribs, as far along as they will reach. In this position ask the patient to inhale and exhale, and go through various movements. Try to distinguish the bone from the contracted muscle. Then do the same things with passive movements. Assume the position to give a 'cork screw' movement. Place your thumb and fingers on the rib as above. Execute a cork screw movement and various other movements with the patient completely passive. It will be discovered that the movements of ribs are quite complicated. It is probably best to focus your mind on what is happening at the transverse process and the position of their vertebra. Trace back from the points where your fingers lie to these points in your anatomical imagination. To develop an efficient technique, it is not enough to have done this once. It requires you to do this long enough for these actions to become almost subconscious. Rehearse and repeat again with each case that presents difficult features.

DIAGNOSIS

Tucker: Diagnosis of rib lesions is best made where it exists—at the juncture of the rib with the transverse process. The rib is not quite a continuation of the process, but extends out from its upper half in the lower vertebrae. Its center is in the mid dorsals, and its lower half in the upper dorsals. It will be remembered that these facets are inclined, not flat with the spine. They incline upward in the lower ribs, forward in the mid, and downward in the upper vertebrae. A 'lesion' will therefore carry the ribs in these respective directions. In the lower chest, they will be less prominent posteriorly if the lesion is downward, more prominent if the lesion is upward. The reverse is true in the upper chest, and neutral in the middle. An exception is that the curve of the neck of the rib acts to bring the angle to greater prominence in any lesion from second or third to ninth or tenth ribs. The approximation to the rib above makes a rib seem less prominent. Failure to form a mental picture of this curved neck, in those ribs where it exists, may be responsible for much confusion in diagnosis.

Secondary deviation may be found along the shaft of the rib in the lesion. This may be masked by the tension of the muscles, especially in inspiration. In general, a rib that is up at the transverse process will be down in front, with its tip pointing at a greater angle. Its inferior border will be palpable behind, and it will not be parallel with the ribs above and below. If the lesion is downward at the transverse process, its tip will point more up than its fellow ribs. Its inferior border behind will be half concealed and its upper border may be palpable.

If the vertebra to which it is attached is in lesion, upward on the right, then the right rib will be raised as the transverse process is raised. The rib will turn on the process and assume a position as if the rib itself is in lesion upward. On the opposite side, this is the reverse. If the actual lesion occurs between the rib and transverse process, this tends to offset the deviation.

Tucker's Rib Technique #1

EXAMPLE: 8th rib elevated on the right
PHYSICIAN: Standing behind the patient
PATIENT: Seated

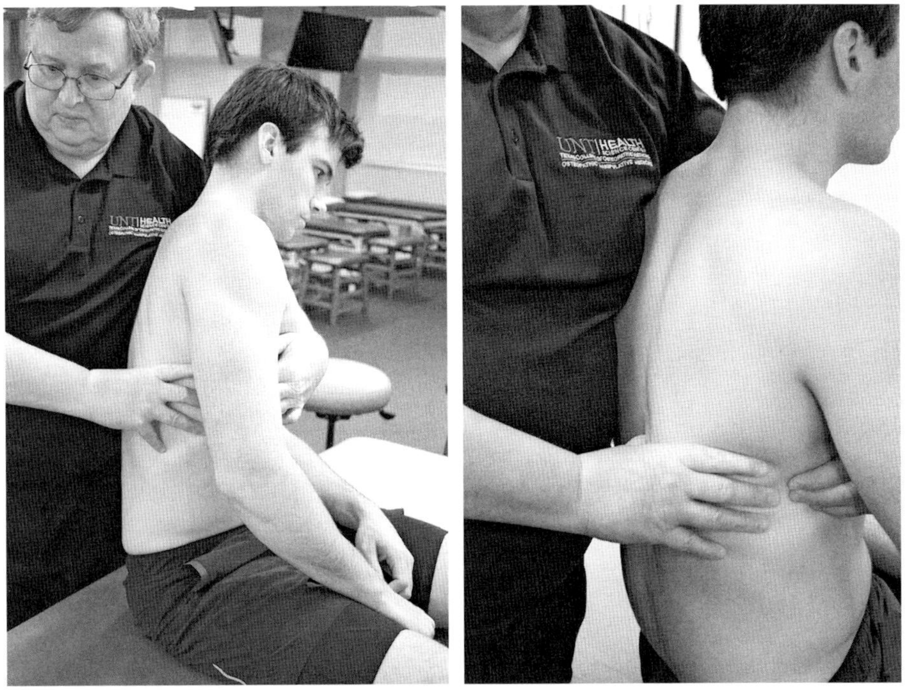

STEPS 1 – 4

1. Place your right hand on the patient's left shoulder
2. Facing right, place your left axilla over the patient's shoulder. Your left arm and hand pass around the patient's body and under the patient's right elbow. Place your fingers on their 8th rib in front of the axillary line
3. Place your right thumb on the 8th rib as near the transverse process as possible, with your fingers as far along their rib as possible. (Your long finger is in contact with the bottom portion of their rib)
4. With your right thumb and fingers carry the patient's rib away from the transverse process enough to overcome the catch or wrinkle that is holding it in dysfunction
5. With your left fingers on the front of the patient's rib press down, in and centrally, overcoming the resistance of the intercostal muscles. Acting through the curved spring, carry the rib still further away from the transverse process. Pressure back and in on the front ends of the rib makes a fulcrum of your thumb in the back. This tends to gap not only the articulation at the transverse process, but also that at the head of the rib. These movements act to tense all muscles, to gap open the joint at the top, and with the pressure of your thumb carry it back to a normal position
6. Then execute a 'cork screw movement' a time or two
7. Bow their spine convex to the right to complete side-bending of the 8th segment, at the same time rotating the patient to the left to the complete limit of their rotation. Alternately bow their ribs

Tucker's Rib Technique #2

EXAMPLE: 8th rib elevated on the right
PHYSICIAN: Standing behind the patient
PATIENT: Seated

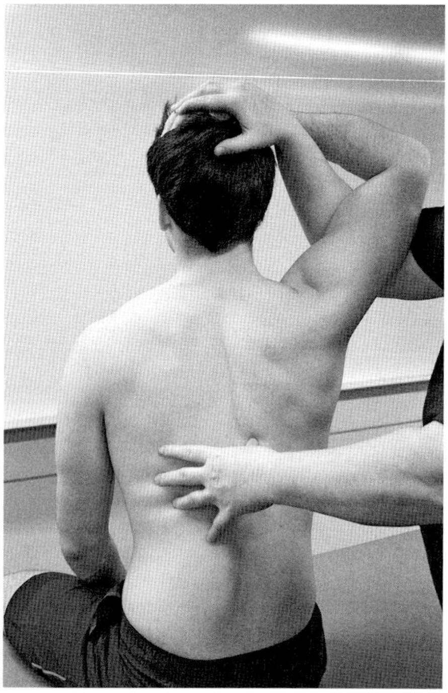

STEPS 1 – 2

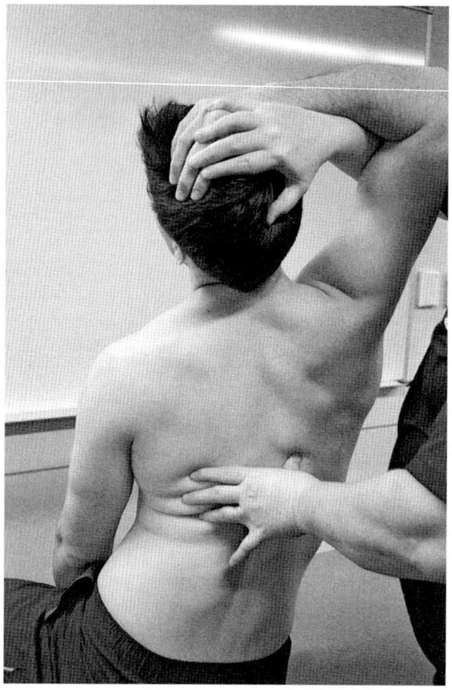

STEP 3

1. Ask the patient to place their right hand on top of their head (at the highest point)
2. Pass your right arm under the patient's axilla (supporting it) and placing your hand on top of the patient's hand which is on their head
3. Place your left thumb on the patient's rib as near the transverse process as possible. Press to the right and forward with your left thumb, while carrying the vertex of their head to the left and slightly backwards
4. Lift their axilla to the full limit of side-bending—convex to the far right end of the extension of the segment in dysfunction

Tucker: Their neck should not be turned sharply nor bent sharply, as is the natural tendency. It should be bent as little as possible. The focus of the motion should be on the lifting of their ribs and the bowing of the spine. Their head should be slightly turned to the right to increase the separation between the transverse processes.

Tucker's Rib Technique #3

EXAMPLE: 8th rib elevated on the right
PHYSICIAN: Stands beside the patient on their right side
PATIENT: Seated

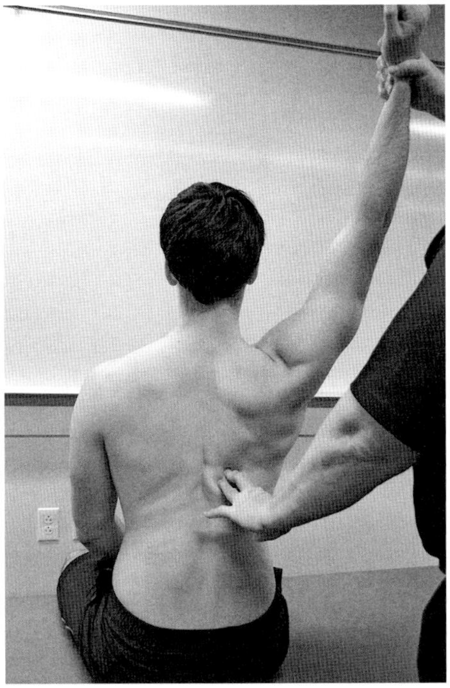

STEPS 1 – 3

1. Place the fingers of your left hand under the angle of the patient's 8th rib, ready to press upwards and towards the patient's head
2. Grasp the patient's right wrist with your right hand, and carry it directly up in the axillary line with a slight pressure backwards to the limit of motion
3. Ask the patient to inhale deeply. At the same time press upward with your left hand towards their head with your finger on their affected rib

Tucker: The effect of this arm position is to carry the rib to the upper limit of motion on the transverse process. While the front end is held down, the rib is controlled by the tensed serratus magnus muscle. This gives it an angle, at the top limit of its motion, which causes the rib to assume as nearly as possible the position of the lesion, or the position it was in when it became a lesion. All of the surrounding tissues are exerting tension on the rib to move it towards normal. Deep inhalation by the patient helps in this effect. Slight lifting with your finger is thus often able to release it from the current 'catch'.

4. Hold your hands and the patient's anatomy in that position for a brief second while the ligaments stretch. Then reverse all the anatomical positions
5. The patient's right hand is brought forward, in front of their shoulder, and carried to full extension over their head. The pressure of your finger on the patient's rib is changed to move the rib towards their feet, and their breath is released all at once. This tends to raise the front end of the rib and lifts the tubercle on the transverse process over the catch and towards 'normal.'

Sutherland's 4th to 10th Ribs Technique

PHYSICIAN: Seated on the side of the patient's dysfunction
PATIENT: Seated

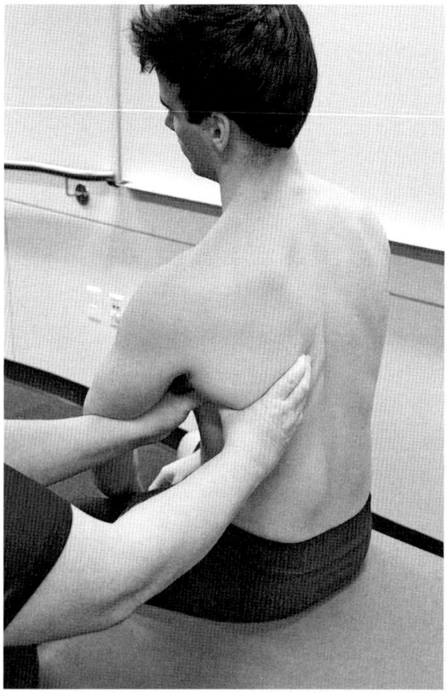

STEPS 1 – 3

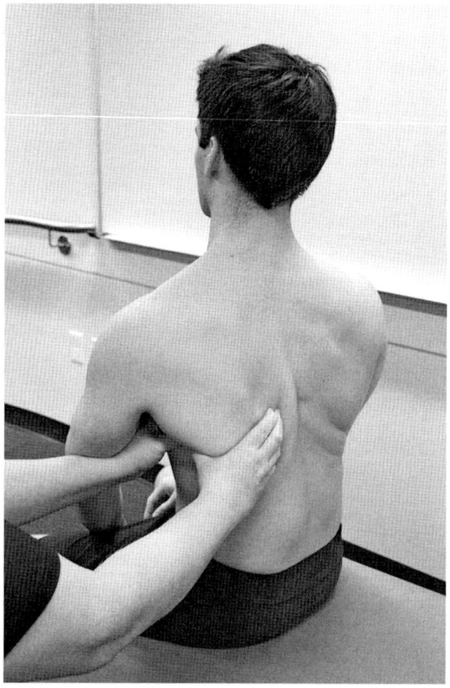

STEPS 4 – 6

1. Your thumbs are placed on the mid-axillary line of the patient's rib
2. The middle finger of one of your hands is on the posterior angle of their rib pointing towards their spine
3. The middle finger of your other hand is on the anterior end of the shaft of their rib towards their sternum
4. Ask the patient to lean towards you. The patient's rib is held to prevent it from moving
5. Ask the patient to hold their head erect and not turn their neck as they turn their body slowly. This carries the patient's opposite shoulder posteriorly
6. The patient inhales and holds their breath in

West's 6th to 10th Ribs Technique, Seated

EXAMPLE: Rib 10 right
PHYSICIAN: Standing behind the patient
PATIENT: Seated on the table

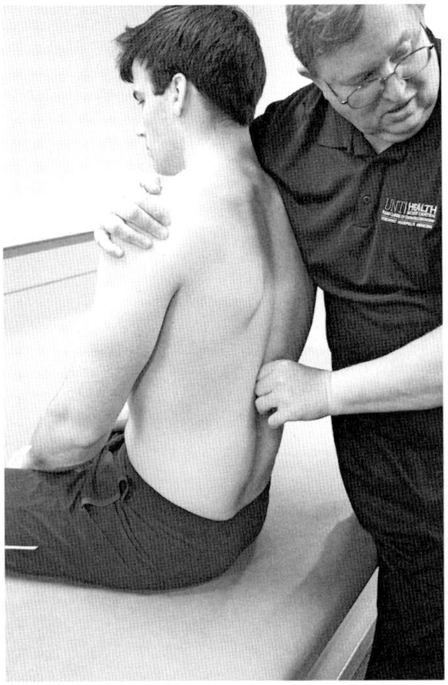

STEP 1

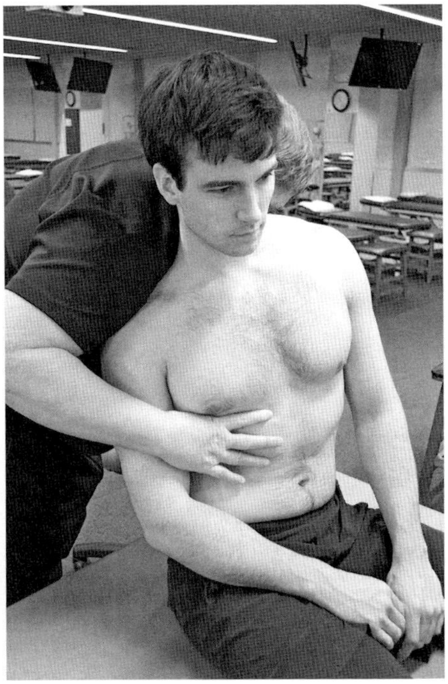

STEP 2

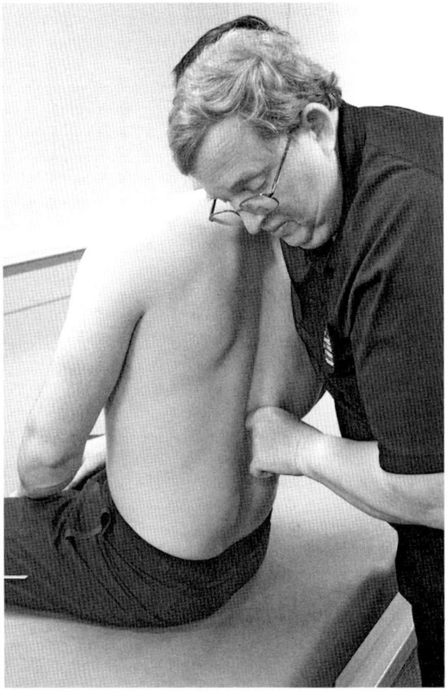

STEPS 3 – 6

1. The physician places their right axilla over the patient's right shoulder
2. The physician places their right thumb on top of the patient's right 10th rib anteriorly and fingers under the 10th rib anteriorly
3. The physician places their left hand between the angle of the 10th rib and the transverse process posteriorly
4. With their axilla the physician rotates the patient's right side backwards while maintaining pressure on the posterior portion of the patient's rib
5. The physician moves the anterior portion of the patient's rib up or down as needed
6. The physician asks the patient to forcibly exhale

West's 6th to 10th Ribs Technique, Side Lying

EXAMPLE: Rib 10 right
PHYSICIAN: Standing behind the patient
PATIENT: Lying on their left side

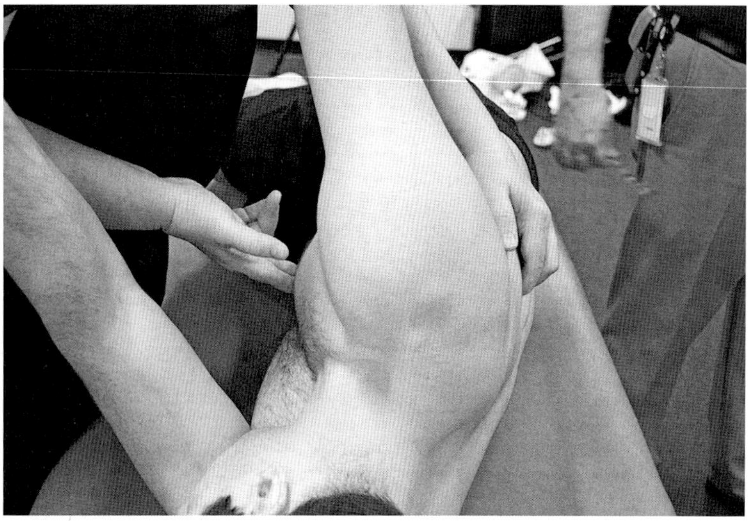

STEP 2

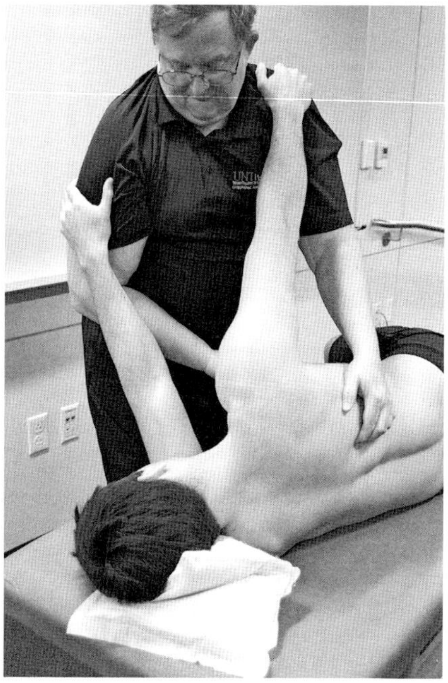

STEP 3

1. The physician places their left arm under the patient's right axilla and grasps the posterior region of the patient's right shoulder
2. The physician takes their left hand and places their fingers and/or thumb on the 10th rib between the head of the patient's rib and the posterior angle
3. The physician's right hand (fingers/thumb) is on the sternal end of the patient's 10th rib
4. The physician stands up and stretches the patient's arm upwards
5. The physician's hands press the anterior and posterior aspect of the patient's ribs together
6. Ask the patient to release the physician's shoulder
7. The physician's right hand grasps the patient's right elbow and then presses down with a sweeping motion backward with the patient's shoulder

Sutherland's Two Techniques for Rib Dysfunctions Associated with Hyper Extension of the Thoracic Vertebrae

Lippincott: During a traumatic injury the rib can be literally subluxed. This occurs when the thoracic spine is in extension and twisted causing a side-bending with the convexity on the side of dysfunction. The rib head is caught in a depression between the bodies of the vertebrae caused by separation of the demi-facets. This prevents flexion and bending toward the side of dysfunction and is painful. The pectoral muscles can pull the upper ribs out when the spine is in extension. Also, the ribs can be pushed forcibly out of place.

▶ TECHNIQUE ONE

PHYSICIAN: Standing behind the patient
PATIENT: On their side with their dysfunctional side up

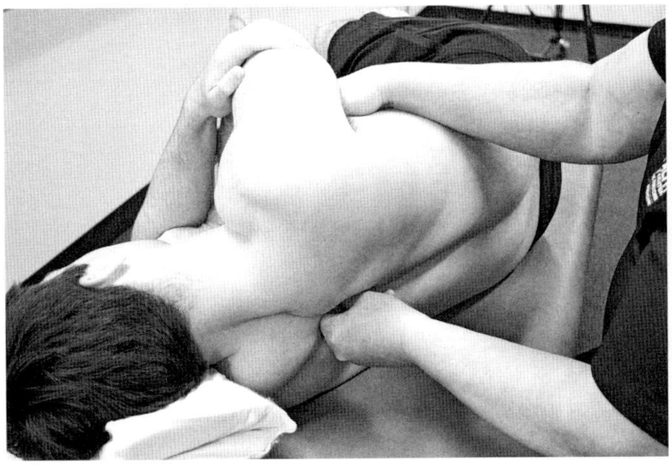

STEPS 1 – 3

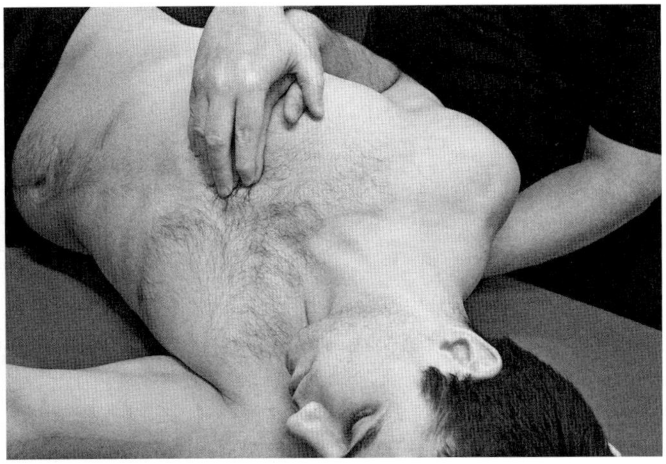

STEPS 2 – 5

1. Stand behind the patient and partially flex the patient's body
2. Facing the head of the patient, take your hand nearest the patient and draw the sternal end of their rib posteriorly
3. Your other hand lifts the dysfunctional spinous processes of their two vertebrae towards their head. This moves the costo-transverse articulation anteriorly and should leverage the head of the rib out of the depression between the demifacets
4. Ask the patient to rotate their upper shoulder posteriorly
5. This position is held while the patient holds their breath in either inhalation or exhalation. Ask the patient to take a deep breath in first. If it softens, then hold it. If it becomes tighter, then tell the patient to exhale slowly. When you feel the rib softening ask the patient to hold their breath at that point. This usually occurs at the beginning of exhalation

TECHNIQUE TWO

PHYSICIAN: Standing behind the patient
PATIENT: Seated with elbows on the table

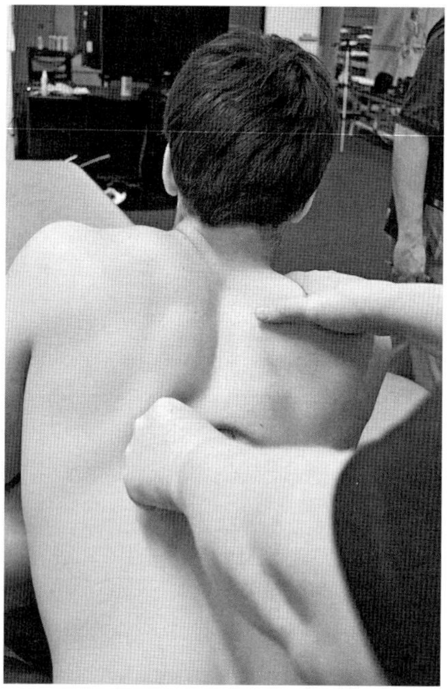

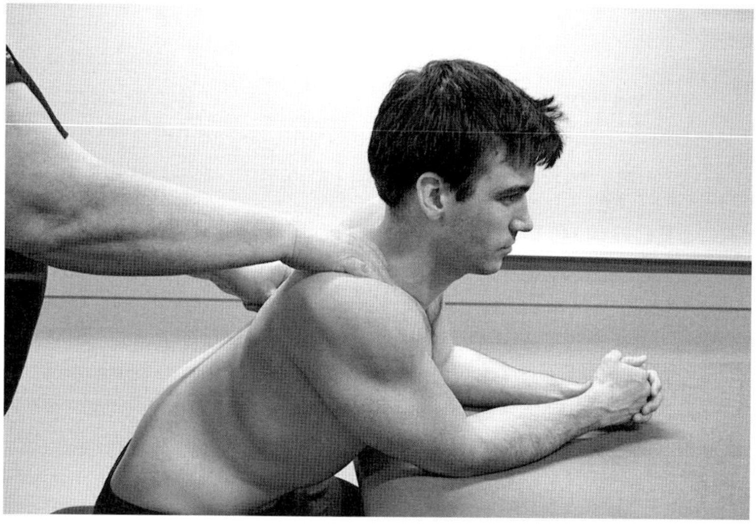

STEPS 1 – 5

1. Ask the patient to lean on their elbows and push down. This gaps the demi-facets and releases the rib head
2. Place your hand on the shoulder of the patient's affected side to increase the spinal extension
3. Your thumb and knuckle/finger of your other hand rotate the bodies of the patient's vertebrae away from the head of the rib
4. This position is held while the patient holds their breath in either inhalation or exhalation. Ask the patient to take a deep breath in first. If the rib softens, then hold it. If the rib becomes tighter then ask the patient to exhale slowly
5. When you feel their rib releasing ask the patient to hold their breath at that point. This usually occurs at the beginning of exhalation. The ligaments are then tensed to a point of balanced tension

Sutherland's Technique for the Floating Ribs 11 and 12

PHYSICIAN: Seated beside the patient
PATIENT: Seated

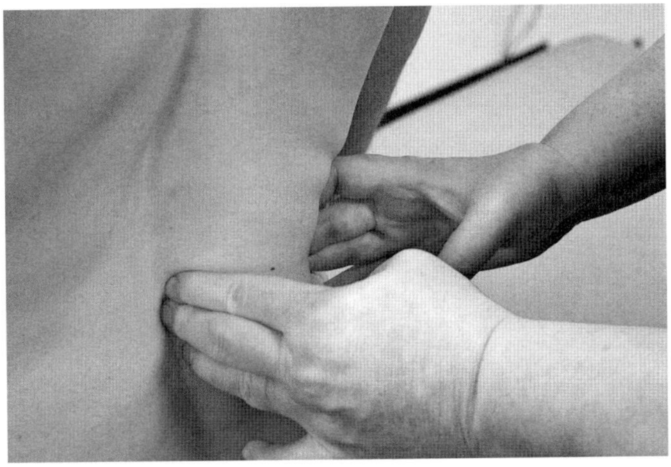

STEPS 1 – 3

1. Place the thumb of one of your hands on the tip of their 11th or 12th rib
2. Place the fingertips of your posterior hand at the patient's costo-tranverse junction
3. Place the fingertips of your anterior hand on the tip of the patient's rib
4. Have the patient hold their head erect and not turn their neck as they turn their body slowly. This carries their opposite shoulder posteriorly
5. The patient inhales and holds their breath in

Wales' Technique for Treating the 11th and 12th Ribs

PHYSICIAN: Seated beside the patient
PATIENT: Supine

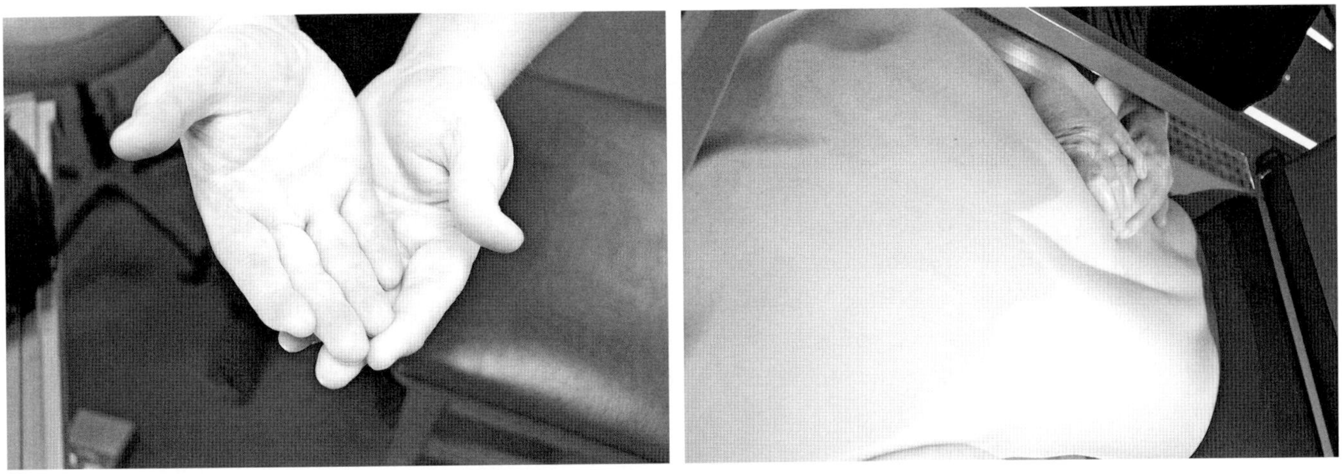

STEPS 1 – 2

1. Place the fingertip of your index finger on the patient's spinous process and the fingertip of your long finger over the nail of your index finger

2. Add traction and find a point of balanced tension

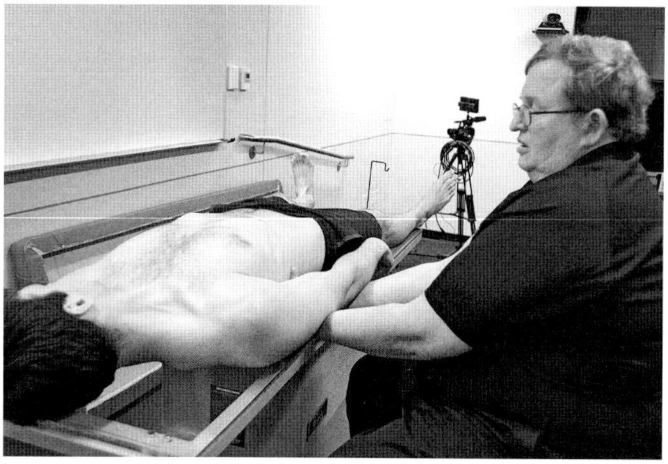

STEPS 3 – 4

3. Ask the patient to turn their head opposite to the side you are treating. For example, if you are treating the right 11th or 12th rib, ask the patient to turn their head to the left
4. Ask the patient to dorsiflex their foot opposite to the side being treated. For example, with right 11th or 12th rib dysfunctions ask the patient to dorsiflex their left foot

Wales: I'm interested in only one thing—using the rib as a handle for putting traction on the thoracic costal arches. If it does the ribs some good that's a bonus. Now the costal arch stabilizes the posterior wall of the abdomen. This arch also stabilizes the thoracic abdominal junction and the crurae of the diaphragm that are attached to the anterior longitudinal spinal ligament at approximately the level of the first and second lumbar bodies. They are called crurae because the diaphragm is essentially a transverse fascia septum with muscles intertwined at the edges. They are attached to the inside of the lower ribs. The crurae of the diaphragm are attached to the anterior longitudinal spinal ligament at the uppermost lumbar region. They cross over the aorta as it becomes the abdominal aorta. The cisterna chyli is right beside it. All the lymph of the lower half of the body is brought through the cisterna chyli including the abdominal lymph. From there it goes into the thoracic duct and empties into the left subclavian vein. Three quarters of the lymph of the body goes into the left subclavian vein. The other quarter goes into the right lymphatic duct and into the right subclavian vein, and this is how the interstitial fluids get back into the venous system.

You can see that with getting the lymphatic system working the patient is getting a complete systemic treatment. And I can feel this action. It was Dr. Sutherland's idea that the cisterna chyli is the center of the lymphatic system. It's a hydraulic system and the cisterna chyli is the center. When you do the lymphatic pump with a manual action on the front of the thorax, you are stimulating the vasomotor around the 2nd thoracic vertebrae by the heads of the second ribs, and that isn't a bad thing to do.

These "just start to float," and these ribs are moving with the patient's breathing on the transverse processes of the 11th and 12th ribs. This is my clinical experience. I don't consider that I'm actually getting the body's lymphatic pump working till I feel it working. Even if it takes some time, I think I'm performing a manual operation which is valuable and necessary.

The costal arches are attached to the arcuate ligaments. These are really concentrations of fascia, which make an arch over the quadratus lumborum. The medial arcuate ligament goes over the psoas to blend into the crura of the diaphragm and the anterior longitudinal spinal ligament. Additionally, you have the lateral arcuate ligament on each side attaching to the 12th rib. This whole area across the posterior abdominal wall at the bottom of the rib cage is connected to the diaphragm and attached to the inside of the lower ribs. This is an area that is valuable and important to address as the main cause for treatment for a number of reasons. When the crura of the diaphragm has released the tension or drag, you will feel the diaphragm on the side you are working on ascend into the thorax with exhalation.

This particular operation can be used for a number of clinical situations, starting with pyloric spasm in newborn infants. It will also relax the sphincter of Odi and help with digestive processes so that the gallbladder and pancreatic ducts will drain and the liver will begin to move more freely in its space under the dome of the diaphragm. This procedure may be all that's necessary to get all these viscera across this part of the trunk free of drag. They will then be able to move normally with the diaphragm during ordinary respiration

Tucker's Floating Ribs (11th and 12th) Technique

The eleventh and twelfth ribs are simply joined to the pedicles of their respective vertebrae, posterior to the bodies, and at some distance from the transverse processes, which are very short. They stand as it were erect, without other bony support or limitation.

In these two ribs all movements are possible, limited only by the ligaments and muscles that attach to them. Of these the capsular ligaments are the most restrictive, but have no effect on the varieties of motion possible. Ligaments doubtless attach to the transverse processes, and should be studied. The fascia of the intercostals is poorly represented. The most effective of the ligamentous limitations, however, is the intercostals' aponeurosis. In the twelfth rib, this extends down and in to the costal process of the first lumbar, and above, up and out to the eleventh rib. It draws the rib down and in, from the middle third, and up and out from the spinal end.

DYSFUNCTIONS

Tucker: Any movement sufficiently extreme to carry the base away from its articulation on the pedicle may create a lesion. The tensions that hold the rib to its base draw not directly to that base, but a quarter of the way towards the spine. When strained beyond its normal articulation with the base, these tensions so draw the rib against the articular surface that in trying to return to normal a 'wrinkle' may be made. This wrinkle may be maintained as a lesion.

The lesion may be in any direction from the base. The most usual direction is upward and forward, produced by blows from behind and below (almost the only blows that reach it). Or by wrenches in which the shoulder is twisted backward on that side. In this movement the tension of the abdominal muscles acting mostly on the tip, draw the rib down and forward. The ligaments to the eleventh rib, together with the intercostal muscles, draw the rib upward near the head. The combined tensions gap open the upper part of the articulation, twist the rib, slide it upward in the twisting, and leave it as a lesion [dysfunction].

DIAGNOSIS

Tucker: Diagnosis of the dysfunction of this rib is made by comparison with the opposite side, with the ribs above, with the average normal, and by sensitiveness and visceral disturbances traceable to it.

For those ribs, particularly the twelfth, exact technique is perhaps the most difficult to apply of all parts of the body. This is on account of the absence of bony leverage by which to draw the rib away from its point of engagement.

Tucker's Floating Ribs Technique #1

EXAMPLE: Right 12th rib
PHYSICIAN: Stands behind and to the right side of the patient
PATIENT: Kneels on the table, with their feet over the edge, and sitting back on their heels

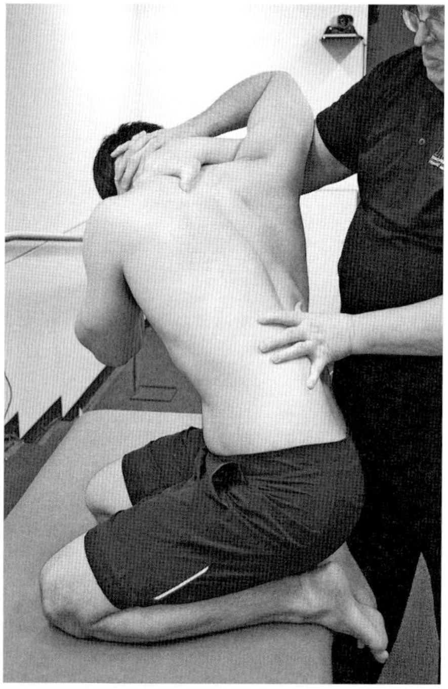

KNEELING ON TABLE

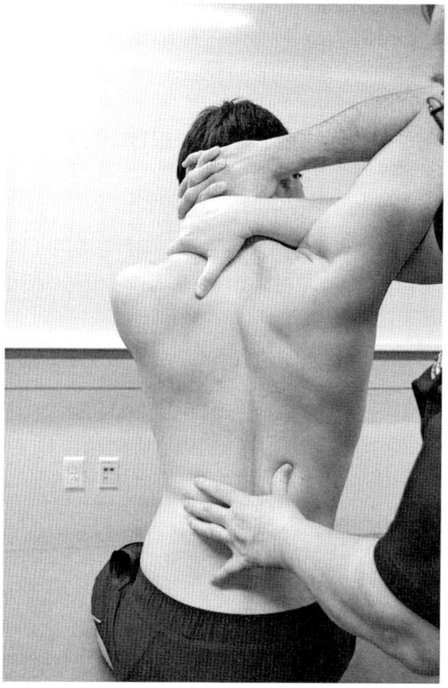

SEATED

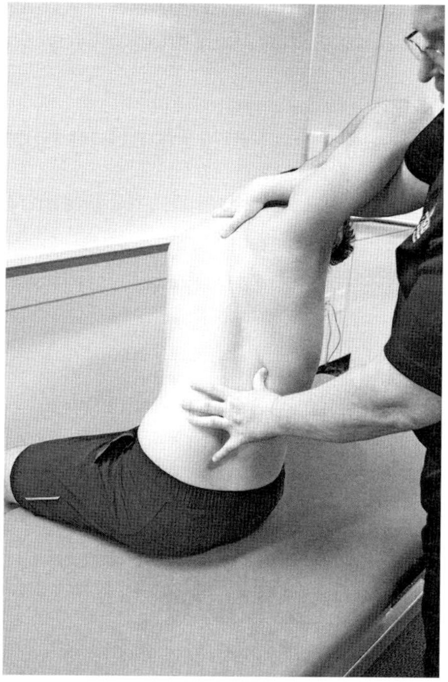

STEP 3

1. Ask the patient to clasp their hands behind their neck
2. Pass your right hand under their right axilla and place your hand over the clasped hands of the patient. Place your left thumb on the 12th rib as near to the rib head as possible, between the 11th rib if the lesion is upward and below if the lesion is downward
3. Swing the patient's spine to the right, so that they sink on the table and onto their heels to their right. Support their weight with your right hand and arm under their axilla. Keep their neck as near the mid-line as possible
4. Ask the patient to take a deep breath in (inhale) and hold their breath

Tucker: In this position the spine is bent to the right to the limit of its motion, the 12th rib is drawn up at its outer extremity by the intercostal muscles tensed by the raising of the patient's arm. The intercostal aponeurosis below, acting on the center of the rib, acts as a fulcrum. Your thumb is pressing forward, outward and downward, to move the rib head back to its normal position.

Tucker's Floating Ribs Technique #2

PHYSICIAN: Stands behind the patient
PATIENT: Seated on the table

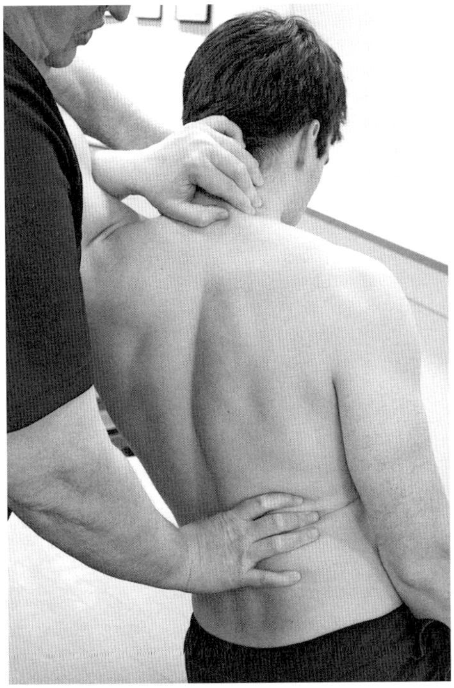

STEPS 1 – 3

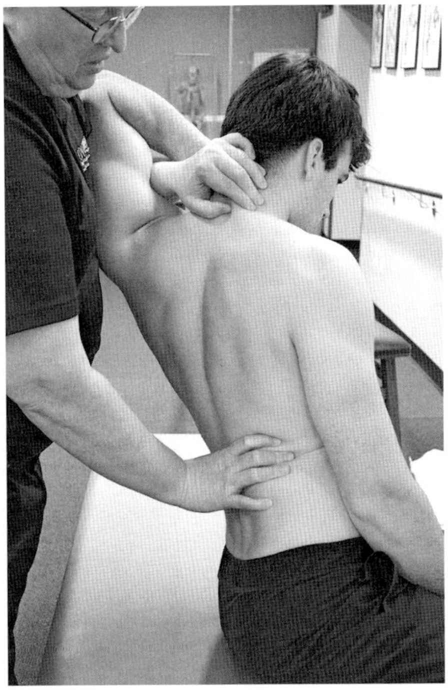

STEPS 4 – 8

1. The patient places their left hand behind their neck
2. Place your left hand under the patient's left axilla and over the patient's hand at the back of their neck. Your forearm is supporting their axilla
3. With your right hand press forward on the 11th thoracic vertebra until the spine is in full extension
4. With your right thumb on the head of their rib as above, produce a side-bending motion to the right. Keep the patient's neck as near to the mid-line as possible, and focus all motion at the 12th rib
5. Complete with extension and complete lateral flexion. Add some rotation until the dysfunction is felt to have released
6. Ask the patient to take a deep breath and hold their breath in
7. If the rib hasn't released, the physician may then press downward on the patient's neck, while carrying their spine suddenly into flexion. Maintain side-bending rotation and constant pressure with your thumb

8. Alternate extension and flexion until complete correction is made

Tucker: In all of these forms of technique, deep inspiration may be of some assistance. In deep inspiration the intercostal muscles are tensed, drawing up and towards the spine. The diaphragm is also tensed, drawing up and on the tip of the rib and transversely across the body.

6

Techniques for the Lumbar Region

Tucker on the Lumbar Spine

The purpose for the student should be to form a mental moving picture of the normal bone and the bone in 'lesion'.

A lumbar vertebra stationary in the mid-position is balanced over the core of the intervertebral disc, the weight of the body pressing down in front of this core, and the pull of the muscles drawing down from behind. Over this center of balance, axis of motion, or fulcrum of leverage, flexion and extension occurs by relaxation and contraction of the spinal muscles. This occurs by sliding out (flexion) and in (extension) of the articular surfaces, and by compression and decompression of the remainder (front part) of the disc.

LIMITATION TO MOTION

Tucker: Limitation to the proper motion of extension occurs from the tensing of the anterior longitudinal ligament and possibly, (rarely if ever) of the disc itself. Also by bony contact (through intervening tissue) of the lower edge of the upper articular process of each joint (inferior articular process of the vertebra above) with the lamina of the bone below. The capsular ligaments, loose enough to allow of free flexion and rotation, are probably loose enough to play little part here, or even to allow separation as noted below.

Further motion can occur only by the separation of the articular surfaces and further stretching of the anterior ligaments. This, however, can only occur if the bony contact permits sliding. The ligament then acts as a radius of this further motion, and gives rise to a secondary motion. It draws down the anterior edge, allowing the whole bone to move posteriorly with the separation of the articular surfaces. Into this vacuum thus produced the capsular ligament may be forced by atmospheric pressure, especially at the lower edge. The lesion is thus produced, which (except in warped conditions) in all likelihood corrects itself. The forces tending towards normal are overwhelming, and there are no forces, except position, helping to maintain the lesion. When maintained, it is an extension or approximation lesion. Approximation lesions (except in warps and secondary to separations above or below) are rare.

Limitation to the proper motion of flexion is from the tensing of the posterior longitudinal ligament, the interspinous ligaments and the capsular ligaments, and from compression of the disc in front. The disc is the softer of these, so the chief checking influence is the ligaments behind. Of these ligaments, the ligamentum flavum (posterior surface of the spinal canal) consists of yellow elastic fibers, and is highly elastic, being at the same time close to the axis of motion. The interspinous ligaments are not disposed longitudinally, but pass forward from the top and bottom of each spinous process at about 45 degrees. As in all cases uniformly throughout the whole body, they lie radially to the motion of the bones they hold (longitudinally to the direction of tension, radially to the direction of motion) so they're tense at all times. At the limit of their motion, a very slight stretching will allow comparatively great further motion, with increase in tension in proportion to the degree that they are inelastic.

Beyond this point further motion can occur in cases of violence by the stretching of these ligaments. A change in the angle of motion occurs, though to a very slight degree, limited by the shape of the articular surfaces. The upper half of the articulation (inferior articular process of the upper bone) passes beyond the edge of the lower, assumes an angle with it, and receives an indentation from its upper edge. Meanwhile, it is being driven against it with great force by the stretching of the interspinous and other ligaments, all of which force the bony contacts against each other and increase the dent, and serve to retain it in that position as a 'lesion'. There is gapping of the lower part of the articulation, and compression of the disc.

This secondary motion with a lesion we believe rarely occurs in the median line, although median lesions, i.e., separation lesions, are sometimes noted. The reason for this is that in the median line all of the ligaments are at their most favorable angle and all are acting together. This tends to prevent the occurrence of lesions. When in extreme flexion, however, some other motion, such as rotation or side-bending, occurs. Then these ligaments cease to act together, one or two are easily stretched, and great danger of lesion arises. By the very relation of the articular surfaces, one corner or edge of one side is forced at an angle against the opposing surface. This action makes under heavy pressure, a more acute indentation, from which it may be unable to release itself unaided.

The proper motion of rotation in the lumbar region is in reality side-bending rotation. It is due chiefly to the action of the anterior spinous ligament, which immediately the body of the vertebra has moved from the median line, acts to produce a motion of which it becomes a radius. This draws down the anterior edge and transforms rotation into rotation/side-bending (and we might add flexion also).

From the position of extreme extension, rotation/side-bending is accomplished by lifting of the articular facet on the convex side. Since even in this extreme position, indeed, especially in this extreme extension, the anterior ligament also acts, and any rotation becomes rotation/side-bending. The result is that the articulation on the convex side is not only lifted, but moves forward. On the opposite side (still at the lower limit of motion) the vertebra moves back and twists. This brings the lower edge of the inferior articular process (upper of the two vertebrae in each joint) on the convex side against the vertebral facet surface on that side, with indentation and possibly lesion. A lesion in this position is comparatively rare, except from continuous warping with weakening of ligaments. The reason for this is that there is not a sufficient edge on the articulation, and no sufficient stretching of the elastic ligaments in this position, to maintain the angular pressure against the facet surface. Such lesions usually correct themselves. From the position of extreme flexion, rotation does not occur (except from a yielding of all elastic tissues). From this position, side-bending occurs by the recession of one articular facet surface.

This, however, immediately becomes rotation/side-bending. This occurs by the depressing of the facet articular surface of the concave side, with sliding back on the facet concave side, and forward and in on the convex side. Torsion occurs on both sides. The least exaggeration of this motion causes a change in the angle of motion, which immediately brings the lower edge of the upper articular facet surface on the convex side into contact with the opposing articular facet surface of that side, with indentation and possibly lesion. As a person recovers from such a position, unless he recovers the rotation before he recovers the flexion, the lesion is very likely to persist. The concave side of the lesion moves towards normal, increasing the angle and the indentation on the convex side. The weight of the vertebral body descends and fixes it thus. There is no normal tension here leading to correction, which does not also serve to maintain the lesion. The majority of lesions (except warp lesions) are of this character. They may be compared quite accurately to a bureau drawer which has become jammed.

Rotation in the median position is transformed almost immediately into rotation/side-bending through the action of the anterior longitudinal ligament. The motion is radial around this ligament in respect of side-bending. As to the vertebral rotation, it is radial around a point posterior to the articular facet surface, even perhaps to the tip of the spine itself. Examining and experimenting with the actual bones makes the forming of a mental picture of this motion easier. Across the top of the body of each lumbar vertebra, near the back, is found a shallow groove which just about fits your fingertips. This groove is curved and concave backwards. Its curve is sharpest in the 3rd vertebra, less and less in the 4th and 5th and also in the 2nd and 1st. This curved groove points fairly accurately to the center of rotation of the vertebra above. It is the groove through which the core of the intervertebral disc moves as each bone rotates on the vertebra below. The difference in the arcs of these grooves verifies the work done by the vertebral motions referred to in reference to the centers of rotation of the lumbar vertebrae.

The cores of the intervertebral discs then become important. These cores are found nearer the posterior margins of the discs. They are more solid than the rest of the disc, and act on the principle of ball bearings. They are therefore necessarily fulcra for all motions of the bodies on each other, except that of rotation. In rotation they themselves move, making the groove. In equilibrium of the body the line of weight passes in front of them in the median line.

The pull of the muscles is behind the vertebral body, but also (through the transverse processes) on either side. All act downwards, so that this vertebral core is the teeter of the balance. In flexion and extension it is the teeter, the axis of motion, until limitation to motion arises at some other point. In side/bending the core is also the axis of motion, which passes through the core antero-posteriorly. If the limit of motion occurs at some other point, then of course that limitation forms part of the axis of motion. The axis therefore passes through the core to the point of limitation. But in rotation it is merely a ball bearing on which the bone rolls. The vertebral body above immediately passes from its central position over the core and tilts, and hence also side-bends. It also carries this core with it, as in a ball bearing joint (since the core is fastened to the base above as well as to the surface below), hence the rolling motion of the rotation/side-bend. But we must not forget that the core is also squeezed to the convex side by the pressure from the inclined plane of the base above. This qualifies this motion, bringing about the greatest possible amount of effective side-bending producible with the least possible extension of muscular tissue (as is universal in the body).

In rotation/side-bending from the median position, the articulations on the concave side slide in (extend) before those of the convex side slide out (flex). Why? This is due chiefly to the action of the intervertebral disc. The disc is immediately squeezed to the convex side as soon as there is any tilting of the surface. Hence, without raising the convex side, it lowers the concave side. Remember also that the muscles that maintain the balance of the vertebra are in action continuously, and any change that involves contraction or shortening of a muscle is likely to occur first. Rather than one that calls for stretching of the muscle. Again, extension occurs first. The axis of this motion becomes a line drawn through the intervertebral core and the articulation of the convex side, and the axis swings as this core moves.

Around this axis rotation/side-bending occurs first by depression of the articulation on the concave side, doubtless due to the varying distances in different persons and under different conditions. Movement is possible until the limitation to motion on that side is encountered. By elevation of the articulation of the convex side, the axis becomes a line through the core and the opposite articular surface.

This agrees with the results of the work done by the classes referred to, where it was found that the two articulations of the lumbar vertebrae did not have the same center, but that the center of rotation of each was approximately a point posterior to the opposite articular surface. This point was wider in the lowest vertebra, less wide in the upper, and coincides opposite the tenth or the eleventh dorsal, whose discs are so thin as to preclude such motion.

This principle, the moving of one side at a time, is vastly important in the correction of lesions. It enables us to use one side as a fulcrum for the disengagement of the other side. The actual amount of rotation/side-bending in single joints is slight. But as the normal amount of actual motion is slight, so is the amount of excess motion necessary to produce a lesion slight. This motion is just as important as if it were wide.

Tucker's Lumbar Spine Technique #1

PHYSICIAN: Standing behind the patient
PATIENT: Seated on the table

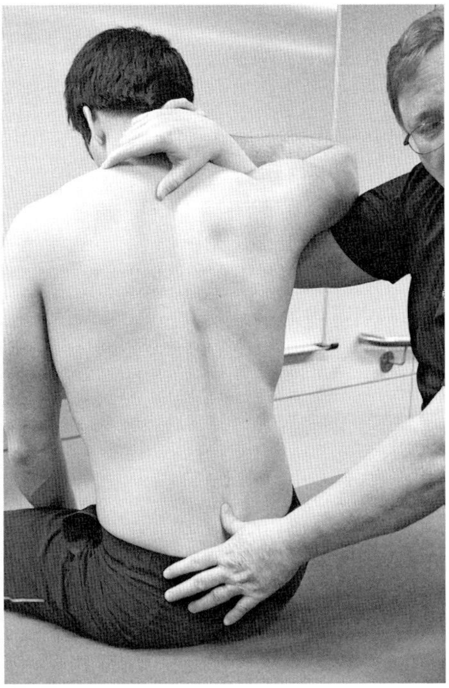

STEPS 1 – 5

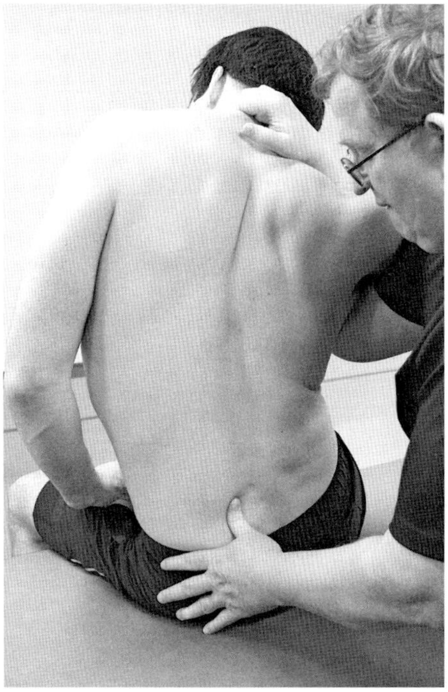

STEPS 6 – 9

1. Place your right forearm under the right axilla of the patient with your hand behind their neck
2. Ask the patient to raise their right arm up at a 90 degree angle and put their hand on the left side of their neck
3. With your left thumb press against the right side of the spinous processes of each lumbar vertebra in turn—beginning with the 5th
4. Keep the patient's shoulders parallel with the edge of the table (no rotation) and parallel with the surface of the table (no tilting), while moving the patient's body and their trunk to the left. This focuses all motion on the vertebra against which the thumb is pressing
5. Translate the patient's shoulders directly to the left, allowing your weight to descend on their right shoulder
6. Lift their right side with their right arm, and at the same time press with your thumb against the 5th lumbar spine so as to carry that vertebra to the limit of its lateral excursion (and introducing side-bending). This requires their right ischium to be lifted completely from the table. All of the side-bending is thus concentrated on the left ischium, and so for each lumbar vertebra in turn
7. When the limit of motion is reached, a definite check to motion is felt. Some further pressure should be exerted to stretch the ligament
8. The costal and transverse processes of the concave or right side have moved far forward and are approximated to each other. Those of the convex or left side are prominent posteriorly and are separated

9. At the limit of side-bending/rotation, or before, there is a strong natural tendency to flex the body as a whole. Note that the limit to pure side-bending is naturally at the costal and transverse processes, at the center of that side. Further motion is possible only by turning one way or the other, with separation of the bodies or of the spinous processes. Nature prefers the latter, with flexion
10. Now if in this position of extreme side-bending/rotation you extend the spine, you will note that the transverse processes on the right side retreat still further. If you flex the spine, you will note that they reappear again posteriorly

Tucker: The mistakes commonly made with this technique are first in drawing the patient back against your hand instead of lifting toward the patient's head with both their hands. The result is that the lesion is increased. Second, the physician may unduly stretch the skin over the spinous processes by allowing your hand to slip upward on the spine, thus causing potential pain to the patient. In very heavy persons some pain may be caused to the physician's wrist unless caution is employed. This is until your wrist has become accustomed to this strain.

Tucker's Lumbar Spine Technique #2

PHYSICIAN: Standing behind the patient
PATIENT: Seated, leaning slightly forward

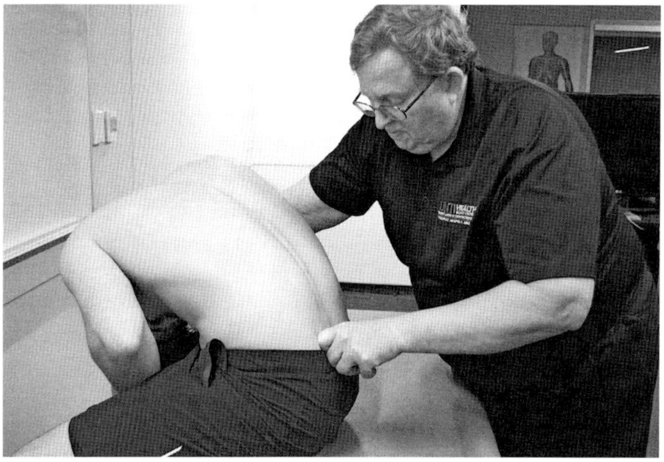

STEPS 1 – 6

1. Pass your right arm under the patient's right axilla and place your right hand on the patient's left shoulder
2. Place the thumb of your left hand on the right side of the spinous process of each lumbar vertebra in turn, in such a way as to feel two spinous processes at the same time
3. Place the fingers of your left hand on and between the transverse processes of these same vertebrae
4. Swing the patient's shoulders side to side to produce normal rotation/side-bending. Note the motions of the spinous and transverse processes
5. Rotate their shoulders and raise their right shoulder up by pressing down on their left shoulder at the same time as the patient rotates their body. The total amount of

vertebral excursion is observed to be very much less

6. Alternately, place the knuckle of your left 1st finger on the left side of the spine on the transverse process. Your thumb extends across the vertebra to engage the right transverse process before executing the same movement

Tucker's Lumbar Spine Technique #3

EXAMPLE: L5 RRSL
PHYSICIAN: Standing behind the patient
PATIENT: Seated

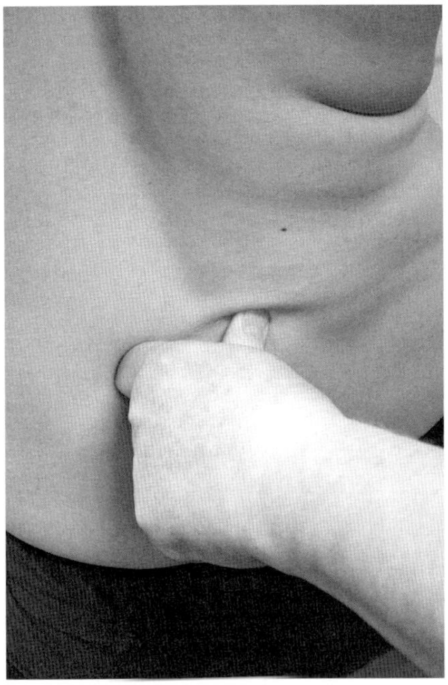

STEP 1

STEPS 2 – 5

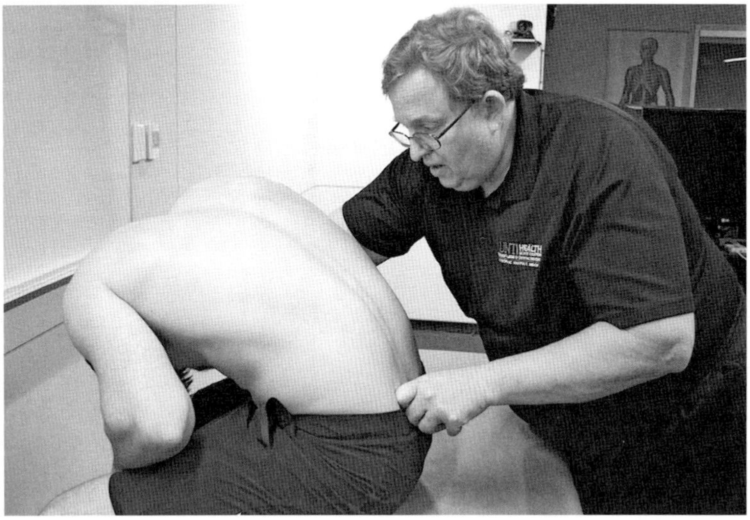

1. Place your left thumb against the prominent side of the spinous process of their L5, the right side since it is rotated right. Anchor the knuckles of your first finger against the opposite side of the vertebral spinous process below. This is the lower of the two vertebrae in lesion
2. Pass your right hand under the patient's right axilla and grasp their left shoulder
3. Ask the patient to flex their spine, and lean slightly forward
4. The physician supports the patient's weight
5. Press down on their left shoulder until their lumbar spine is bent back into full flexion
6. Rotate their shoulders to the right (forward on left, backward on right). The patient's lumbar spine will move to the left, into full rotation

Tucker: At the limit of motion, the left articular facet of the dysfunctional vertebra reaches a fixed point. It is restrained by capsular and other ligaments. At the extreme upper part of an excursion, the facet presses against an opposite articular surface in the direction of forward and to the left. Further motion in this direction, acting against this surface as a fulcrum, draws the right articular surface (the one in lesion) backward, also upward and to the left—and disengages it. The physician produces such motion by further rotation with firm pressure downward on their left shoulder. Lift their right shoulder if necessary, while exerting appropriate pressure with your thumb against the vertebra in lesion.

Tucker's Lumbar Spine Technique #4 "The Corkscrew"

PHYSICIAN: Standing behind the patient
PATIENT: Seated

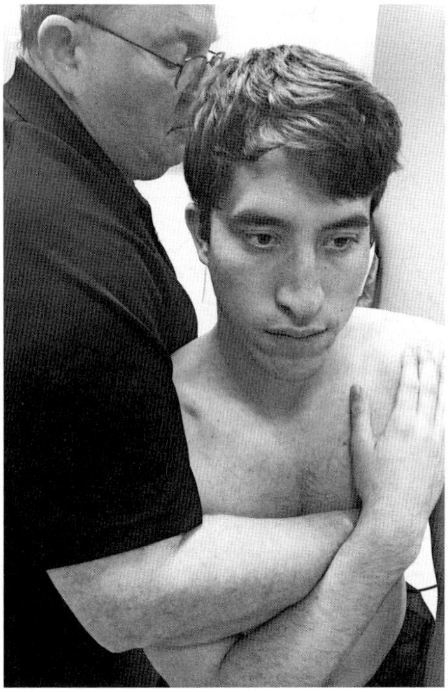

STEPS 1 – 2

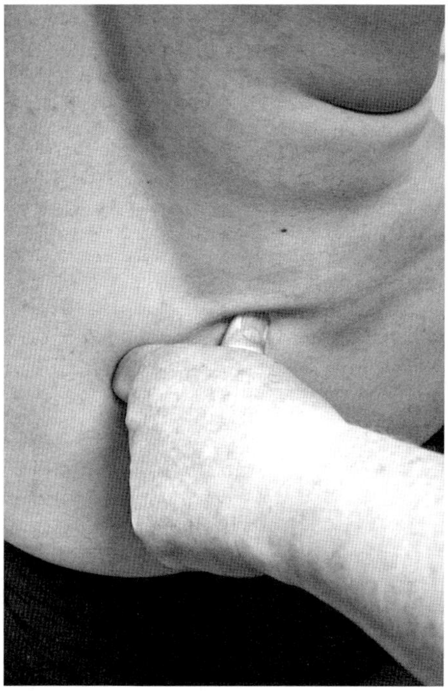

STEP 3

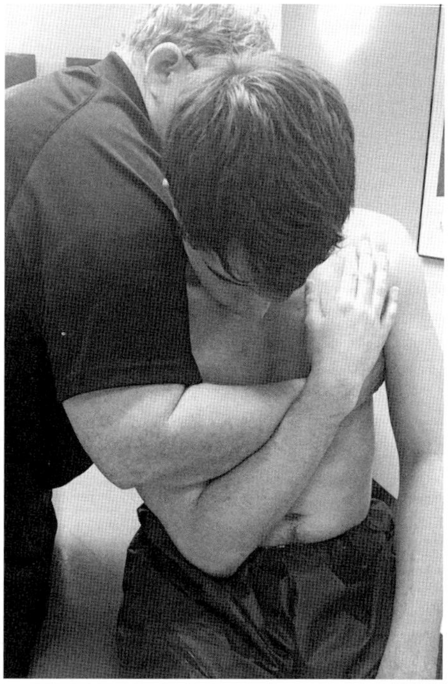

STEP 4

1. Place the patient's left hand on their right shoulder
2. Place your axilla over the patient's right shoulder and under their hand. Pass your right arm under the left elbow of the patient, against their chest. Place your right hand under their left axilla, grasping their left shoulder from beneath
3. Your left thumb rests against the right side of the spinous process of the dysfunctional vertebra, and the knuckle of your first finger against the left side of the vertebra below. Prepare to exert pressure forward and from side to side
4. Draw the patient towards you (standing at the rear and to the right of the patient). With your elbow pressing against the patient's chest, push the spine back into full flexion

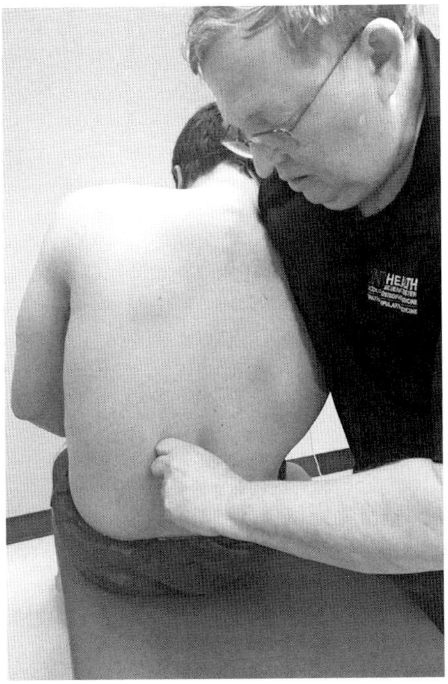

STEPS 5 – 6

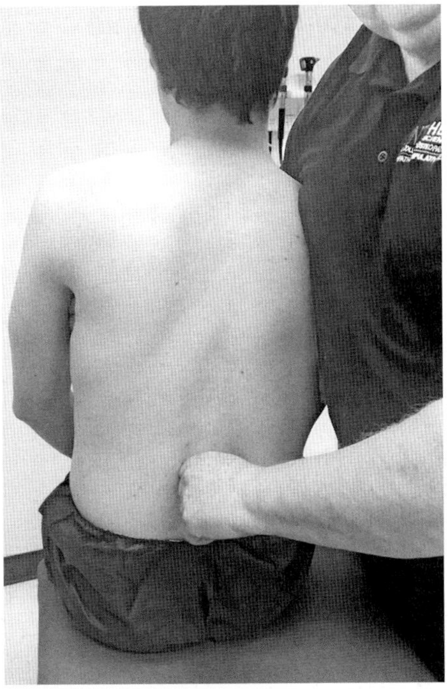

STEP 7

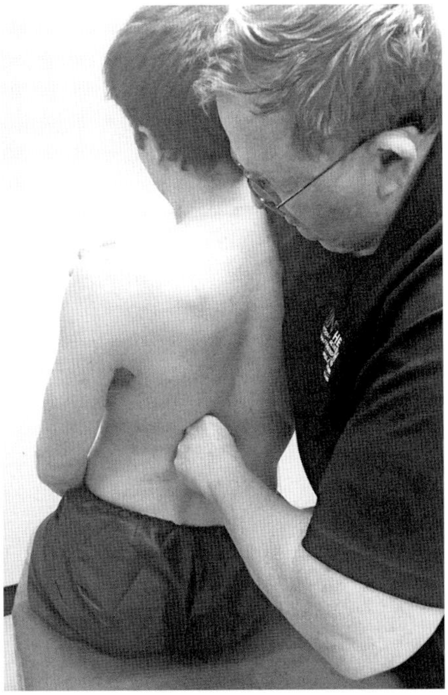

STEP 8

5. Turn the vertebra in flexion into side-bending to the left by pressing down on their right shoulder while lifting the left shoulder. Press the vertebra with your thumb to the left
6. Add extension to the vertebra in side-bending by pressing down on their right shoulder while lifting on the left. Press also with your thumb towards the left
7. Turn the vertebrae in side-bending into extension by pressing forward with your thumb while their shoulders are retained in a mid or neutral position
8. Take the lumbar spine from extension into side-bending to the right by lifting their right shoulder. Press down on their left shoulder, thus drawing their lumbar spine to the right
9. Repeat this sequence more rapidly until you are sure that the patient is thoroughly relaxed. Then turn the patient gradually more and more to the right to limit of their flexion and rotation. The corkscrew motion is maintained until their dysfunctional vertebra is freely moving

Sutherland's Lumbar/Sacral Region Technique

EXAMPLE: L3 RLSR
PHYSICIAN: Seated beside the patient
PATIENT: Supine

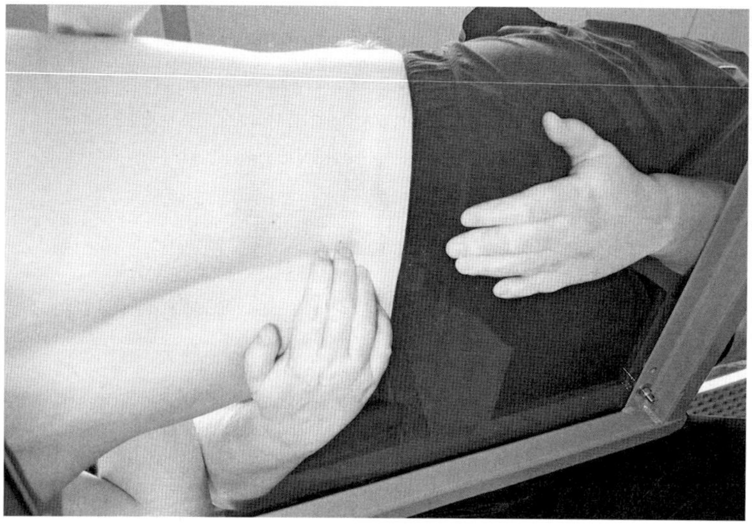

STEPS 1-3

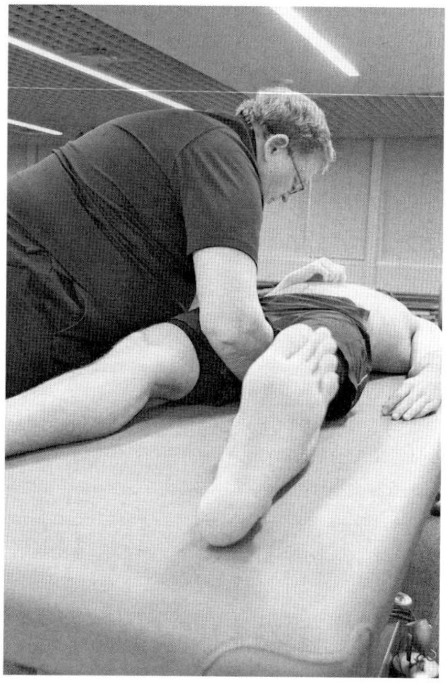

STEP 6

1. Slide one hand under their lumbosacral junction. Feel how their sacrum is moving with their breathing—or not moving as the case may be
2. Place your long (middle) finger on the opposite spinous process of their L3 from where you are seated
3. Their spinous process moves as the patient breathes more to the left and less to the right
4. Now press on the other side of the spinous process and pull it toward you to observe whether or not the vertebral body will move to the left. It shouldn't
5. What you want to do is balanced ligamentous tension (BLT). You use the spinous process as a handle to turn the body of their 3rd lumbar slightly toward you by pushing or pulling the spinous process in the direction of ease
6. Ask the patient to dorsiflex both feet because this is a midline structure. This causes the lumbar spine to straighten and thus become a little firmer or resistive
7. Ask the patient to inhale and hold their breath in until they are forced to exhale. That uses the crura of the diaphragm to put some 'action' into this region
8. After their exhalation have the patient release their feet and breathe normally
9. Re-check

Wales on the Thoracic Lumbar Junction

Now the next thing I want you to observe is the thoraco lumbar junction. That is the last two thoracic vertebra and 1st and 2nd lumbar vertebra. The trunk, ribs and arcuate ligaments are along the costal arches, which are attached to the inside of the 12th ribs. They go from the tip of the 12th rib to the transverse process and arch over the quadratus lumborum muscle. The medial lumbar costal arch arches over the iliopsoas muscle and blends in with the diaphragm. This in turn blends with the medial lumbar costal arch on the other side. There are these five arches across the posterior abdominal wall and they are a really important part of the postural mechanics in this region. The lumbars have a direct influence upon the anchoring and the stability of the diaphragm, but the musculature of the diaphragm is attached to the inside of the lower ribs and it domes up to the central tenting. It is a fascial septum with the muscles under there, and a dome on top of the central tenting. The pericardium is placed so that the heart and all its appendages are really a part of the action of the diaphragm.

The diaphragm goes down with inhalation and up with exhalation. Because the diaphragm takes everything it's attached to when moving, there are these numerous attachments to the other surface of the hepatic ligaments. These are the hepatic flexure of the colon, the splenic capsule and the inferior vena cava. The esophagus goes through the esophageal opening to become the stomach with a kind of sphincter action there. The inferior vena cava has its own aperture to take the flow from the lower part of the body up into the thorax and into the right side of the heart. Behind all this there is the stomach, and behind that the pancreas. Over on the side are the kidneys. The peritoneum envelops everything in the abdominal cavity. The omentum is an apron-like structure which protects the abdominal viscera. If "things" aren't attached to the diaphragm, their facial attachments are attached to the spine. The rest sits on and is predominantly in the thorax. There are two pleura containing the lungs and the heart. The pericardium and the heart lung complex are really one organ. Neither one of them can work without the other. The mediastinal fascia is the stabilizing connective tissue partition. It's attached to the inner surface of the sternum, and is also attached to the front of the body of the thoracic vertebrae. It is directly related to these fascial planes, pericardia and pleura.

7

Techniques for the Sacrum and Pelvis

Lippincott: The auricular surfaces of the sacrum and the ilium, covered by cartilage, lie more or less in sagittal planes, but flare anteriorly and inferiorly. Their shape is that of a broad letter "L". The long arm is directed dorsoventrally, and from its anterior end the short arm extends cranially. Roughly following the line of this "L" there is usually a curved ridge on the auricular surface of the ilium, this fits into a groove on the sacrum. They describe an arc around a transverse line running approximately through the spinous process of the first or second sacral segments. The arrangement of the ligaments is such that the sacrum can swing within limits between the ilia, along the line of those ridges. This does not materially change the tension of these ligaments. Meanwhile the ligaments are limiting the tilt of the sacrum, downward and forward at the base, and backward and upward at the apex. This is caused by the weight of the trunk through the lumbar spine when the body is in the erect position. There is a notable absence of muscles between the sacrum and ilia which would normally control the motion of one upon the other.

Doctor Sutherland has called attention to an involuntary movement of the sacrum between the ilia in contra-distinction to the postural mobility of the ilia upon the sacrum. This involuntary motion is associated with what is termed in his cranial concept as the 'primary respiratory mechanism', and concerns a motility of the neural axis. The dural membranes, the cerebro-spinal fluid and the cranial bones and sacrum participate in this movement. The primary respiratory mechanism is fundamental to the pulmonary respiration, the cardiovascular system and the various other systems of the body. So it is not to be confused with diaphragmatic breathing. In the involuntary movement of the sacrum, the base alternately moves cranialward and recedes downward as a part of the primary respiratory mechanism. The inhalation or flexion phase of this movement causes the base to draw upward and the apex to move anteriorly. The sacrum swings on the arc of the L shaped auricular surface, or the ridge and groove described above. Since this movement reduces the anterior convexity of the lumbosacral junction and since it bears no relationship to the movement of the sacrum as the trunk bends forward in the standing position, the term respiratory flexion is applied to it. 'Respiratory extension' of the sacrum takes place when the base is lowered, the lumbosacral convexity is increased, the sacrum swings posteriorly in its arc, and the apex moves posteriorly. Postural or voluntary movement of the ilium upon the sacrum is known as the rotation of the innominate bone anteriorly or posteriorly on a transverse axis through the body of the second sacral segment.

Sutherland's Diagnosis of Respiratory Dysfunctions of the Sacrum

PHYSICIAN: Standing or seated behind the patient
PATIENT: Seated or prone

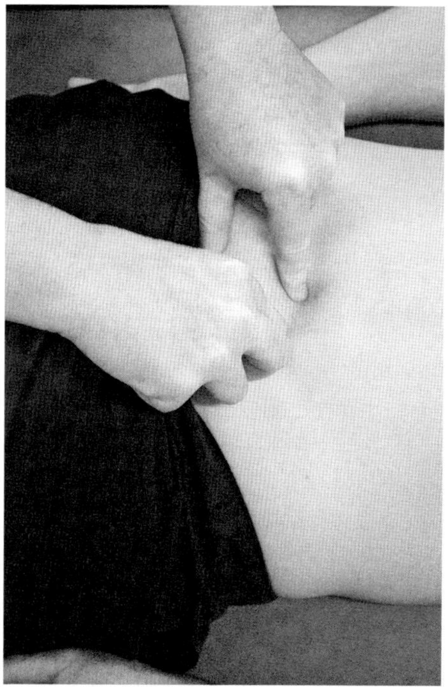

STEPS 1 – 5

1. Place your fingertips on the sacral base and the inferior lateral angles of the patient's sacrum
2. Ask the patient to take a deep breath to accentuate the respiratory motion. Sacral motion or the lack of motion is palpated
3. Flexion dysfunction—limited movement of the sacral base forward and downward
4. Extension dysfunction—limited movement of the sacral base backwards and upwards
5. A unilateral dysfunction is indicated by flexion on one side and extension on the other

Wales' Differential Technique

PHYSICIAN: Seated in front of the patient
PATIENT: Seated

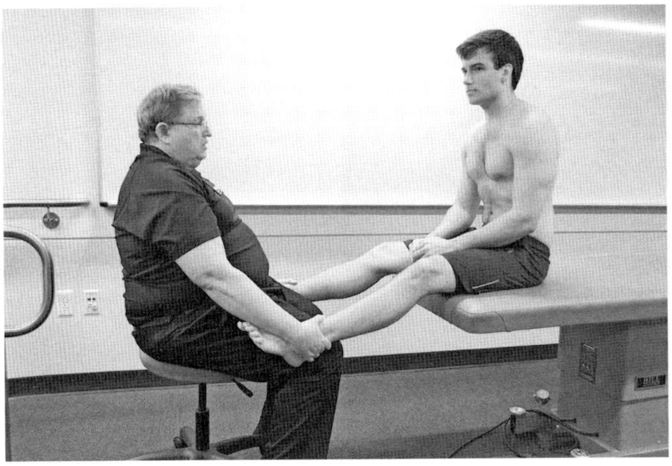

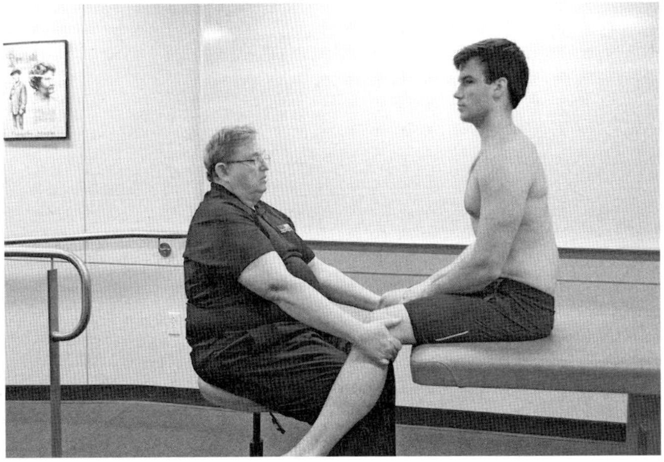

STEPS 1 – 2

1. With the patient seated hold the patient's ankles between 30 and 45 degrees from normal and relaxed in dorsiflexion or alternately hold behind their knees with a firm but not too firm a contact
2. Feel for equality of tension in their lower extremities. Feel for a balance point of disengagement of the patient's hip muscles

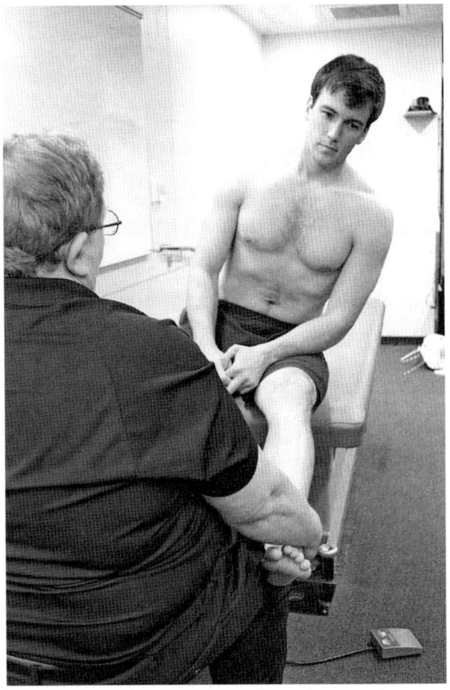

STEP 3

3. Ask the patient to lean to the right until you feel equal tension in both their legs. Hold their legs until the tension eases or balances

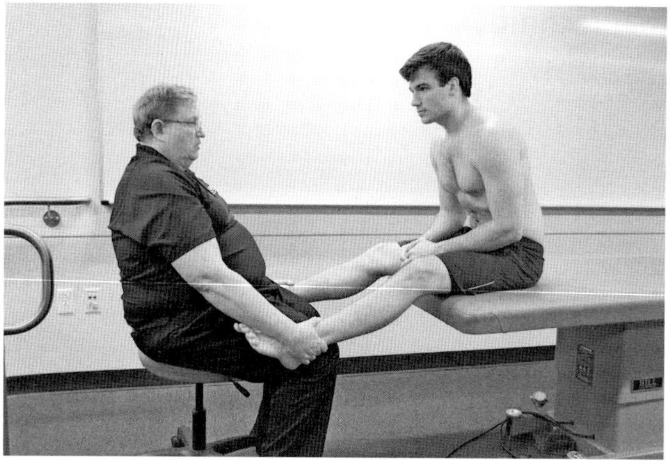

STEP 4

4. Ask the patient to lean to the left slowly until you feel equal tension in both legs. Hold until the tension eases or balances
5. While holding the legs, ask the patient to drop their head down and lean forward, until you feel equal tension in both legs. Hold until the tension eases or balances
6. Next, ask the patient to sit tall until you feel equal tension in both legs. Hold until the tension eases or balances
7. Now ask the patient to take their upper body in a circle while you hold tension on their legs. This reseats all the ligaments in the pelvis

Wales: This technique came out of Dr. Sutherland's inventiveness in 1951. Dr. Althea Miller who practiced in Oakland, California had a woman referred to her who had been in low back pain for years. She had two surgical operations for disc pathology for some reason and they gave her no relief. He saw the patient, saw the problem, and he told Althea that the patient would not be hurt with properly directed treatment. She could use the legs as long levers for turning the innominate bones into a position of balanced ligamentous tension in the pelvis. Using the patient's co-operation, once she'd achieved the balanced ligamentous state, the patient could turn their lumbar spine and sacrum within that framework. Althea didn't have to do it for her. The patient would stay within her own limits.

'It's like the differential gears in the automobile.' Dr. Sutherland stated that the sacroiliac joints function in postural body mechanics, and serve the same purpose as differential gears in an automobile. Now I understand, or I thought I did, that the differential gears in an automobile allow an automobile to turn a corner. Because the wheel on one side is at a different speed than the other, it's accommodated in the middle by the big box (differential). The transmission gears have to be different, so they can turn differently. Well, we're bipeds and we go around different corners. This is Will's idea, the sacroiliac joints have this function in body mechanics. When you have someone with low back pain, and you know you need to reset the sacrum, this is one way to do it. So this technique was called the differential 'technique'. And it is a co-operative effort between the patient and the physician.

There is a direct connection between the patient's hips and your hands. You use the patient's legs as long levers to turn the innominate bones through the acetabulums. These are higher than the tuberosities when the patient is sitting.

Crow: As Dr. Wales put it, "I'm looking at the pelvis through the legs. I move one lever and the other alternately, and then I come back to neutral and ask you to sit tall."

Wales' Pelvic and Lower Extremity Fascial Release Technique

Crow: Dr. Wales used this technique to free the lower extremity fascia, hip capsule and the pelvic fascia.

PHYSICIAN: Standing beside the patient
PATIENT: Supine

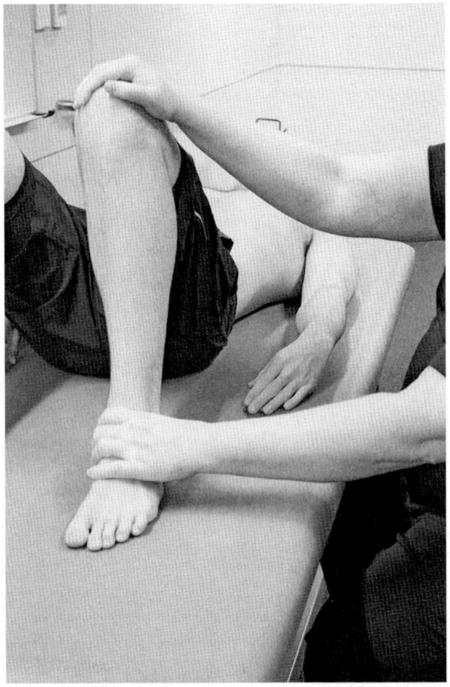

STEPS 1 – 4

1. Bend the patient's knee and place the patient's foot on the table
2. Place your left hand on their left ankle
3. Place your right hand on their left knee
4. Make a very small excursion from one side to the other. This will relax the hip capsule and release their diaphragm, as well as moving the lymphatic fluids through the fascia
5. Repeat this procedure on the other side

Wales' Technique for the Anterior Sacroiliac

PHYSICIAN: Seated at a slightly lower level in front of the patient
PATIENT: Seated on the table

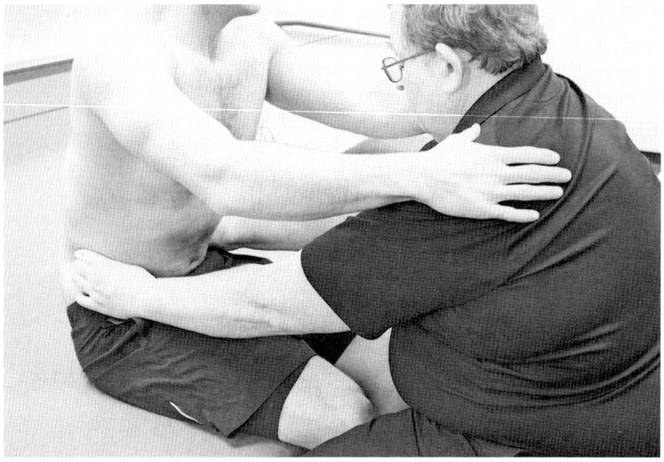

STEP 1

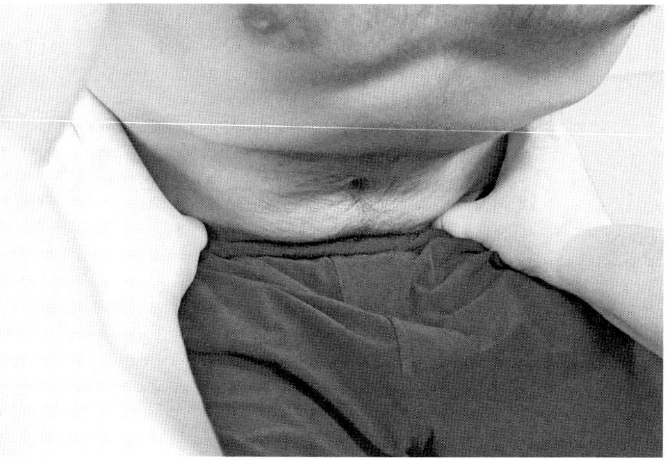

STEP 2

1. The patient places their hands on the physician's shoulders
2. Place your thumbs just inside of their iliac crest and pointing toward the face of their sacrum. There is a potential fascial space at the edge of their quadratus lumborum attachment

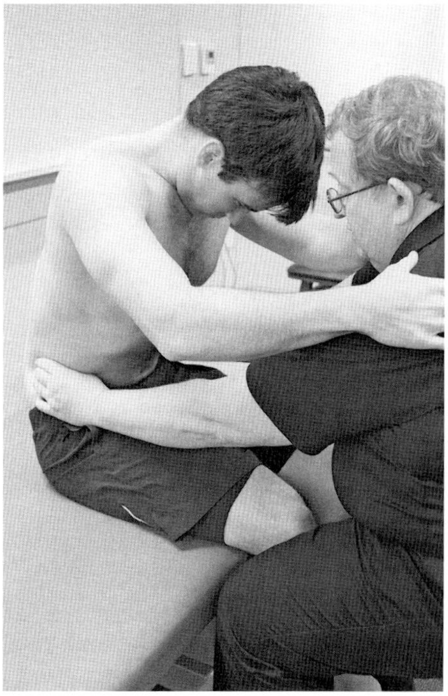

STEPS 3 – 5

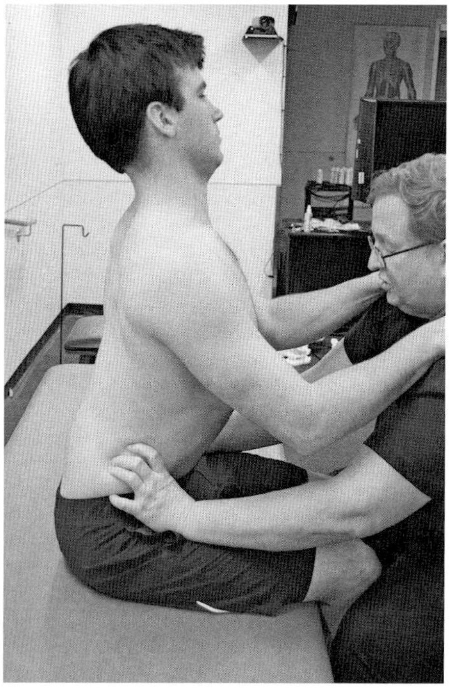

STEPS 6 – 7

3. Hold the patient's knees between your knees
4. The patient leans forward from the hips
5. Ask the patient to drop their head down and forward

6. While holding their head down, ask the patient to arch their back like a cat
7. Next, ask the patient to straighten up, thereby increasing the lordotic curvature

Wales: Now it is not probable that you can actually get the tips of your thumbs in contact with the tips of the sacral ala. But if your thumbs are pointed towards the anterior surface of the sacrum, and you are leaning into your contacts, then the patient is leaning into you with their weight. The physician is balancing the patient's weight around their thumbs and the patient is bearing their own weight. So your thumbs become the fulcrum. As the patient sits up the sacrum resets itself as you let your thumbs come up with the sacral movement.

The story behind this began in 1948 when Dr. Sutherland was in Providence and I had been treating a young woman. I was treating her and failing to get anywhere with her pelvic mechanics. So I asked Dr. Sutherland if there was anything that I could do that I wasn't doing. When I told him how overwrought she was, he said "Well, you do need to release her sacrum. How is it?" I said "Well it's in there and I can't get at it." He said "Did you ever think of pushing it from the front? All you have to do is get in front of it and push." Will did not show me. He just told me what to do, so I just made it up as I went along.

The point is when you ask the patient to sit back and sit up, you, the physician, stay with them and pull their knees together so that the innominates will get out of the way. This technique came to be called 'backing the sacrum into the garage.'

Sutherland's Techniques for the Innominates

Lippincott: Dr. Sutherland said most of these sacroiliac strains occur in the standing position, so why not adjust them in the standing position—this is a standing posture technique. Balanced ligamentous tension you can do with the patient supine, or another position is with the patient prone. Once you have realigned the sacrum in relation to the ilia its involuntary action can follow, but then you want to get the lumbar spine to go with it and you want to rebalance the lumbar joints.

Sutherland's Technique for the Posterior Rotation of the Innominate Diagnosis

EXAMPLE: Right posterior innominate
PHYSICIAN: Standing behind the patient
PATIENT: Seated

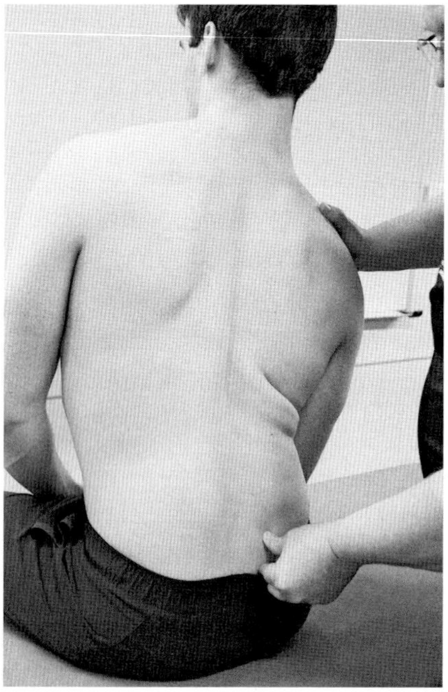

STEP 1

STEP 2–A

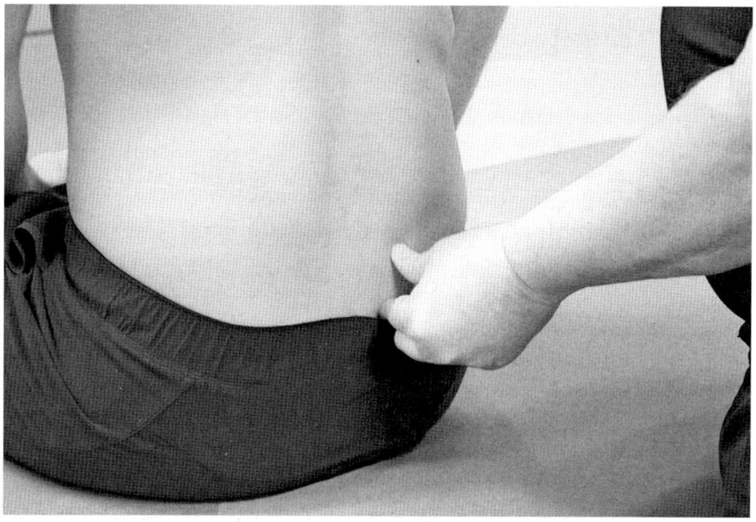

1. Place your hand on the patient's shoulder on the side that you want to test (use your right hand on their right shoulder for their right innominate)

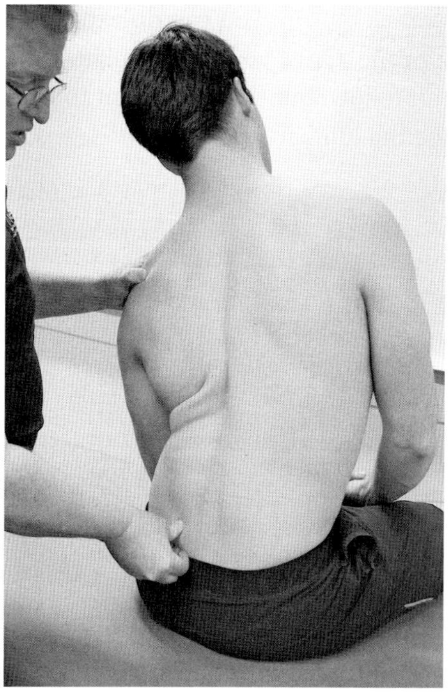

STEP 2–B

2. Place your right thumb on the left side of the patient's sacrum and your right index

finger on their right posterior superior iliac spine (innominate)

3. The motion between the sacrum and their right posterior superior iliac spine is going to be palpated
4. Compress their left shoulder. If the sacral/innominate motion is free as their shoulder is compressed when introducing side-bending into their lumbar spine, and their innominate moves posteriorly, this ligamentous articular strain is a posterior rotation of the innominate bone

Sutherland's Technique for a Posterior Rotation of the Innominate Treatment

EXAMPLE: Left posterior innominate
PHYSICIAN: Seated beside the patient
PATIENT: Standing with their hand on the physician's shoulder

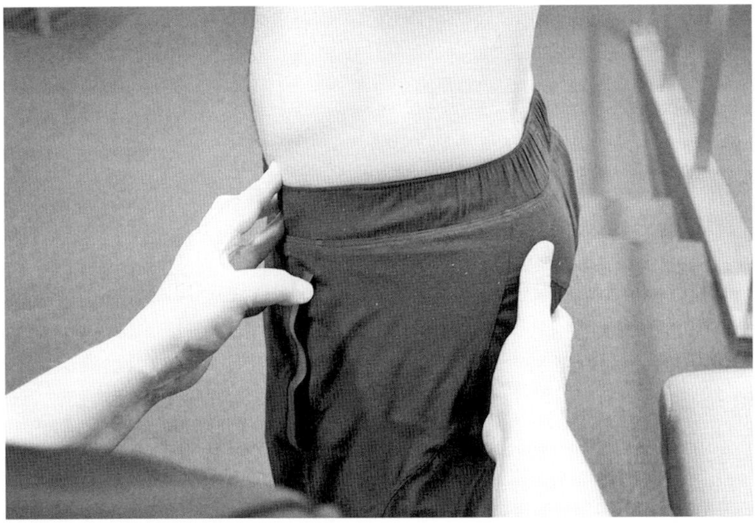

STEP 1

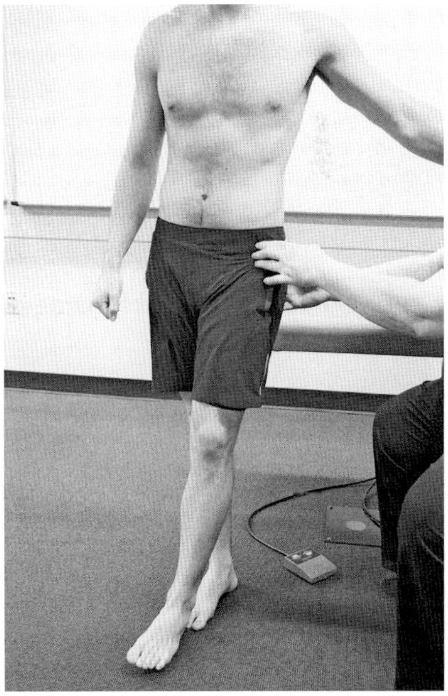

STEPS 3 – 4

1. Hold the patient's left tuberosity in the palm of your right hand and the crest of their left ilium in your left hand
2. Their left innominate bone will be rotated with your hands, anteriorly towards the position of correction
3. Ask the patient to place their left hand on your right shoulder on the side of the dysfunction (patient's right hand on your left shoulder for a right posterior innominate)
4. Their left leg on the side of the dysfunction is crossed in front of their right leg, with their left foot resting on its lateral edge. This will transfer weight from the spine through the sacrum to the right innominate bone. This stabilizes the sacrum and frees the ligaments on the dysfunctional side (left side)

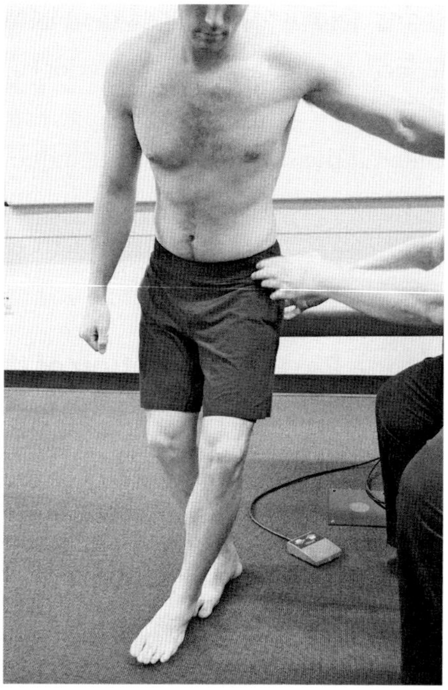

STEPS 5 – 6

5. Ask the patient to flex the weight bearing right knee to about 135 degrees, while keeping their left leg relaxed
6. The physician is moving the patient's left innominate in an anterior direction for correction

Sutherland's Technique for an Anterior Rotation of the Innominate Diagnosis

EXAMPLE: Left anterior innominate
PHYSICIAN: Standing behind the patient
PATIENT: Seated

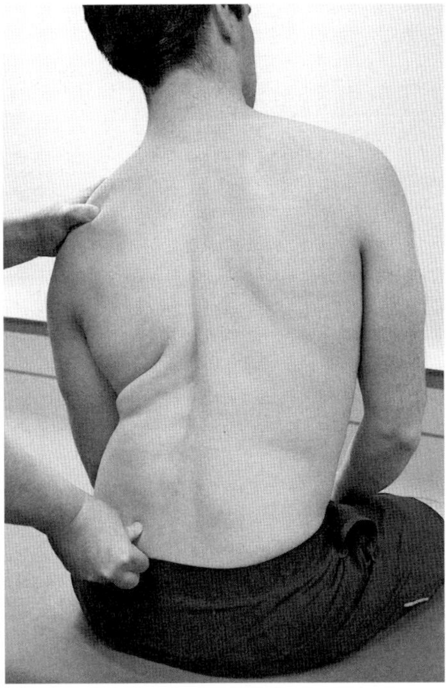

STEPS 1 – 3

1. Place your left hand on the patient's shoulder on the side that you want to test (use your left hand on their left shoulder for their left innominate)
2. Place your thumb on the left side of the patient's sacrum and your right index finger on the posterior superior iliac spine of their left innominate on the same side as your right hand. The motion between their sacrum and their left posterior superior iliac spine is going to be palpated
3. Compress their left shoulder with your left hand. If the motion is free at the posterior iliac spine as the patient's left shoulder is compressed and side-bending is introduced in their lumbar spine, and the innominate moves anteriorly, then this ligamentous articular strain denotes an anterior rotation of their left innominate bone

Sutherland's Technique for an Anterior Rotation of the Innominate Treatment

EXAMPLE: Left anterior innominate
PHYSICIAN: Seated beside the patient
PATIENT: Standing

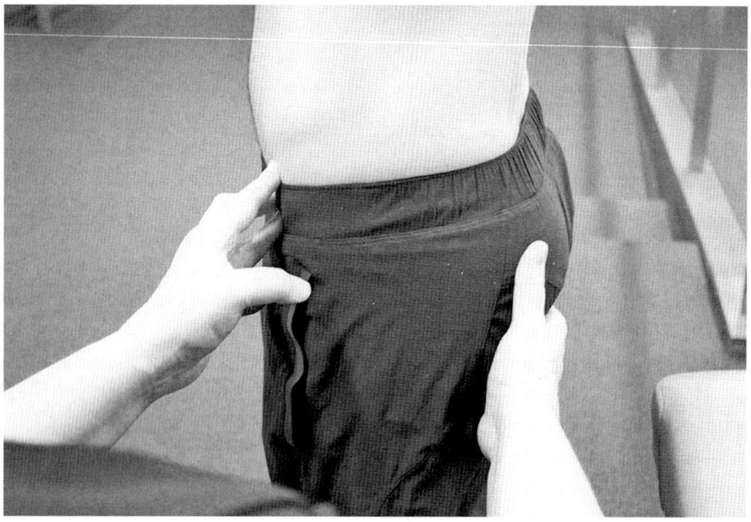

STEPS 1

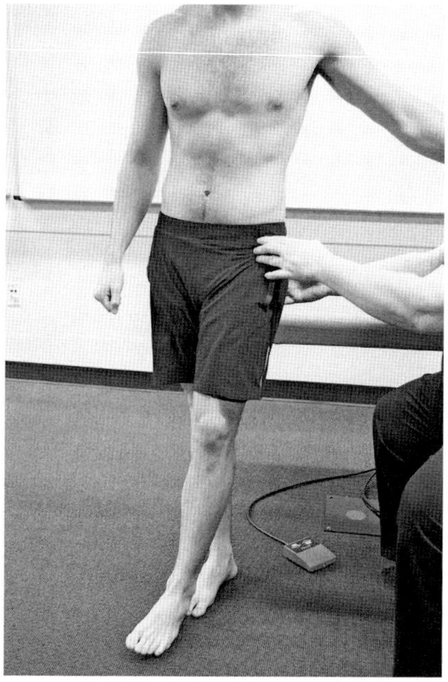

STEPS 3 – 4

1. Hold the patient's left tuberosity in the palm of your right hand and the crest of their ilium in your left hand
2. Their left innominate bone is rotated with both your hands, posteriorly towards the position of correction
3. Ask the patient to place their hand on your shoulder on the side of the dysfunction (their left hand on your right shoulder for an anterior left innominate)
4. Their left leg on the side of the dysfunction is crossed in front of their right leg, while resting their left foot on its lateral edge. This will transfer weight from the spine through the sacrum to the left innominate bone. This stabilizes the sacrum and frees the ligaments on the left dysfunctional side

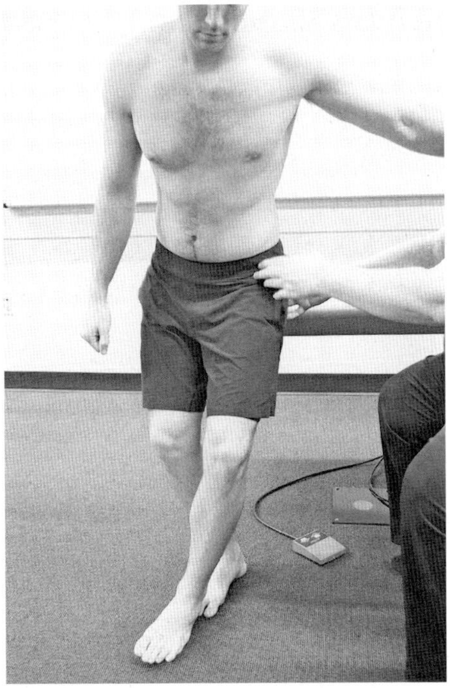

STEPS 5 – 6

5. Ask the patient to flex the right weight bearing knee to about 135 degrees, while keeping the left leg relaxed
6. The physician moves their left innominate in a posterior direction

Wales: It doesn't make any difference if it's an anterior innominate or posterior innominate. No matter what it needs to do, it's going to do it. So you don't have to bother about terminology. You just have to bother about whether you need to do this in order to fix the problem. This is a beautifully simple technique in certain types of sacroiliac strain patterns and complex pelvic patterns. Again, the patient isn't going to hurt themselves. With this technique for resolving sacroiliac problems the patient sometimes experienced pain while I was doing it. This simply fixes it.

THE PUBIC SYMPHYSIS

Liippincott: The symphysis pubis is subject to ligamentous strain, and is frequently associated with sacroiliac dysfunctions. There is an intervening cartilage between the pubes that allows motion to take place. The bones are bound together by strong ligaments, some of whose fibers are diagonally placed. This makes them especially susceptible to strain or imbalance. An unevenness of the superior borders of the pubic bones may be palpated. The inferior ligament, which extends between the inferior rami, is pierced by the urogenital ducts and by a branch of the internal pudic nerve in close proximity to the symphysis. This can be a source of chronic pelvic pain, particularly in women after the birth of a child.

Sutherland's Pubic Symphysis Technique

PHYSICIAN: Stands behind the patient
PATIENT: Lying right lateral recumbent, knees flexed with their back toward you

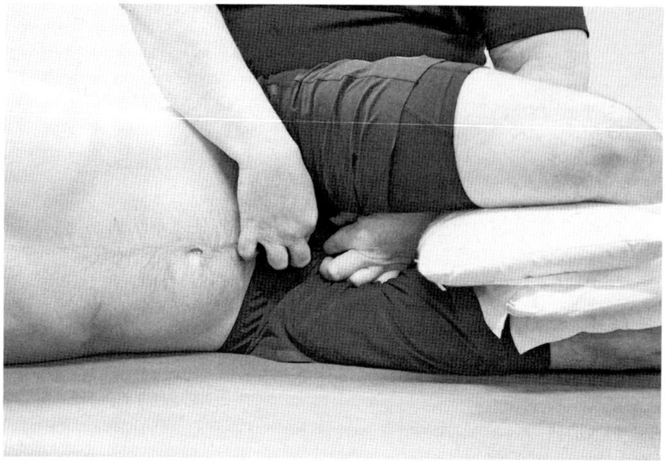

STEPS 1 – 4

1. Place a pillow between the patient's knees
2. The tips of your index and middle fingers or thumb of your left hand (nearest the foot of the table) are placed between their legs, reaching in front of the genitalia up to the inferior border of the symphysis. Your left middle and index fingers are on either side of the cartilaginous pubic joint. This begins the tension on the interpubic ligament
3. The fingertips of your right hand push down on the superior border of the pubic symphysis (bone). This adds tension to the interpubic ligament. The tension may be balanced using the fingers on either hand and applying pressure cephalically or caudally
4. The patient presses their knees together, which helps move the joint

Crow: I have included this technique as originally performed by Dr. Sutherland for completeness. However, I usually choose an alternate way of treating the pubic shears such as muscle energy or the way described below.

Crow's Alternate Pubic Symphysis Technique

PHYSICIAN: Standing beside the patient facing cephalically
PATIENT: Supine with knees bent

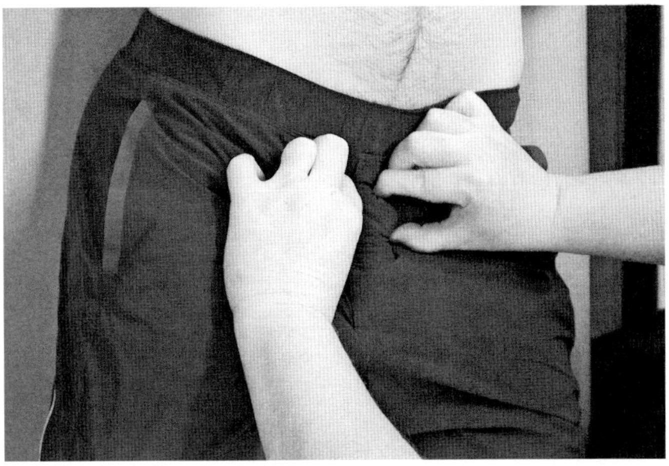

STEPS 1 – 5

1. Place your thumbs on each side of the patient's pubic symphysis below their inferior rami (symphysis border)
2. Place your index finger and middle fingers of both hands on the superior rami to oppose your thumbs on the inferior rami
3. Ask the patient to squeeze their knees together, which will cause tension on their inter-pubic ligament
4. Gently balance tension across the pubic joint to get it free
5. Ask the patient to take a deep breath in and hold it

West's Pelvis Technique

EXAMPLE: Right pelvic dysfunction
PHYSICIAN: Standing behind the patient
PATIENT: Lying on their left side, right side up

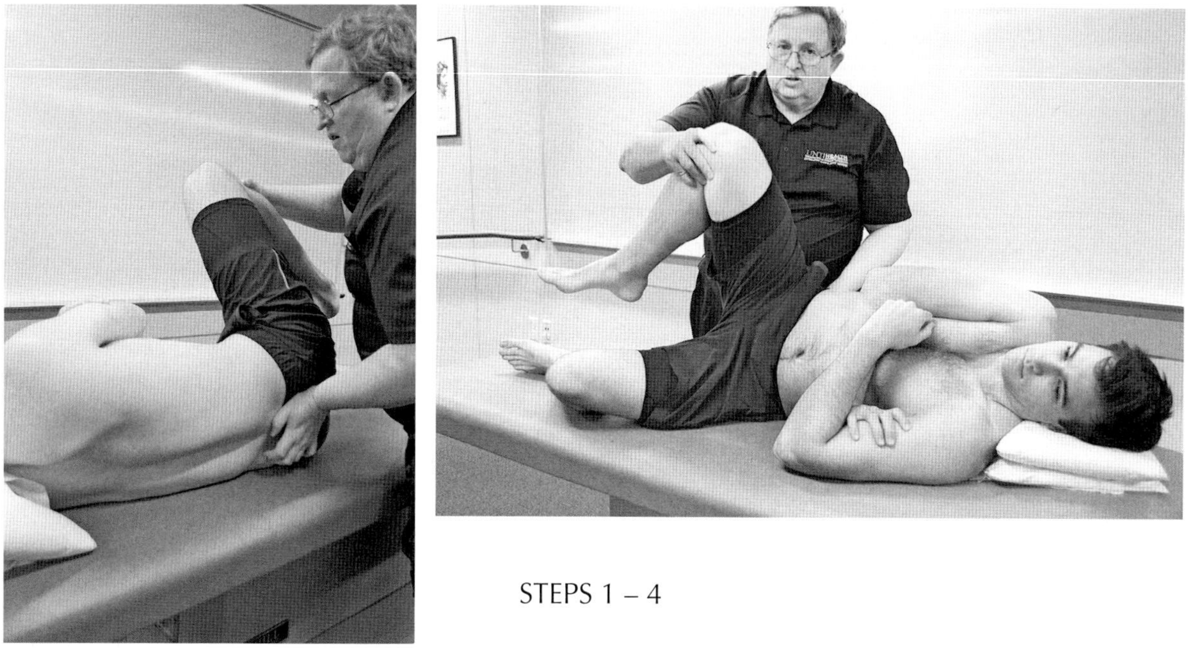

STEPS 1 – 4

1. Ask the patient to flex both knees
2. Place your right hand under the patient's right knee
3. Place your left hand on their right iliac crest to stabilize the patient
4. Circumduct their right leg forward and up, and bring their right leg backward into extension

West's Iliolumbar Technique

EXAMPLE: Right pelvic dysfunction
PHYSICIAN: Standing behind the patient
PATIENT: Lying on their left side, their right side up

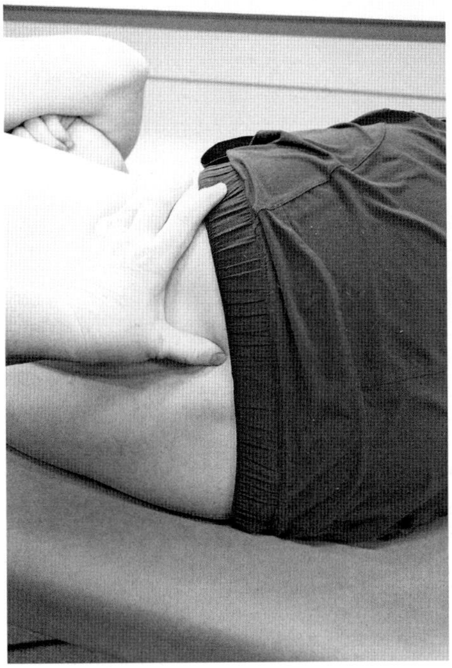

STEP 3

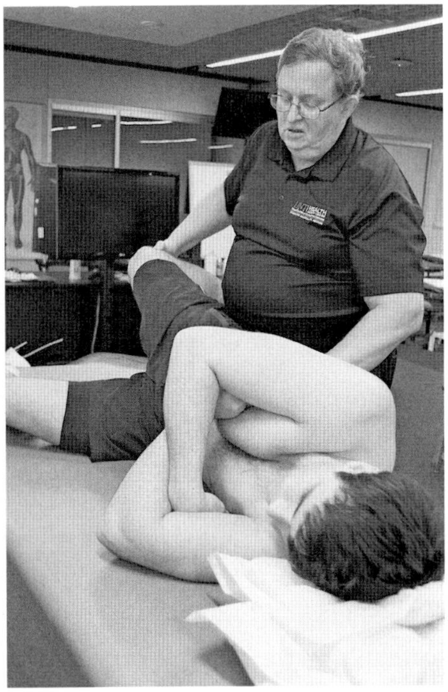

STEP 4

1. Ask the patient to flex both knees
2. Place your right hand under the patient's right knee
3. Place your left thumb deeply into their right iliolumbar ligament
4. Circumduct their right leg and bring the right leg up quickly to their left shoulder across the patient's body

Wales' Coccyx Technique

PHYSICIAN: Standing on the right side of the patient
PATIENT: Prone

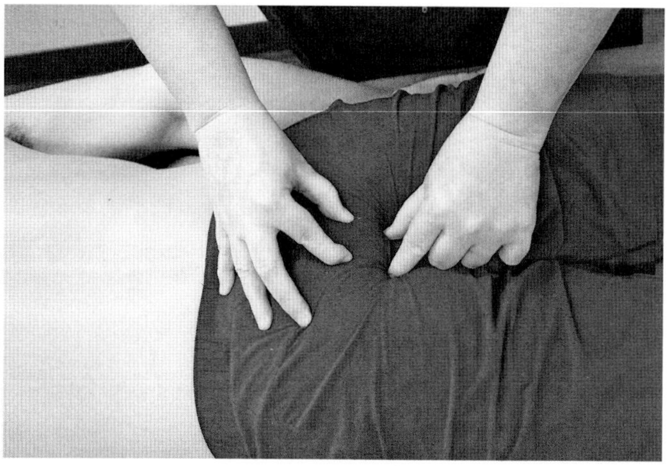

STEPS 1 – 5

1. Place the base of your right hand at the base of the patient's sacrum with your right middle finger at the apex
2. Make a light 'plastic' contact on the dorsum of their sacrum, and then you lean slowly and carefully on the sacrum. You want to feel the sacrum move, and find out how well it moves, and what position it's in
3. Lean into their sacrum and towards their coccyx very carefully with your right hand, so the tension is taken off their sacroiliac ligaments, allowing their sacrum to move freely
4. With your left hand place two fingers (one finger either side) of their coccyx pointing cephalically
5. Add traction with the fingers of your left hand to separate the coccyx from the patient's sacrum and balance their coccygeal ligaments

8

Techniques for the Lower Extremities

Tucker on Treating the Femur and Hip

DIAGNOSIS

Dislocations of the hip and of other joints of the extremities are surgical cases, and are well known and thoroughly described. The principle of correction is traction. A point in the diagnosis of dislocations of the hip is well worthwhile though.

With the patient supine, an assistant stands at the foot of table, grasping the patient's toes and prepared to rotate them outwards and down, then up and inwards (both feet out and down at the same time). The physician places their thumbs on the anterior superior spines of the patient's ilium, and places their hands over the patient's greater trochanter. As the assistant rotates the patient's toes, each greater trochanter describes an arc whose center is the center of the acetabulum in normal hips. This arc is very quickly determined by the curve of the physician's palms. Its position with reference to the patient's anterior superior spine is instantly defined. In dislocations of the hip, their trochanter describes an arc which points immediately to the position of the head of the trochanter bone. The normal arc is slightly more down than up. If the position of the head is on the dorsum of the ilium, the arc will be both up and in. If the position is in the 'thyroid' notch [current terminology is the obturator notch], the trochanter on that side will be correspondingly lower than its fellow, and the rotation will be up and in. If the arc is shorter and more sharply curved than its fellow, it points to a fracture of the neck, or a tubercular destruction of the head of the bone. As soon as the arc is defined under the palm, the position of the head and the length of the neck is instantly defined.

- Lesions of the ligamentum teres are believed to occur. The tendon becomes curled the wrong way and cramped upon itself.
- The diagnosis is obscure—a catch in walking, pains on the inner side of the knee without other lesions of the hip joint.
- The tendon is a development from the transverse ligament, and is originally connected with certain muscles of the thigh.
- May be indicated by pain on the inner side of the knee.

The problem is to stretch the ligament in all directions, relying on the tendency towards normality to restore the ligament to a normal position. Therefore, this must involve carrying the head of the bone around the rim of the acetabulum at the limit of normal tension. From the anterior edge of the notch at the lower anterior corner, rotate the trochanter up, back and around and down to the other side of the acetabular notch. If this does not give relief, rotation in the opposite direction may be tried.

Tucker's Femur and Hip Technique

PHYSICIAN: Standing at the foot of the table
PATIENT: Supine

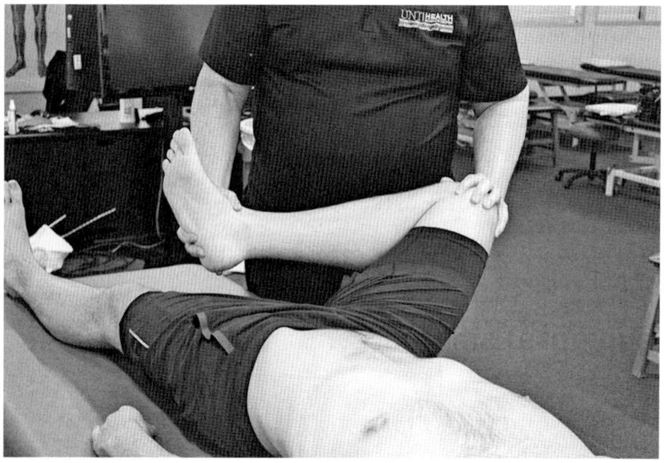

STEPS 1 – 3

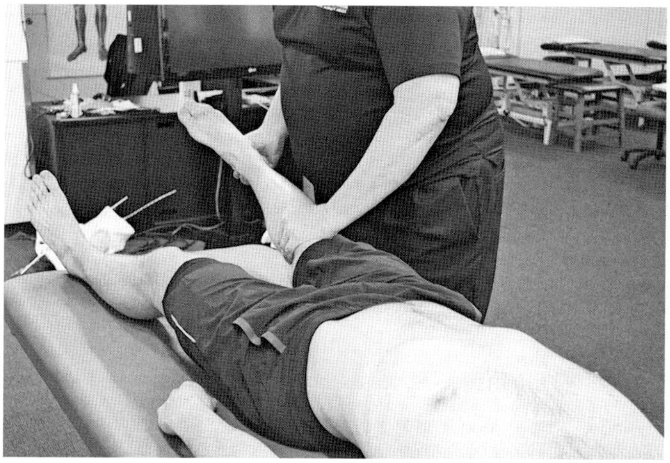

STEP 4

1. The patient's thigh is raised to forty-five degrees, and adducted, with their leg also abducted. This brings the head of the trochanter to the anterior edge of the notch
2. The patient's leg is then abducted, which brings the head of the trochanter to the anterior edge of the acetabulum
3. Their foot and knee are then abducted together
4. This carries the head of the femur to almost the top of the notch

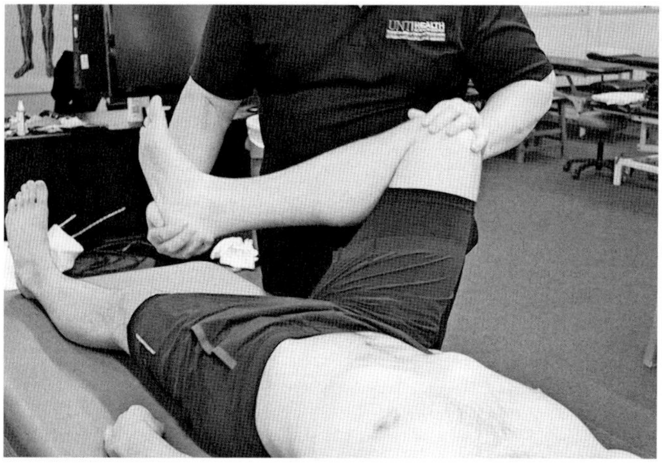

STEP 5

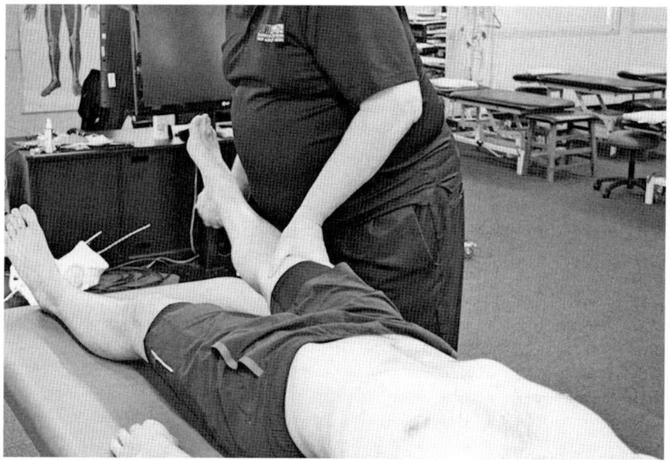

STEP 6

5. The foot is then abducted as the knee is lowered—always at the limit of tension centrally. This carries the femoral head around the upper third of the acetabulum
6. Maintaining their foot in abduction, their knee is then carried up, out, down, and into normal position

Sutherland's Hip Techniques

DIAGNOSIS – METHOD ONE

EXAMPLE: Right hip
PHYSICIAN: Standing facing the patient
PATIENT: Standing

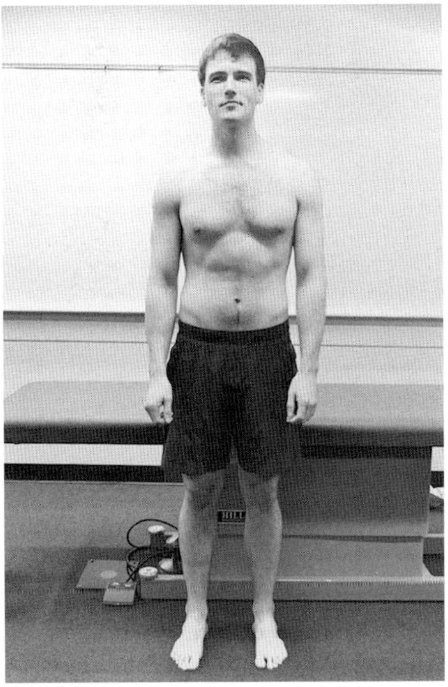

STEP 1

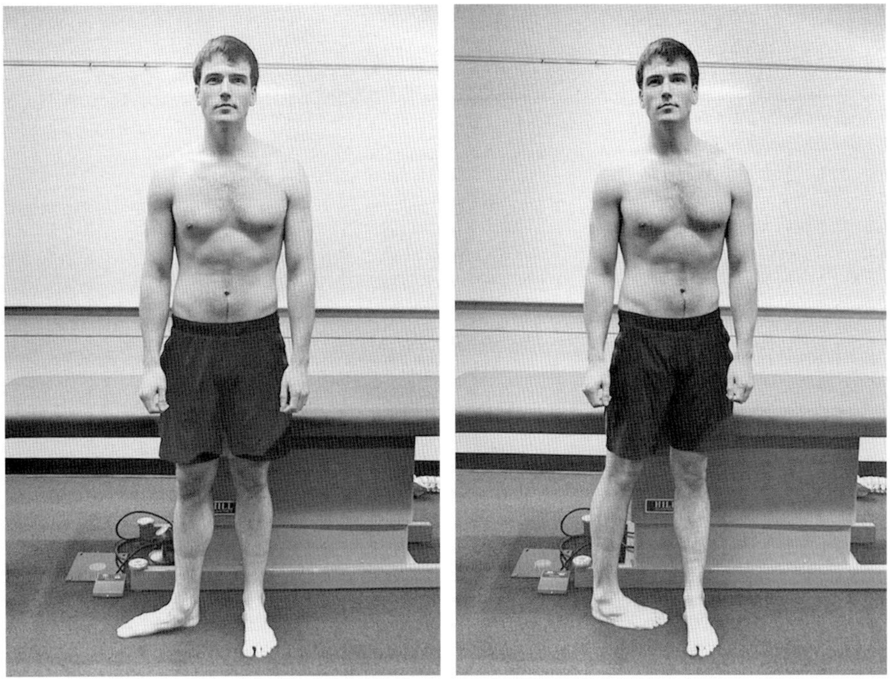

STEP 2

1. The patient stands with their weight on the left foot
2. Without turning their pelvis the patient rotates their right leg and foot laterally and medially to determine the degree of external and internal rotation
3. Comparison of the motion in either direction to the right or to the left side designates the dysfunction

Sutherland's Technique for Internal Hip Rotation – Method One

PHYSICIAN: Seated beside the patient
PATIENT: Standing

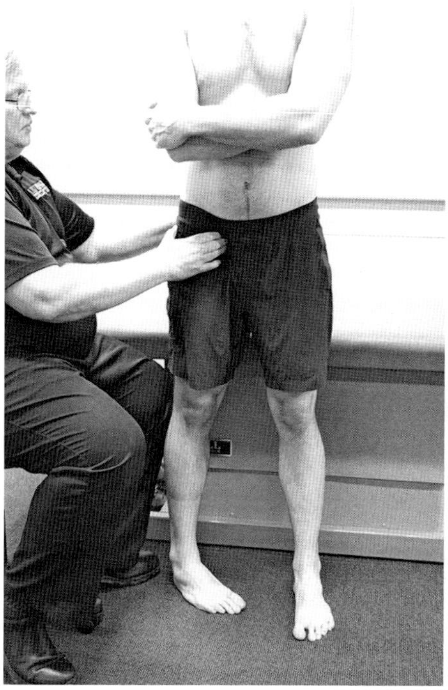

STEPS 1 – 2

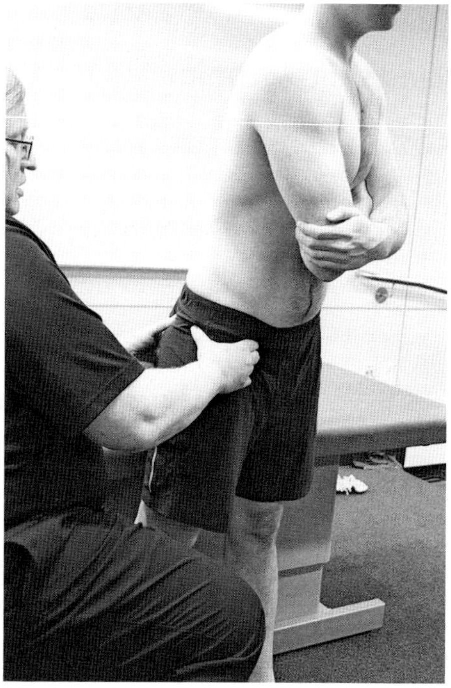

STEPS 3 – 4

1. The physician places one hand on the medial aspect of the patient's thigh with your thumb as close to the femoral head as you can get by pushing the femoral head laterally
2. Your other hand reaches around the back of their pelvis to palpate the motion at the greater trochanter
3. The patient internally rotates their leg and leans forward
4. The patient exhales and holds their breath out

Sutherland's Technique for External Rotation of the Hip – Method One

PHYSICIAN: Seated beside the patient
PATIENT: Standing

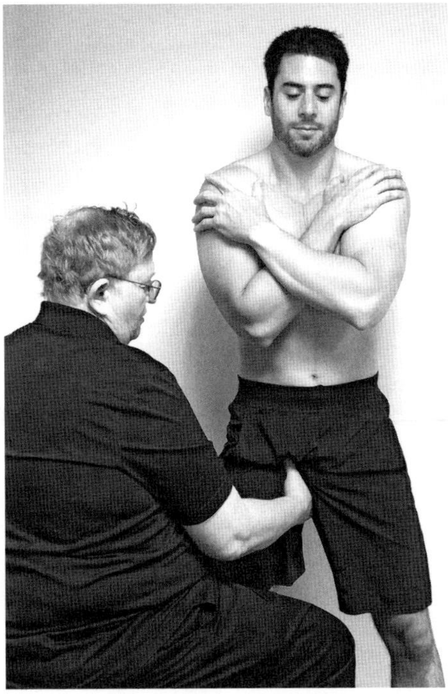

STEPS 1 – 4

1. The physician places one hand on the medial aspect of the patient's thigh with your thumb as close to the femoral head as you can get by pushing the head laterally
2. The physician's other hand reaches around the back of their pelvis to palpate the motion at the greater trochanter
3. The patient externally rotates their leg and leans backward
4. The patient takes a deep breath and holds their breath

Sutherland's Hip Joint Diagnosis – Method Two

EXAMPLE: Right hip
PHYSICIAN: Seated in front of the patient
PATIENT: Seated with their right leg resting over their left knee

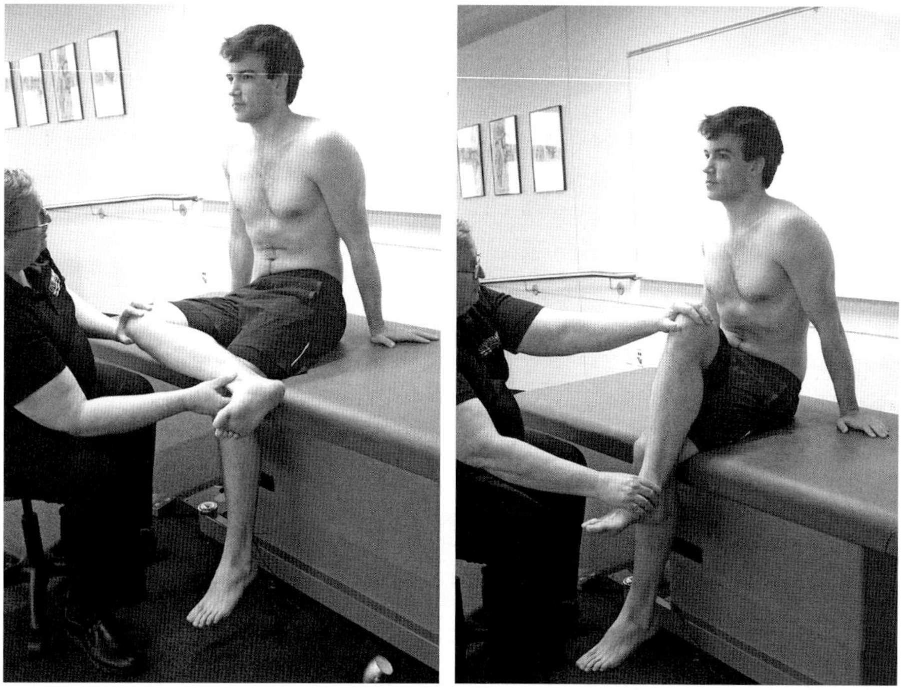

STEP 1

Facing the patient, hold their right leg at the knee and ankle, and rotate their right femur by moving their right leg in either direction over their left knee. Restrictions caused by an exostosis, osteoarthritis or other bony abnormalities are usually indicated by a hard-end feel. Ligamentous articular strains generally have more spring in them

Sutherland's Technique for External Rotation of the Hip – Method Two

EXAMPLE: Right hip
PHYSICIAN: Seated next to the patient
PATIENT: Seated

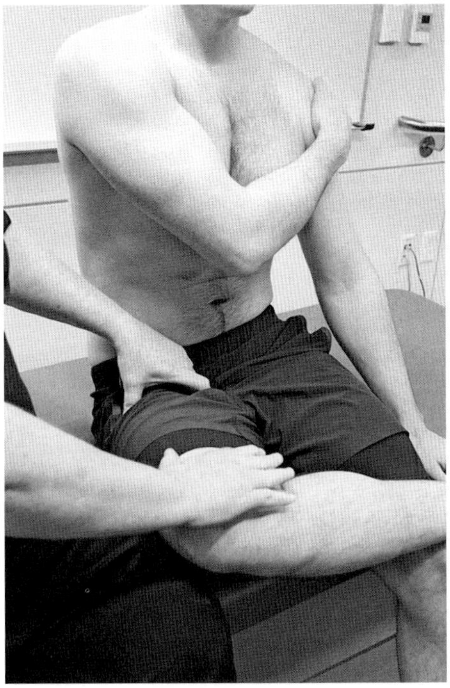

STEPS 1 – 2

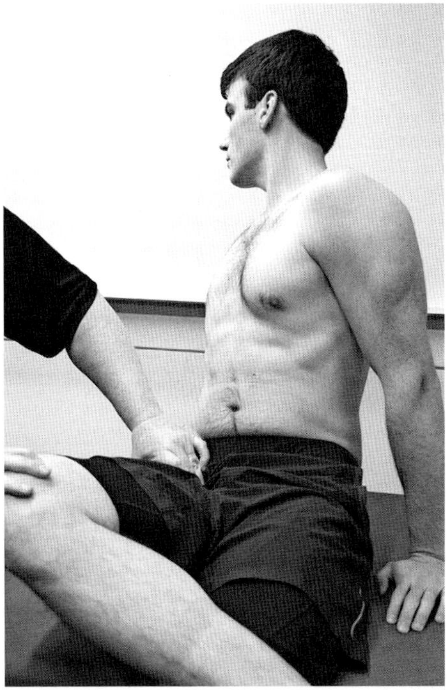

STEPS 3 – 6

1. The patient's right leg is crossed over their left knee, resting on the mid shaft of their fibula
2. Place your left hand on the medial aspect of the patient's right thigh with your thumb as close to the femoral head as you can get by pushing the head laterally
3. Take your left hand and reach around the back of their pelvis to palpate the motion at their greater trochanter
4. Hold the patients right knee laterally and downward with your right hand to exaggerate the movement
5. Ask the patient to side-bend and rotate their body away from their right side and lean backwards
6. Ask the patient to take a deep breath and hold their breath

Sutherland's Technique for Internal Rotation of the Hip – Method Two

EXAMPLE: Right hip
PHYSICIAN: Seated next to the patient
PATIENT: Seated

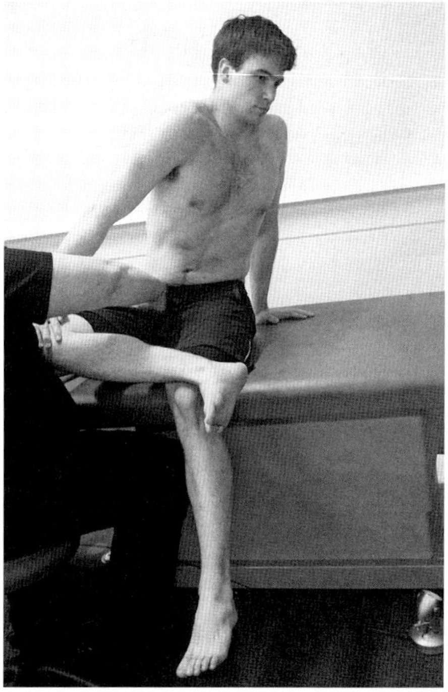

STEP 1

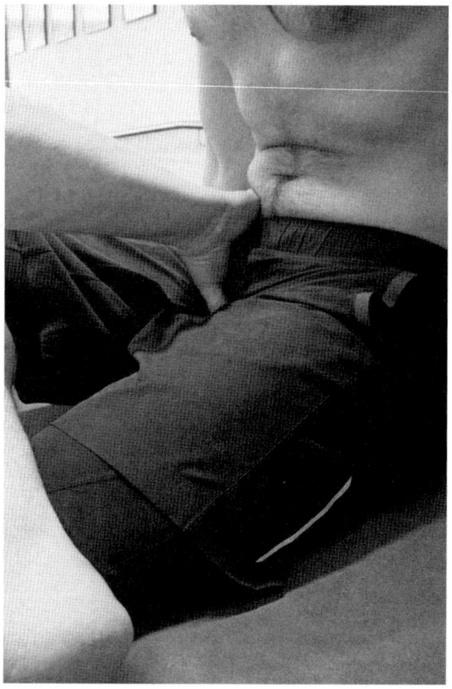

STEP 2

1. The patient's right leg is crossed over their left knee, resting on the mid shaft of their fibula
2. Place your right hand on the medial aspect of the patient's right thigh, with your thumb as close to the femoral head as you can get by pushing the head laterally

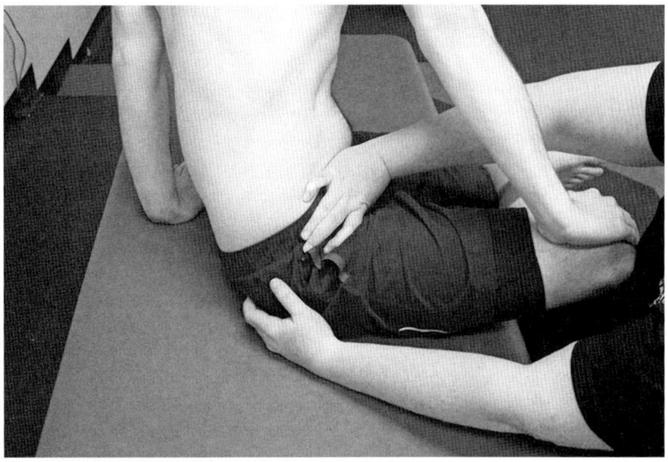

STEPS 3 – 6

3. Take your left hand and reach around the back of their pelvis to palpate the motion at the greater trochanter
4. The patient holds their right knee laterally and downward with their right hand to exaggerate the movement
5. Ask the patient to rotate their body to their left side and lean forward
6. Ask the patient to exhale and hold their breath

West's Sartorius Technique

EXAMPLE: Restricted left sartorius
PHYSICIAN: Standing in front of the patient
PATIENT: Seated

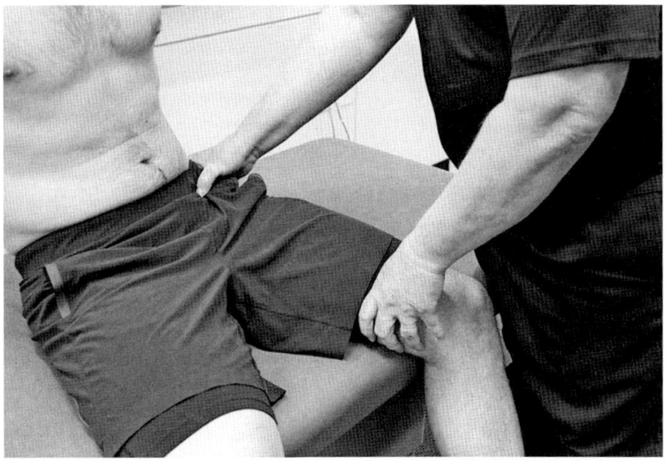

STEPS 1 – 3

1. Place your right hand on the patient's left anterior superior iliac spine
2. Place your left hand on their left sartorius at the edge of their left knee
3. Ask the patient to adduct their left knee while you maintain pressure on both the iliac spine and the sartorius

Sutherland's Tibiofemoral Diagnosis

Lippincott: Tibiofemoral dysfunctions are caused by a sudden or forcible rotation of the tibia in relation to the femur, usually occurring with a side-bending strain upon the knee. In most cases the medial condyle of the tibia has been rotated anteriorly when the foot was turned laterally and the knee bent medially. History of the injury, location of the tenderness, inability to fully extend the knee in most cases, pain and restriction on attempting to reverse the dysfunctional position are indicators. Palpation establishes the diagnosis.

Sutherland's Tibiofemoral / Medial Condyle Technique

EXAMPLE: Tibiofemoral joint
PHYSICIAN: Seated facing the patient
PATIENT: Seated

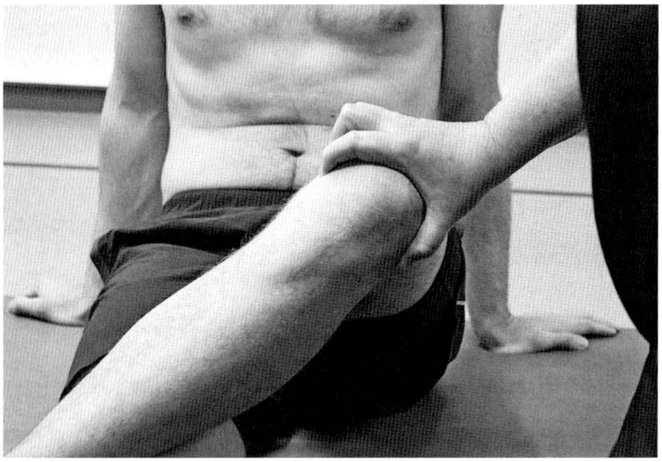

STEPS 1 – 2

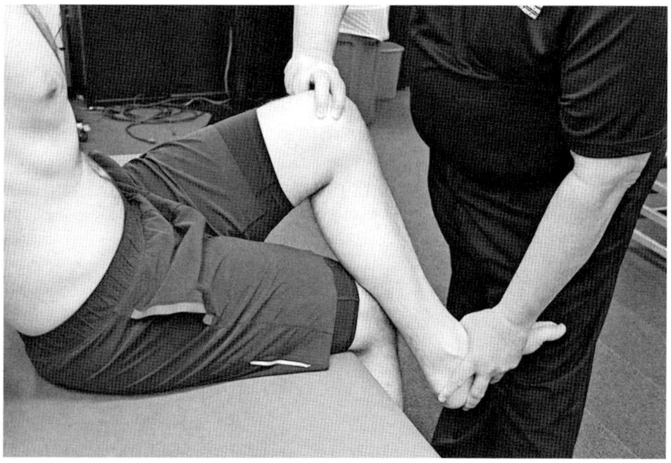

STEPS 3 – 5

1. The involved leg is balanced over the opposite knee
2. Place your right hand on the patient's knee at the tibiofemoral joint line. Your thumb is on the lateral condyle of their left tibia, and one or two of your fingers on the medial condyle of their femur
3. Your left hand grasps their foot—just below the ankle
4. The patient's foot is carried laterally and upward, tipping their knee medially and downward. This tenses their medial collateral ligaments
5. Their tibia is rotated externally or internally by your left hand at their foot—to the point of balanced tension
6. The patient is asked to resist the turning of their foot, and the result of that effort is to glide the medial condyle of their tibia back towards normal

Sutherland's Tibiofemoral / Lateral Condyle Technique

EXAMPLE: Tibiofemoral joint
PHYSICIAN: Seated facing the patient
PATIENT: Seated

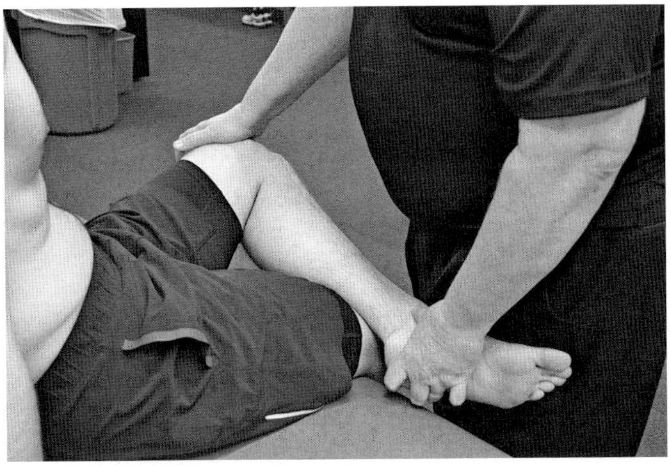

STEPS 1 – 6

1. The involved leg is balanced over the opposite knee
2. Place one hand on the patient's knee at the joint line, with your thumb on the medial condyle of the tibia and one or two fingers on the lateral condyle of the femur
3. The other hand grasps the foot, just below the ankle
4. The knee is carried laterally and downward, tipping the foot medially and upward. This tenses the collateral ligaments
5. The tibia is rotated externally or internally by your hand at their foot to the point of balanced tension
6. The patient is instructed to resist the turning of his foot and the result of that effort is to glide the lateral condyle of the femur back into place

Wales' Fibula Technique

EXAMPLE: Left fibula
PHYSICIAN: Seated facing the patient
PATIENT: Seated

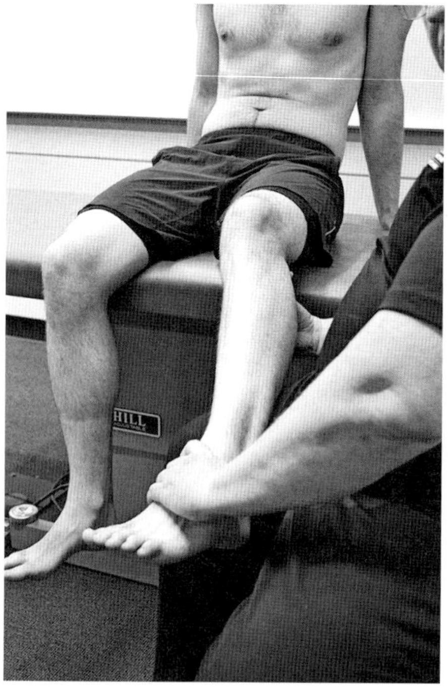

STEPS 1 – 2

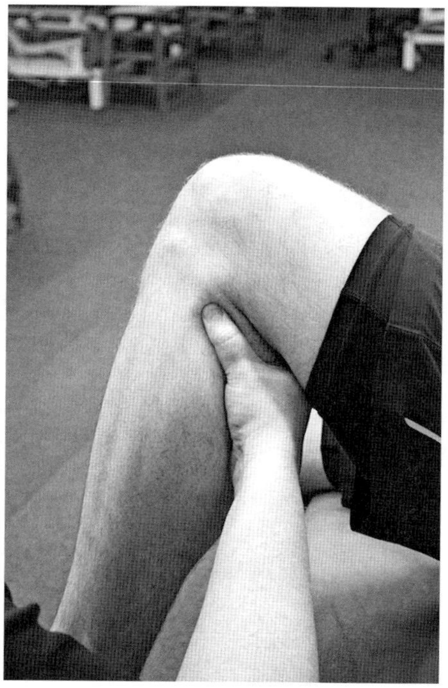

STEP 3

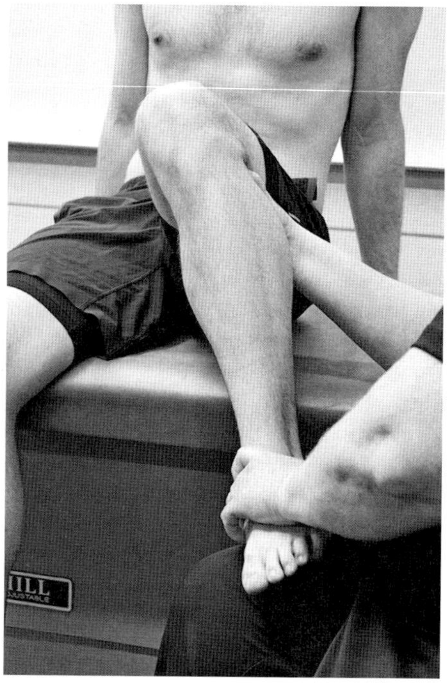

STEPS 4 – 5

1. The thenar eminence of your left hand is underneath the patient's left lateral malleolus
2. The patient's left foot rests on top of the physician's right knee
3. Your right hand comes up behind the proximal head of their fibula
4. Balance the tibiofibular interosseous membrane by pulling their left lateral malleolus posteriorly and moving the left fibular head anteriorly
5. Hold this position of tension. This is not exactly the same thing as balanced ligament tension, because you are using direct action

Wales: The patient is sitting on the table and I sit in front of them. I can look at the patient and I can pick their feet up. The first thing I do is to let my thenar eminences fall along their lateral malleoli. Once I do that I have information as to the position of the fibula. If the fibula is forward I run right into it. If it's back, I can make that distinction. The fibula moves in relation to the ankle mortise. This is a physiologic part of our anatomy. If we are on an uneven surface the heel bone may rock.

The ankle bone has no muscular attachments. If they adjust on the sub-talar surface and the calcaneus rides backwards, the fibula comes forward in the ankle mortise. This allows the ankle joint to become a universal joint in which the hind foot can move around without necessarily losing support. You don't simply break your leg. The fibula and tibia have a joint that functions like a fulcrum. The lateral malleolus goes backward as the proximal end of the tibia comes forward, and this gives the ankle mortise its stability. The tibiofibular interosseous membrane operates this, and it's supposed to spring back when it comes forward. It comes forward as a safety factor, but it doesn't always go backward right away.

Wales' Tibia Technique

PHYSICIAN: Seated facing the patient
PATIENT: Seated with legs dangling off the table

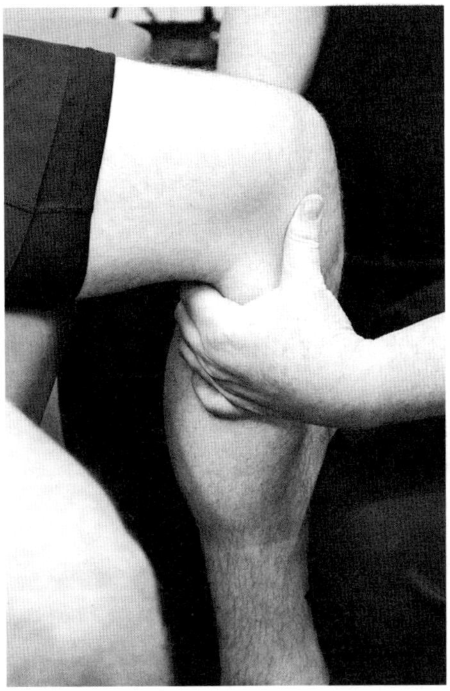

STEPS 1 – 5

1. Wrap your thumb and fingers around the proximal end of their tibia with the patient sitting. Their legs are off the side or end of the table
2. The physician picks up the fibula – thereby gapping it a little
3. The physician leans forward into the fibula which carries it backward, or leans back, which carries the fibula forward to a point of balanced tension
4. Then with the other hand rotate the tibia externally. The tibia comes back to neutral going at a speed that the patient's joint will permit. The physician then takes the tibia into internal rotation and then back to neutral

Wales' Subtalar Joint Technique

EXAMPLE: Right subtalar joint
PHYSICIAN: Seated facing the patient
PATIENT: Seated

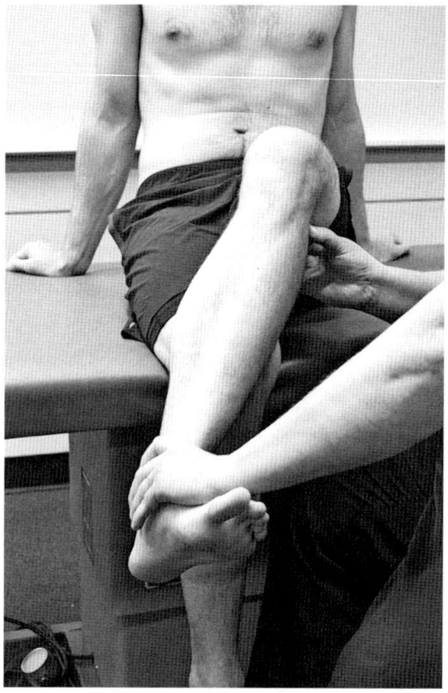

STEP 1

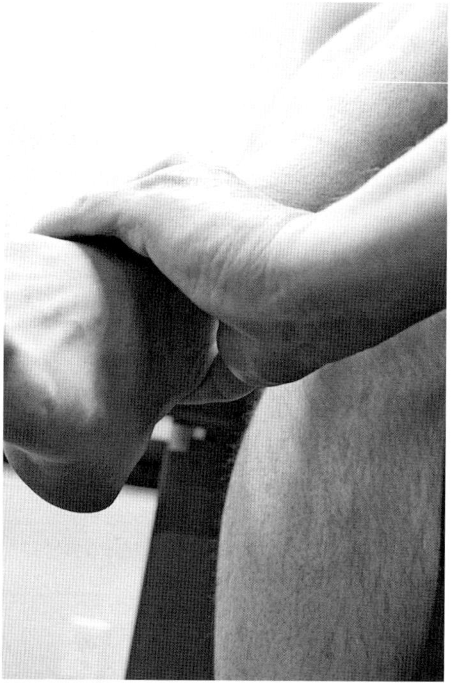

STEP 2 – 4

1. The patient sits with left leg, near the ankle, over their right knee
2. The physician holds both ends of the patient's left fibula anteriorly with your fingers to the point of balanced tension of the patient's ligaments
3. Ask the patient to dorsiflex and externally rotate their left foot
4. Ask the patient to draw their left leg backward and away from you as you hold the fibula anteriorly with your fingers

Wales: Think about the subtalar joint, the bottom of the talus and the top of the calcaneus as a very particular kind of joint. The subtalar joint has very short ligaments, but they extend for quite a long distance considering the whole surface range. Between the joints is fat, and fat at body temperature is liquid. Dr. Sutherland referred to that as the "roly poly" that the body is supported by at the bottom. The heel bone can glide backwards, and the Achilles tendon will accommodate it. The calf muscles will be a little thicker and tighter. However, when the heel bone does that, it puts tension on the plantar fascia and musculature, and you have patients who complain of pain in the front surface of the heel bone. That's no attachment. It's just because their attachment went away and spread out the tension in their foot. So it's important to get the tibiofibular interosseous membrane at a point of ease, and the fibula in a proper relationship to the ankle mortise before you treat the hind foot.

Wales' Tarsal Arch Technique

Crow: This technique usually follows the fibular correction.

PHYSICIAN: Seated
PATIENT: Seated

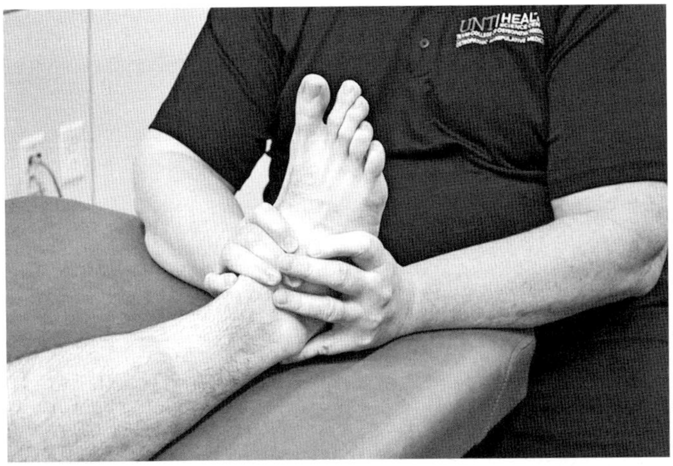

STEP 1

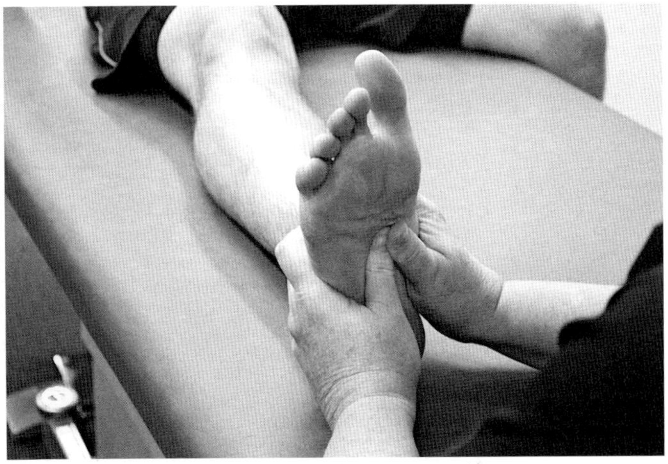

STEP 2

1. Your fingers are interlaced over the top of the patient's foot, and your crossed thumbs on the plantar surface
2. One of your thumbs holds the internal cuneiform and your other thumb on the cuboid to spread the arch apart and exaggerate the transverse flattening to the point of balanced tension

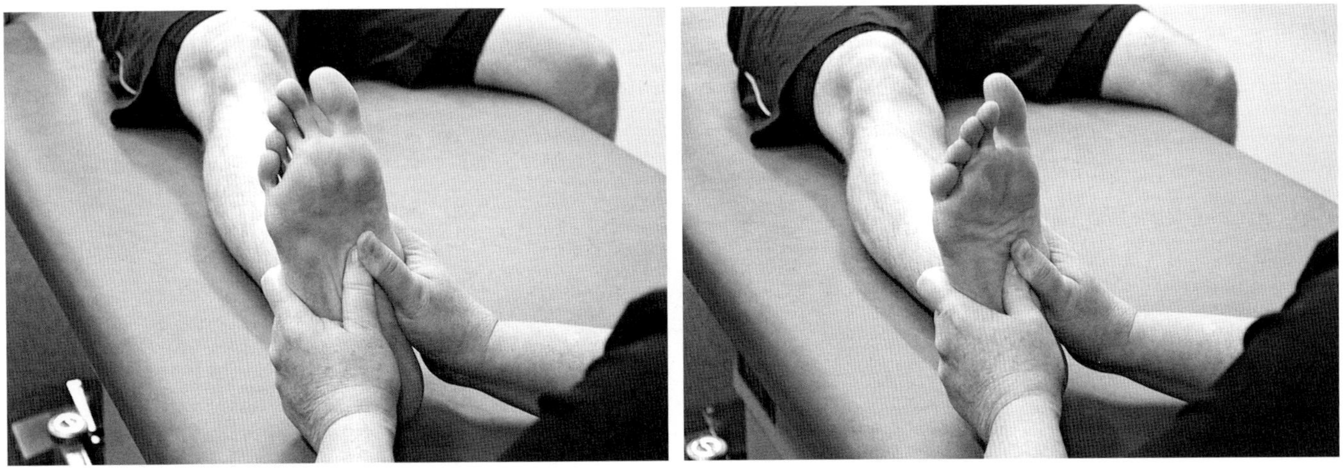

STEP 3

3. The patient, with their foot in plantar inversion, dorsiflexes and then plantar flexes their foot against the resistance of your thumbs

Wales' Talus, Calcaneus, Tarsal Arch Technique

PHYSICIAN: Seated
PATIENT: Seated with their leg and foot on the table

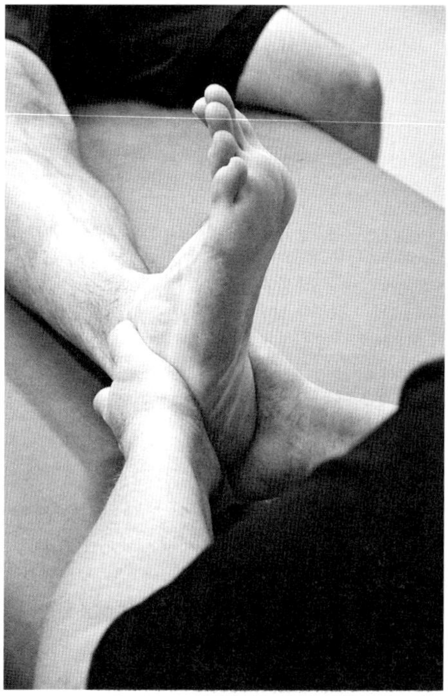

STEP 1

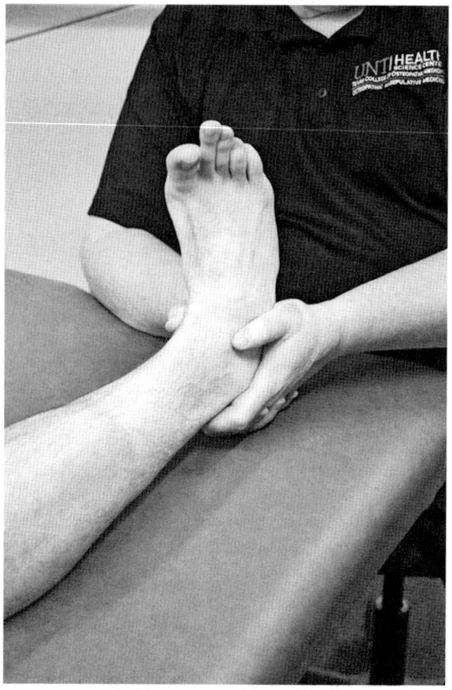

STEPS 2 – 3

1. Interlace your fingers behind the patient's heel
2. With your palms hold the talus and calcaneus firmly in a position so that their ankle is in extension at the ankle joint
3. Ask the patient to dorsiflex, invert and evert their forefoot against the resistance that you provide

Wales' Comment on Feet

Now people complain of feet hurting. They complain of corns and calluses and something called Morton's toe. I believe this is sometimes referred to as Morton's neuroma, and maybe there is a neuroma in some instances. But the weight of the foot goes on to the heel and onto the ball of the foot, and then goes under the big toe. This acts as a big lever which throws you forward and you catch yourself with your other foot. The heel bone and ball joints serve you, and bear your weight. That way you advance by rising and falling again. We walk on surfaces that are not compatible with our skin, so we wear shoes. Shoes have to fit in order for the foot to work properly.

When I started in practice, I treated feet. I treated feet the way my feet were treated. I accomplished some benefits to my patients, but when I got acquainted with Dr. Sutherland's foot technique I was absolutely ecstatic because he understood the foot as a ligamentous articular mechanism. There are particular problems in the mechanism which go to produce painful feet, and I'm not talking about orthopedic problems. I'm talking about functional mechanical dysfunctions of the foot—actually in the mechanism of the whole lower extremity. In any event, the problem with painful feet starts with the leg. Whenever the foot hits the uneven surface of the ground this wobbles your heel bone and the foot tends to fly backwards underneath the ankle bone.

There is a talo-calcaneal ligament on the undersurface of the ankle and on the superior surface of the heel bone. It has parallel lines to the short ligamentous fibers. Between these two rows of ligamentous fibers is fat and at body temperature fat is liquid.

Dr. Sutherland's concept of the function of fat was that this fat provides a guarding relationship. Any time your heel bone is unstable the lateral malleolus goes forward and consequently the heel goes backward. This creates a universal joint out of the ankle mortise. It prevents you from breaking your leg. It's supposed to come back, this tibiofibular interosseous membrane. It's supposed to spring the fibula back to where it was with the lateral malleolus in the back and the proximal head forward held by the biceps femoris. There is some ligamentous relationship with the knee capsule here, too. The fibular collateral ligament of the tibia is quite decidedly free in childhood. It has to be in order for the legs to grow. Sometimes the fibular collateral ligament gets twisted up. Sometimes in a football game some runner comes up against another and slams into the player. It's an external force in this region, which rotates the fibular collateral ligament.

The foot bears weight and absorbs shock, and has a prehensile gripping action from the era when it was a claw. Anything that spreads the ankle mortise is going to make the relationship between the ankle bone and the heel bone in the hind foot unstable.

Now there is a joint with mechanical significance between the hind foot and forefoot. It's called Chopart's joint. It really is two joints which are in the same plane. It's the joint between the calcaneus and the cuboid, and the talus and the navicular. Then you have the role of the cuneiforms. The inner longitudinal arch is the shock absorbing arch. It is the spring in the foot. One-fifth of the weight that hits the heel bone is directed into it to stabilize the shock absorbing mechanism. Now when the fibula goes back proximally the heel bone comes forward distally. The talus wobbles around on top of the heel bone and the heel bone glides backward. The talus is stabilized by the Achilles tendon, which comes from the calf muscles.

When there's friction between the foot and the shoe you get a corn. When there's friction between the toes you get soft corns. When the distal heads of the metatarsals drop too much, the spring, or flexion in the heel, the functional arch, isn't working. You then get plantar warts or talus warts. Then, if you don't have enough toe room your big toe gets pulled medially.

As I was taught, the functional mechanics of the foot do not take on a particular individual characteristic until the foot has grown into the teenage years. Children's feet are just what they look like. They are prehensile. They grasp the ground. They work like baby's feet. Then of course, they get into shoes and they grow. At some time as they approach adulthood, one characteristic becomes more dominant. We have the inner longitudinal arch dominant, or the outer longitudinal arch dominant, or the tarsal arch dominant. A flexible foot type is the result of the inner longitudinal arch being dominant. It has more joints than bones. It is the shock absorbing arch. It is more flexible. It works better if it's in an inflare type of shoe. The outer longitudinal arch is low slung. It is a weight bearing arch. It has more bones than joints. It is a rigid type of foot that works best in an outflared type of shoe last. If this tarsal arch is the dominant feature of a particular foot the prehensile action is more active. That type of foot works better in a shoe that works with the foot much as a glove works with the hand. It allows the prehensile action to work, but it requires quite a bit of toe room and requires a straight last. Shoes and feet don't always go together. So besides the complaints that go with bunions you have the complaints that go with callouses and corns.

Wales' Morton's Neuroma Technique

PHYSICIAN: Standing
PATIENT: Seated with one foot on the table

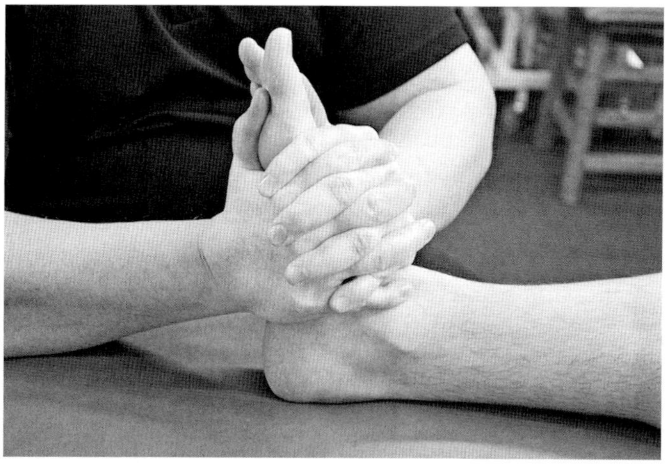

STEPS 1 – 3

1. Interlace your fingers and place the patient's tarsal arch between your palms
2. Squeeze their tarsal arch between your palms and that should pop the keystone (navicular) up
3. Check to see if their cuboid has come down
4. Check the 4th and 5th metatarsals, and also between the metatarsals to see if the pain is gone
5. If the pain is still present, gap the 4th metatarsal by pulling on the related 4th toe
6. Repeat with the 5th metatarsal

Wales: You also have what is called a Morton's toe or Morton's neuroma. The pain is under the 4th metatarsal phalangeal junction. The 4th toe is often sprung up and the callous is under this joint. There is a sesamoid bone under the ball of the great toe. There may be a sesamoid bone in the fascia under the metatarsal arch. There is an arch here, it is just not a true arch. It's how the foot happens to form where the tarsal bone is in space. There may be a plantar wart or simply a plantar callous if the heads of these middle metatarsals drop down enough to create some friction with the shoe. If the cuboid twists on its long axis it takes the proximal end of the 4th and 5th metatarsals with it, and if it drops medially it disturbs the tarsal arch. The arch doesn't support it. This takes the 4th toe down, and the 5th toe is then riding on top of it, and that is painful whether there is a callous under there or not. There are nerves that go between all these bones and so this hurts. So your patient has a pain, especially when they are weight bearing under the 4th metatarsal pharyngeal joint. If you remove the 'pinch' it stops hurting, and I've been able to do that any number of times for a number of people. I don't understand how I can cure a neuroma with one treatment. The thing is, when the cuboid is turned on its long axis, I figure it's really the length of the foot. It's almost as acute as its name implies, but if it's turned so that the cuboid is dropped medially it takes the 4th or 5th metatarsals with it and their toes. Then it breaks the continuity of this outer longitudinal arch so it doesn't work too well. The patient is then inclined to get more weight bearing in the middle of the foot.

Now the shock absorbing arch wasn't made for weight bearing. So it gives way and everybody wants to turn away from painful action so they pronate the foot. That opens up the tarsal arch. The external cuneiform and the middle cuneiform drop, and they don't have anything to take them back where they came from. So some people call that a flat foot. What is needed is a restoration of the mechanics of the tarsal arch.

Wales' Bootjack Technique

EXAMPLE: Left foot
PHYSICIAN: Standing at the end of the table
PATIENT: Seated with their left foot on the table

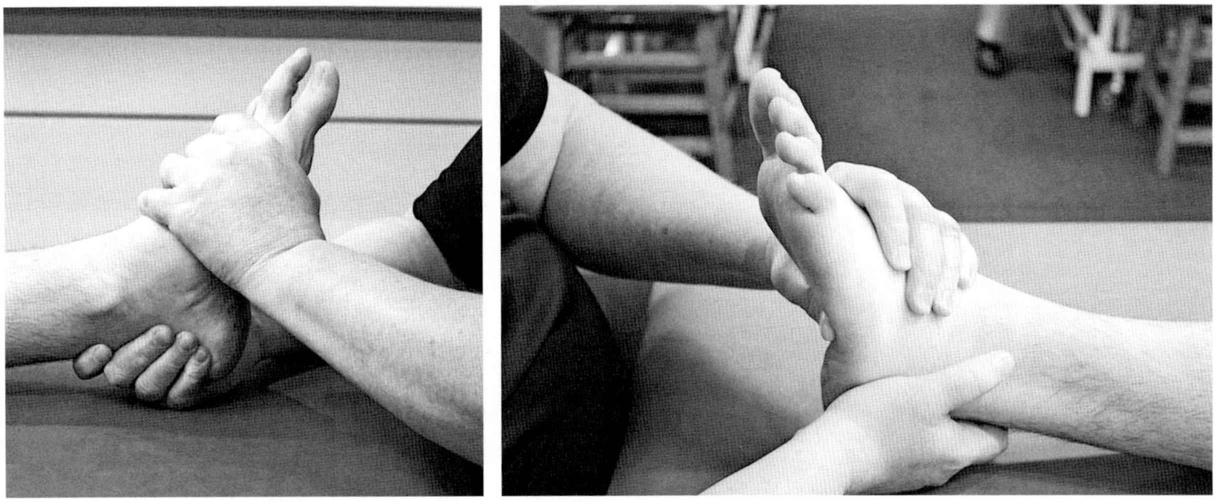

STEPS 1 – 3

1. Place your right hand under the patient's left calcaneus—pulling it towards you

2. Place your left hand over their forefoot
3. Pull their left forefoot towards you
4. Their subtalar joint should come free—recheck motion

Wales' Bunion Technique

EXAMPLE: Left foot
PHYSICIAN: Standing
PATIENT: Seated with their left foot on the table

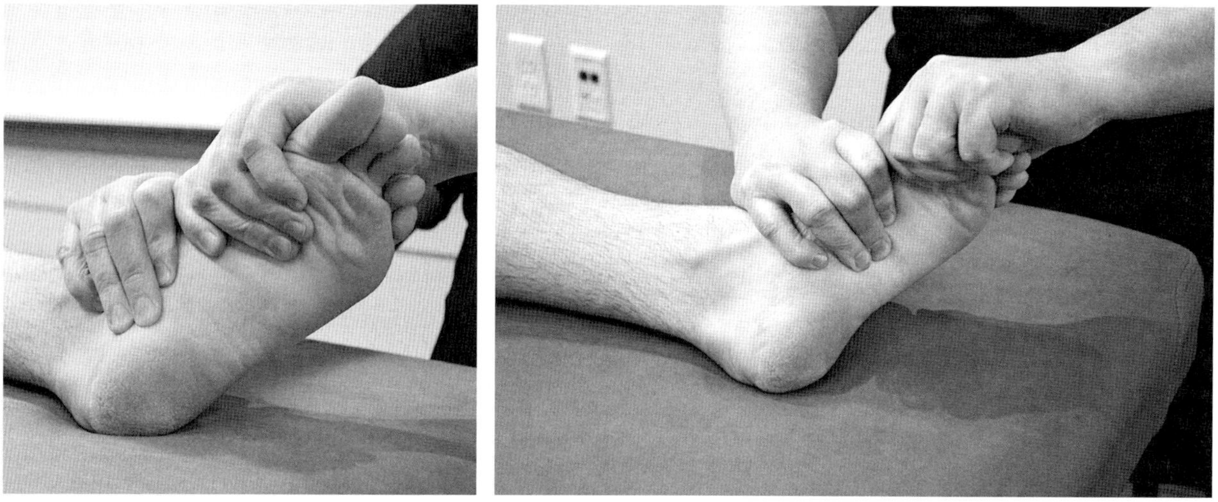

STEPS 1 – 2

1. Place your left hand over the tarsal head of the first metatarsal of the patient's left foot
2. Place your right hand on their navicular
3. With your hands twisting in opposite directions separate the joints

Wales: All you do with a bunion itself, a really flourishing bunion, is practically a dislocation. So you can hang on to the distal end of the 1st metatarsal, take the big toe in the other hand and lift it. You lift it where it is. If it's up here, it's 'out' here. You get a proximal separation between the surfaces of this joint. Then you just hold it there. Its normal fascia will realign things unless these bones are changed in shape.

Crow's Ankle Sprain Technique

PHYSICIAN: Seated at the foot of the table
PATIENT: Seated with their foot on the table

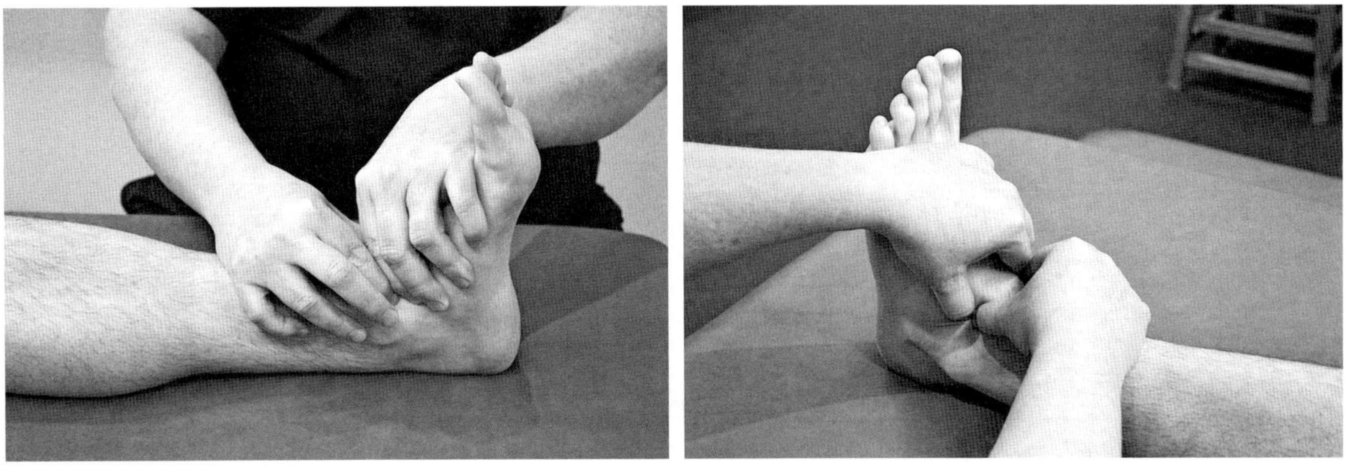

STEPS 1 – 2

1. Place your thumbs on the patient's anterior talofibular ligament and compress the patient's foot
2. Ask the patient to dorsiflex their foot
3. The physician places their thumbs on the talocalcaneal ligament with their fingers on the dorsal surface of the patient's foot
4. The patient dorsiflexes their foot as pressure is applied by the physician to the tibiofibular syndesmosis (anterior ankle ligaments)
5. After their tibiofibular syndesmosis softens, place your thumb and forefingers on the lateral ligaments, and on the deltoid ligament on the medial side
6. With your other hand reach behind the patient's heel and invert their ankle until the ligaments are held in equal tension
7. When the ligaments have softened, return their ankle to a neutral position
8. Remember to free the fibula and interosseous membrane afterwards or the patient may have difficulty with balance

Wales' Fibula and Interosseous Membrane Release Technique

PHYSICIAN: Seated in front of the patient
PATIENT: Seated

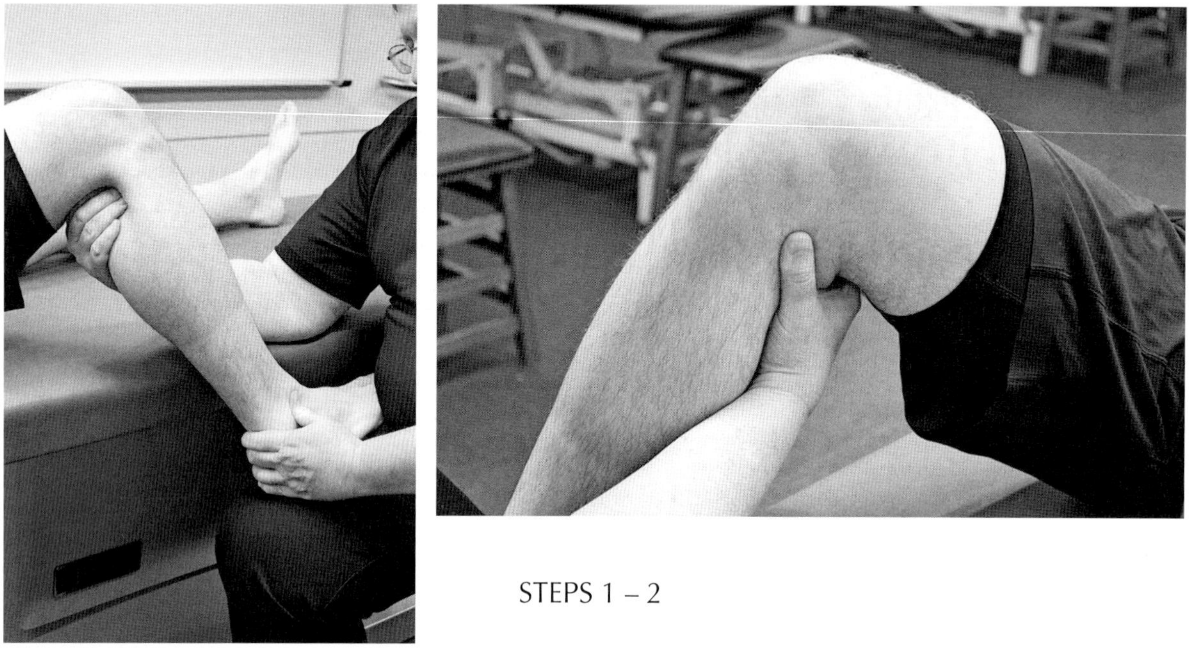

STEPS 1 – 2

1. Place the patient's foot on your knee, place one of your thenar eminences on their lateral malleolus with your fingers on their calcaneus
2. Place your other fingers on the fibular head
3. Push the lateral malleolus with your lower hand and pull the proximal head until you find that the interosseous membrane has been released from tension. This will permit the fibula to move

Wales: Well, the first thing I do with a foot is to consider the leg-ankle-foot as a whole region. Between the tibia and the fibula is an interosseous membrane. The fibula is attached to the tibia above the ankle, so we have the ankle mortise. This is a kind of fulcrum. The long arm of the fibula will move back and the lateral malleolus will move forward if the calcaneus is unstable. That is a provision for walking on the uneven surface of the earth. The calcaneus will glide backward when the fibula comes forward, and the talus will function as a universal joint instead of a hinge joint. So the first thing I do to address the hind foot mechanism is to balance the tibiofibular interosseous membrane with the fibula itself. Now underneath the talus and on the top of the calcaneus the talocalcaneal ligamentous attachment has two layers.

Wales' Outer Longitudinal Arch/Cuboid Release Technique

EXAMPLE: Left foot
PHYSICIAN: Seated facing the patient
PATIENT: Seated

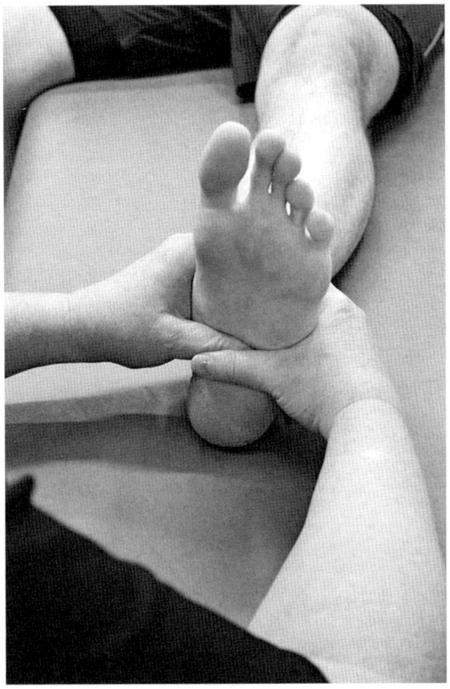

STEPS 1 – 4

1. Hold the dorsal surface of the patient's left foot with your left hand
2. Place your right thumb under the proximal head of their 4th and 5th metatarsals
3. Press their 4th and 5th metatarsals upwards until you feel a ligamentous balance in relation to the hind foot and forefoot
4. Let the weight of their foot (heel) go down a little bit so you get some traction and separation between the metatarsals and the cuboid

Wales: The outer longitudinal arch, which is the weight bearing arch, takes up most of the weight from the heel to the ball of the big toe. The 4th and 5th metatarsals articulate as one joint with the cuboid. I feel this whole outer longitudinal arch in action all the way from the calcaneus through the cuboid to the 4th and 5th metatarsals. It's going from back to front and back again. The inner longitudinal arch is obviously at a higher level. Once its weight is stabilized it assumes its true shock absorbing function. Consequently, as the inner arch is higher than the outer arch we have a true tarsal arch with a keystone. That's the external cuneiform which is wedge shaped. There are no muscles attached to these bones in relation to each other. It's a true architectural arch with a keystone. It's the keystone that's dropped. Even with that, it's still wedge shaped. The cuboid is part of the arch, and the navicular is at the other end.

Wales' Dropped Navicular/Cuneiform (Keystone) Technique

PHYSICIAN: Seated facing the patient
PATIENT: Seated

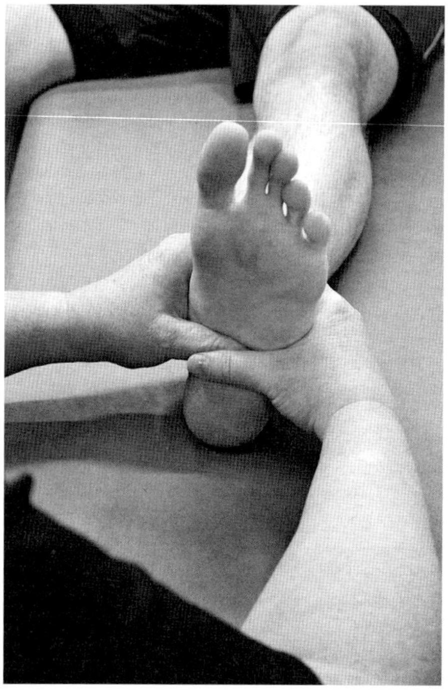

STEPS 1 – 4

1. Place your thumbs on the plantar surface of the patient's foot under the navicular (the keystone)
2. Interlace your hands across the dorsal aspect of their foot
3. Ask the patient to plantar flex their foot so it will spread the tarsal arch and the cuneiform will pop up because it's wedge shaped and the arch will make room for it
4. Then ask the patient to alternate between plantar flexing and dorsiflexing their foot

Sutherland's Foot Technique per Wales

PHYSICIAN: Seated
PATIENT: Seated with their right foot over the edge of the table

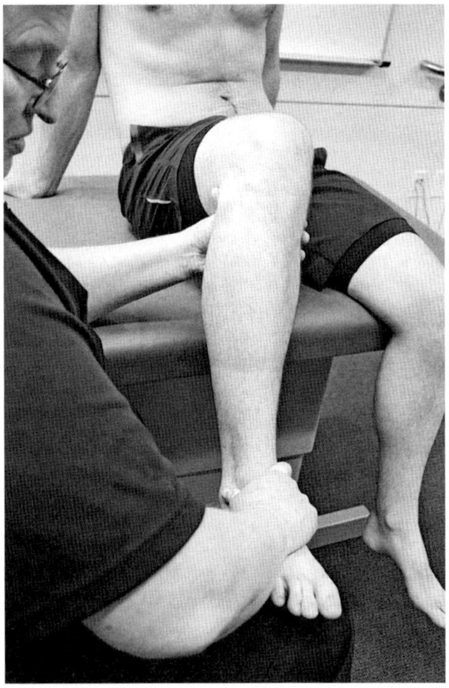

1. Place your right thumb in front of the lateral malleolus of the patient's right foot
2. Take your left hand and get under the proximal head of their fibula
3. Press their lateral malleolus outward and posteriorly
4. Press the fibular head anteriorly and inwards
5. Ask the patient to slightly dorsiflex their foot

Cochrane's Foot Exercise

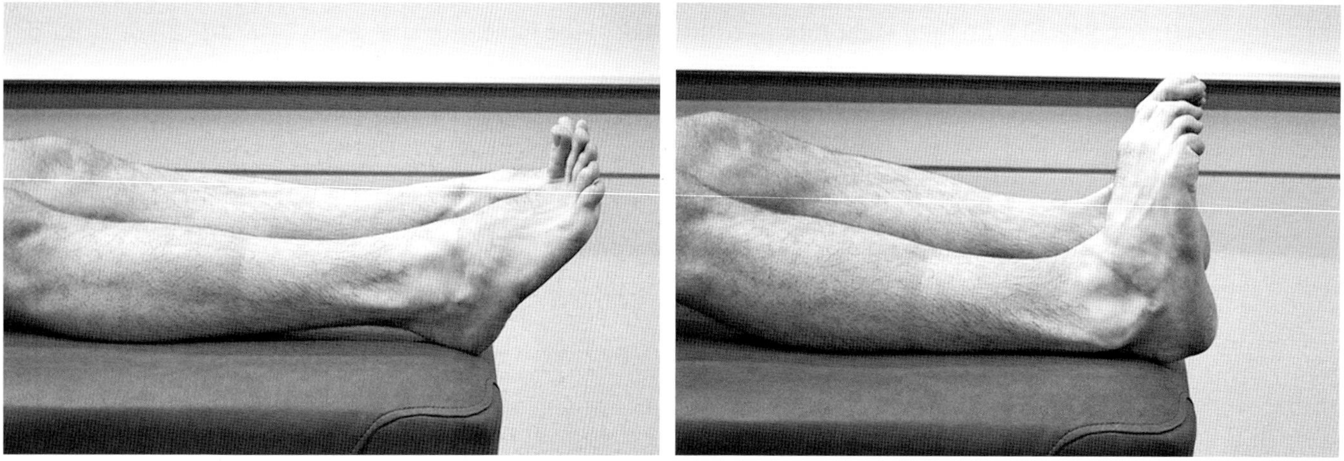

THE EXERCISES

Wales: Now I'm going to have you do an exercise which I learned from Dr. Cochrane, who was an earlier osteopath. She had worked out something which she called 'Physio Synthesis'—motion exercises which patients can do at home. This one was for the feet and went like this. You plantar flex the whole foot and while you're holding the foot down you dorsiflex your toes. Then, holding that position you dorsiflex the whole foot. Then you plantar flex your toes. That's the payoff. When you do the last plantar flexion it brings all the plantar muscles into action and it is sometimes a jolt to the whole foot mechanism.

Wales on Short Leg Syndrome

We have the short leg syndrome that we talk about. Standing x-rays are made by some radiologists to confirm whether or not one leg is anatomically shorter than the other. If it is anatomically shorter than the other then a lift for the shorter leg is indicated. But if it appears to be a shorter leg but it isn't anatomically shorter, then the result is because of the postural mechanics and the hip mechanics. Heel lift therapy is therefore contraindicated.

I like to pick the feet up when the patient is supine with my thenar eminences on the lateral malleoli, and wait for the hip capsules to relax. Then I lean backwards, which puts straight traction on their legs and through the femurs on to their psoas magnus muscles. These muscles originate in the lower thoracic vertebrae. When the soleus is tight and contracted, not working symmetrically with the other, it makes a difference to the legs and how they operate. The iliopsoas muscle below connects with the ilius inside the ilium. They make a joint tent which goes over the pubic arch to the lesser trochanter on the femur. Consequently, our legs hang more laterally back. What you want to know, especially with any problems below the waist, is whether the soleus muscle is a problem.

When anybody is sitting you want to know whether the obturator internus is a problem. What I observe is whether this traction that I apply is symmetrical. I don't know any way to discover certain non-symmetrical situations except to test as you go. I place a pillow under the thighs for the purpose of relaxing the lumbar region.

Wales on Psoas/Soleus Contraction

If the psoas is contracted on one side, what do you find with the legs? If it's a chronic contraction of the psoas, there is a tendency for the whole pelvis to rotate around the other leg. If the soleus muscle is contracted, even if it's an old story (injury) and it isn't giving any pain signals now, the distance between the origin and the insertion is shorter on one side than it is on the other. Consequently, the shorter soleus can be the cause of lumbar spine, lumbar sacral and sacroiliac problems. They have simply responded with postural mechanics to the fact that the soleus is shorter. That's all there is to it. The thing to do when this is the problem is to deal with the soleus. But the patient complains that where they feel the pain is in the psoas.

9

Techniques for the Upper Extremities

Wales: As far as the upper extremity is concerned, the only bone to bone connection is the sterno-clavicular articulation, and that is only with the clavicle and manubrium. There is also a joint between the manubrium and the body of the sternum. The shoulder girdle is comparable to a Dutch yoke that is sitting on top of the rib cage. A Dutch yoke is a piece of wood that goes over the shoulders, with a hole carved out for the neck. On the ends of the piece of wood are cables with which someone carries heavy buckets. The clavicle is a strut which holds the shoulder joint lateral so the arms can swing. Therefore the problem with the upper extremity starts right here. The clavicle is one bone with which we move both ends at once. It is stabilized by the acromio-clavicular ligament which is attached to it at the back. The shoulder joint has a wide range of motion. It is like a large ligamentous capsule, and it permits both external rotation and internal rotation of the arms. The humerus then articulates with the forearm, with the ulna and its process fitting in close to where the motion gets started.

Problems related to the upper extremity are stiff neck, torticollis, painful shoulder, tennis elbow, brachial neuralgia, brachial neuritis, and paresthesias of one sort or the other. Also, carpal tunnel syndrome, Dupuytren's contracture of the tendons in the palm, arthritis, and Colley's fracture. It's amazing how many people, if they think they're going to fall, think that they're going to help themselves by putting their arm out. In the orthopedic realm you can have a dislocated shoulder.

This dislocation is with the head of the humerus through the capsule of the shoulder joint. The inferior dislocation is the most common dislocation of the shoulder and the easiest to get back, but that doesn't prevent it happening again. Then we often have edema and problems with the fingers.

TUCKER ON THE CLAVICLE

The motion of the sterno-clavicular joint is wide in many directions, but narrow as to range. It bends forward or is drawn back or up as the shoulder blade is driven forward. It rotates as the shoulder rotates. It may slide in and out on the manubrium.

The size of the end of the bone indicates the amount of pressure it sustains, and the size of the ligaments indicates the amount of tensile strain they bear.

Warp lesions of the clavicle are very frequent. Real lesions doubtless occur, but it is not easy to distinguish between the two.

DIAGNOSIS

Tucker: Diagnosis of lesions of the clavicle is made by comparing the two sides, and is by no means positive. The two sides may differ much in size. It may be assumed, however, that the less prominent side is in lesion if either side is. There are few forces drawing the clavicle forward.

Tucker's Clavicle Technique

EXAMPLE: Right shoulder
PHYSICIAN: Standing with your right thigh resting on the table next to the patient's right shoulder
PATIENT: Supine with their right shoulder next to the physician

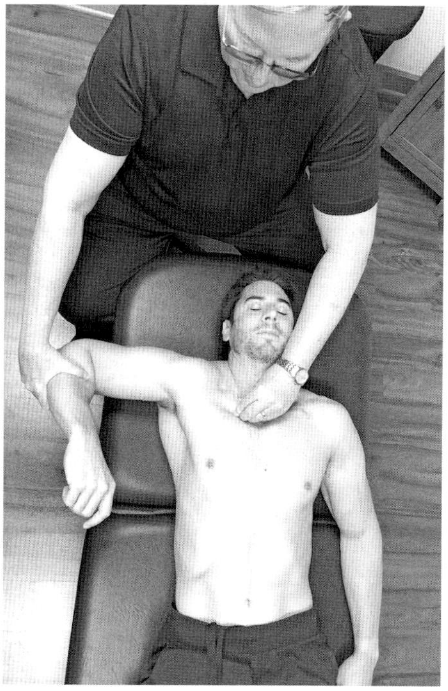

1. Lift the patient's right shoulder on the right side onto your right thigh so that their right shoulder blade rests on your right thigh
2. Press down on their right shoulder and right arm to stretch the ligaments of their right clavicle
3. Place the fingers of your left hand under their right clavicle and lift towards the ceiling
4. Draw their right elbow backwards with your right hand and up to the limit of rotation posteriorly towards their head
5. Then bring their right elbow superiorly and towards their head. Then swing the elbow down towards the physician's feet, using your right thigh as the fulcrum

Tucker: The tissues under the clavicle are very sensitive and easily bruised. It is necessary to find the point at which pressure will cause the least pain. This point is usually at the juncture of the inner third with the middle third of the clavicle. The fingers must be neither pressed too far in—barely enough to produce upward pressure, nor lifted up with too much power. The leverage over your thigh, the drawing of the joint out, up, and rotating it backward, does most of the work of restoration. Lesions of the cartilages of the ribs are sometimes found. These cases are probably surgical.

Sutherland's Clavicle Technique

EXAMPLE: Right clavicle
PHYSICIAN: Stands in front of the patient
PATIENT: Seated with their left arm resting on the physician's right shoulder

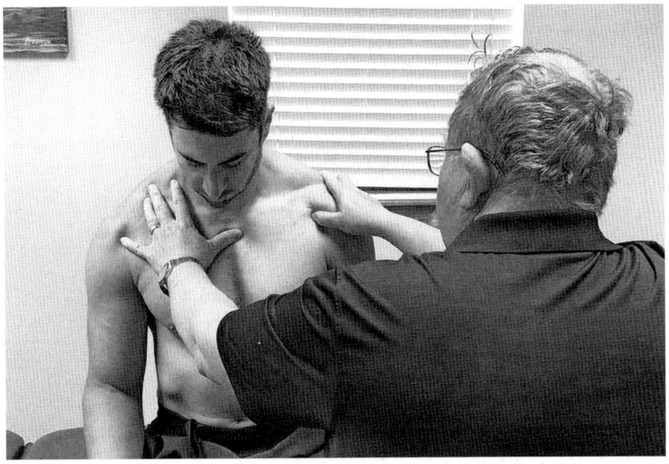

STEPS 1 – 4

1. Place your left thumb at the patient's right sternoclavicular junction and your left middle finger at their right acromioclavicular junction
2. The patient leans forward onto the physician's thumbs
3. The patient rotates their left shoulder backwards
4. The patient takes a deep breath and holds their breath

Wales' Depressed Clavicle Technique

EXAMPLE: Right clavicle
PHYSICIAN: Standing in front of the patient
PATIENT: Seated

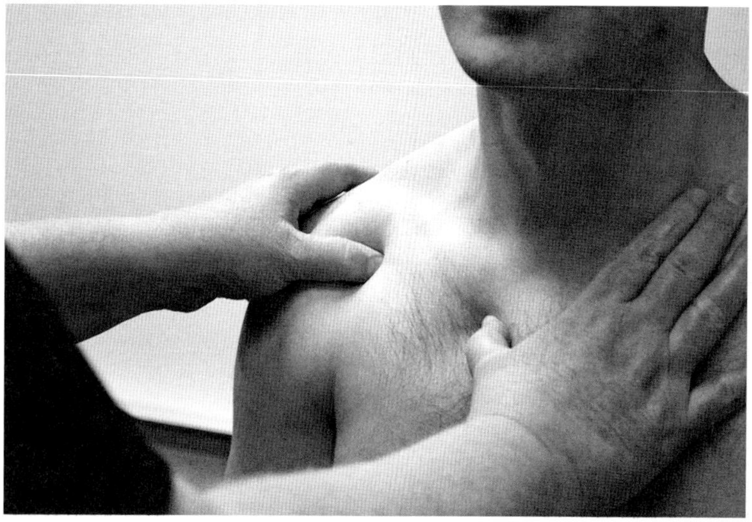

STEPS 1 – 3

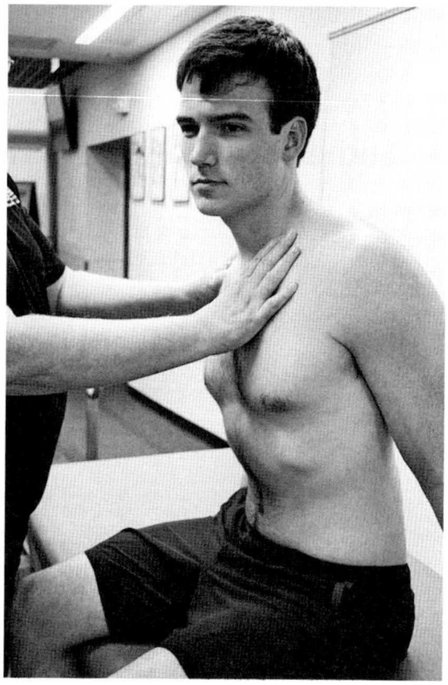

STEPS 4 – 6

Crow: The acromioclavicular ligament is going to be the fulcrum around which both ends of the clavicle will move.

1. Place your right thumb under the patient's right clavicle junction near the sternal end
2. Place your left thumb under their clavicle at the acromioclavicular end
3. Ask the patient to bend straight forward from the hips with all their weight onto your thumbs
4. When that has stabilized the field operation, ask the patient to carry their left shoulder backwards. That takes their left clavicle and the manubrium away from their right clavicle
5. Ask the patient to take a deep breath in and hold it. The right clavicle will slide back into place
6. Ask the patient to now sit up straight

Wales: When the patient bends forward from the hips, you must have a wide base with your own feet. Let your knees bend so you can support your patient's weight. This stabilizes the field of force application. This way the clavicle is actually stable before you ask the patient to carry their other shoulder backwards. The patient carries the other shoulder backward, and the patient's breathing does the treating. The clavicle is acting like a seesaw around the acromioclavicular ligament.

Wales' Clavicle Technique #2

EXAMPLE: Right clavicle
PHYSICIAN: Standing in front of the patient
PATIENT: Seated

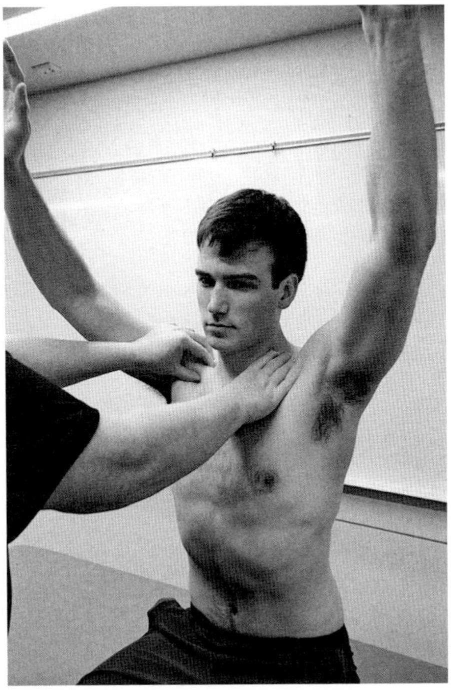

STEPS 1 – 4

Place your left thumb on the patient's right sterno-clavicular junction

1. Place your left thumb at their right acromio clavicular junction
2. Ask the patient to lean forward and place their weight on your thumbs
3. Ask the patient to move their left shoulder backward to move their manubrium away
4. Then ask the patient to raise both their elbows backwards or downwards to about 90 degrees

Tucker's Shoulder Joint Technique

Tucker: Lesions of the acromial end of the clavicle are occasionally found. One end of the joint may be used as a lever to adjust the other, and then the technique reversed if necessary. This articulation is parallel to the sagittal axis of the body, and at right angles to the articulation at the sternal end. This is in order to permit those motions of the shoulder blade, not permitted at the sternal end.

EXAMPLE: left Shoulder
PHYSICIAN: Standing behind the patient
PATIENT: Seated

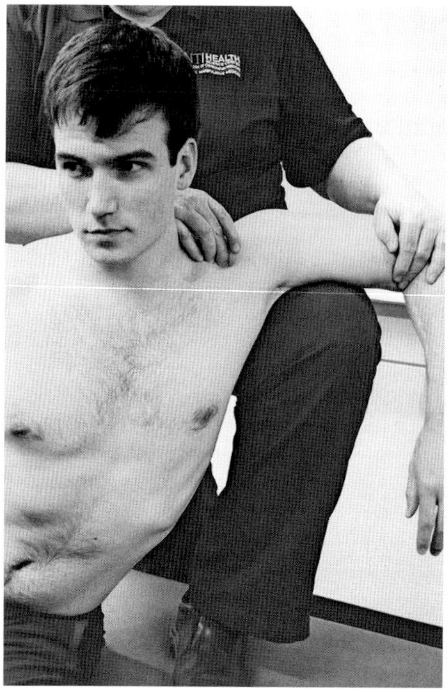

STEPS 1 – 5

1. Place your left foot on the table and left knee under the patient's left axilla
2. Move your left knee with their left axilla away from the body of the patient until part of their weight is resting on your left knee. There is tension away from the median line. Your left knee under their axilla presses equally against their left humerus, tending to gap any lesions. Your knee is also against their left scapula, tending to close the scapula and thus pry open their shoulder joint
3. Lift their left shoulder and their shoulder blade will gap their acromio-clavicular joint. If the posterior end is in dysfunction, turn your left knee to point towards their median line, carrying with it their left scapula. This makes a fulcrum of the anterior end of the clavicle and gaps open the posterior end of the clavicle
4. Press down on their left acromial process as needed, or move their right arm and scapula as needed to reduce the dysfunction
5. If the anterior end of the clavicle is in dysfunction, turn your left knee to point outward from the median line. This gaps the anterior end of the clavicle. Press down on their left acromial process or left clavicle as needed while adding rotation of their left arm and left scapula to reduce the dysfunction

SUTHERLAND'S HUMERUS DIAGNOSIS

Lippincott: Freedom of rotation of the humerus in the glenoid cavity is tested with the arm at an angle of 45 to 90 degrees laterally from the body with the elbow flexed.

Sutherland's Technique for the Internal Rotation of the Humerus

EXAMPLE: Right shoulder
PHYSICIAN: Stands on the right side of the patient
PATIENT: Seated

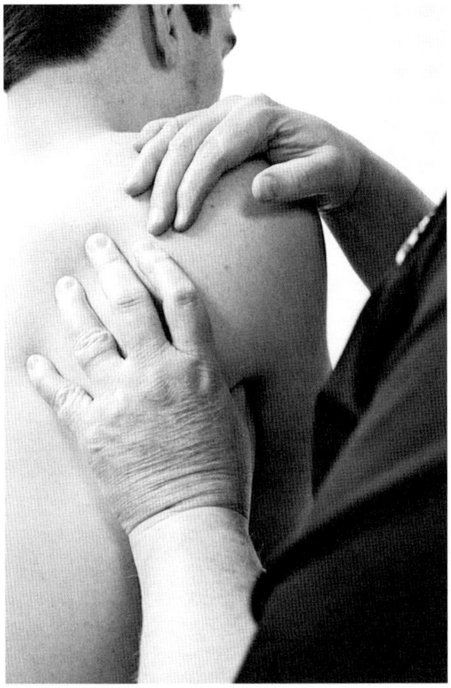

STEPS 1 – 2

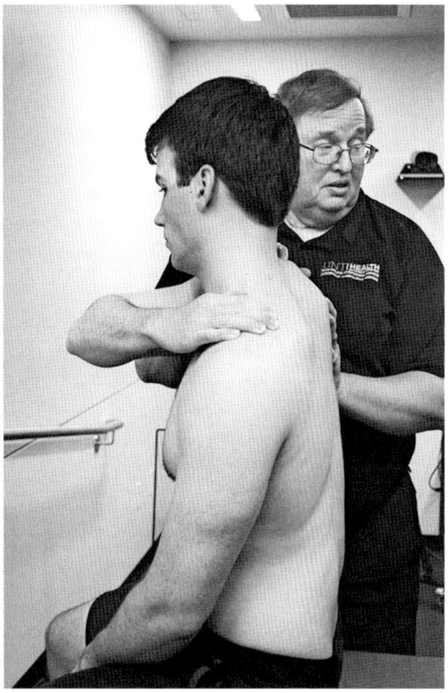

STEP 3

1. Place your right hand on top of the patient's right shoulder joint
2. Your left hand is under their right axilla against their ribs, with your left thumb in as close to the head of their right humerus as possible
3. The patient places their right hand on their left shoulder and holds their left shoulder
4. Ask the patient to elevate their right elbow. This draws the lower end of their right humerus across their chest in order to disengage the head of the humerus
5. The patient then moves their left shoulder posteriorly while still holding their left shoulder with their right hand
6. The patient inhales and holds their breath

Sutherland's Technique for the External Rotation of the Humerus

EXAMPLE: Right shoulder
PHYSICIAN: Stands on the right side of the patient
PATIENT: Seated

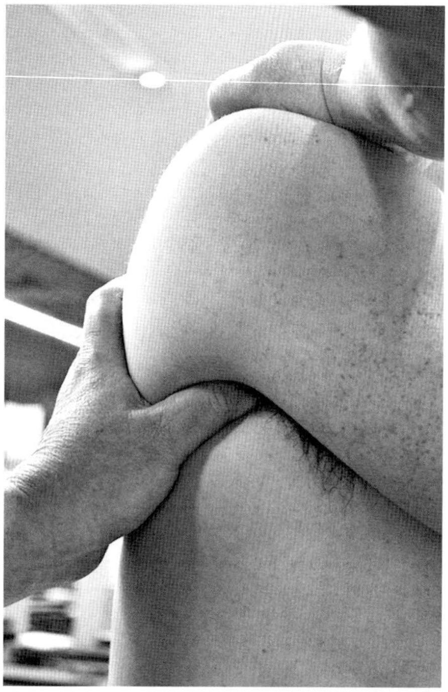

STEPS 1 – 2

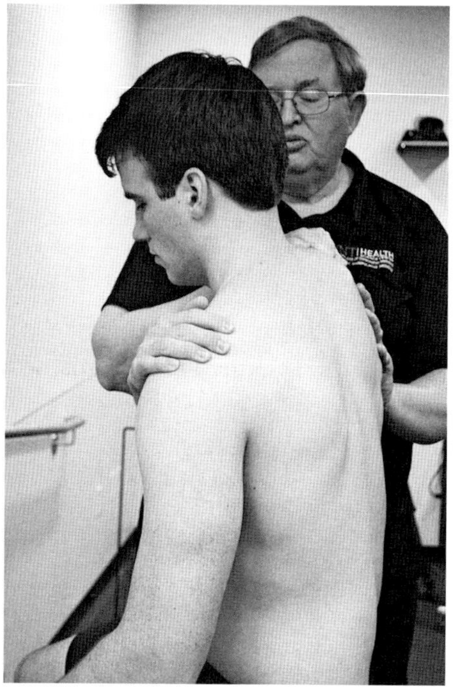

STEPS 3 – 6

1. Place your right hand on top of the patient's right shoulder joint
2. Your left hand is under their axilla, against their ribs with your left thumb in as close to the head of their humerus as possible
3. The patient places their right hand on their left shoulder and holds their left shoulder
4. Ask the patient to lower their right elbow
5. The patient then moves their left shoulder posteriorly while still holding their left shoulder with their right hand
6. Patient exhales and holds their breath out

Tucker's Technique for the Bicipital Tendon

The long bicipital tendon is often found to have slipped out of its groove, stretching or rupturing its retaining ligaments, and is now lying close to the coracoid tendon of the biceps.

DIAGNOSIS

Tucker: Inability to raise the arm in front or behind the back, or laterally beyond a certain point. Soreness over the bicipital groove and a relaxed state of the outer half of the biceps muscle.

DIFFERENTIAL DIAGNOSIS

Tucker: This condition must be distinguished from inflammation of various portions of the shoulder and from rheumatoid arthritis, which commonly shows itself first in this area. Rheumatoid arthritis often simulates this lesion very closely. Other symptoms of rheumatism, or of diseases allied to rheumatism, aid in the diagnosis.

TECHNIQUE

Tucker: The problem is to bring the groove as close to the present position of the tendon as possible, to reposition the tendon into the groove. Hold the tendon thereby fixing the shoulder in an inverted position until the tissues have resumed their normal tone.

EXAMPLE: Right shoulder
PHYSICIAN: Stands on the right side of the patient
PATIENT: Seated

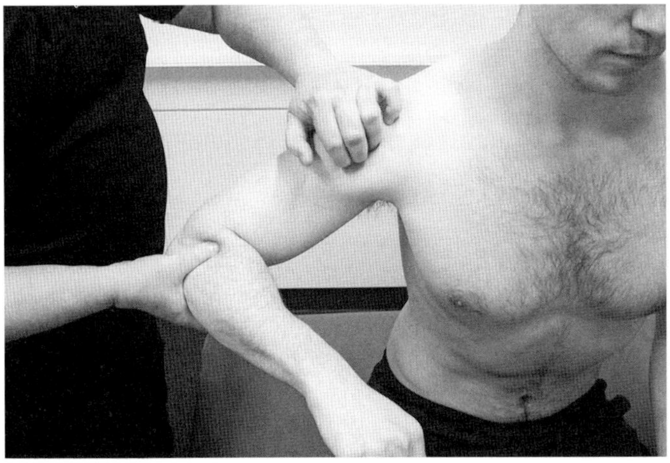

STEPS 1 – 3

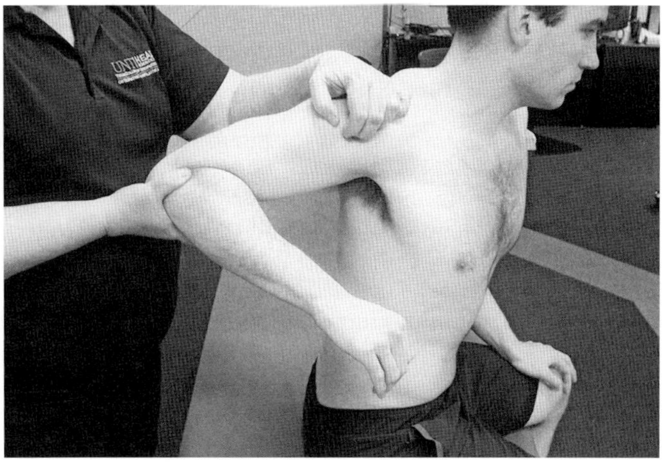

STEP 4

1. With your right hand grasp the patient's right arm at the right elbow, with their right forearm flexed to relieve tension on the right biceps
2. Lift the patient's right arm to about forty-five degrees, rotating their right forearm down as far as possible

3. With the fingers of your left hand locate their biceps tendon and lift the tendon into the groove
4. Rotate the patient's right arm backwards with a lift of their right forearm
5. An adhesive bandage or ace wrap may be applied to hold the shoulder back and the arm everted as much as possible. Keep it there for a week or ten days

Wales' Shoulder Diagnosis and Technique #1

EXAMPLE: Left shoulder
PHYSICIAN: Standing in front of the patient
PATIENT: Seated

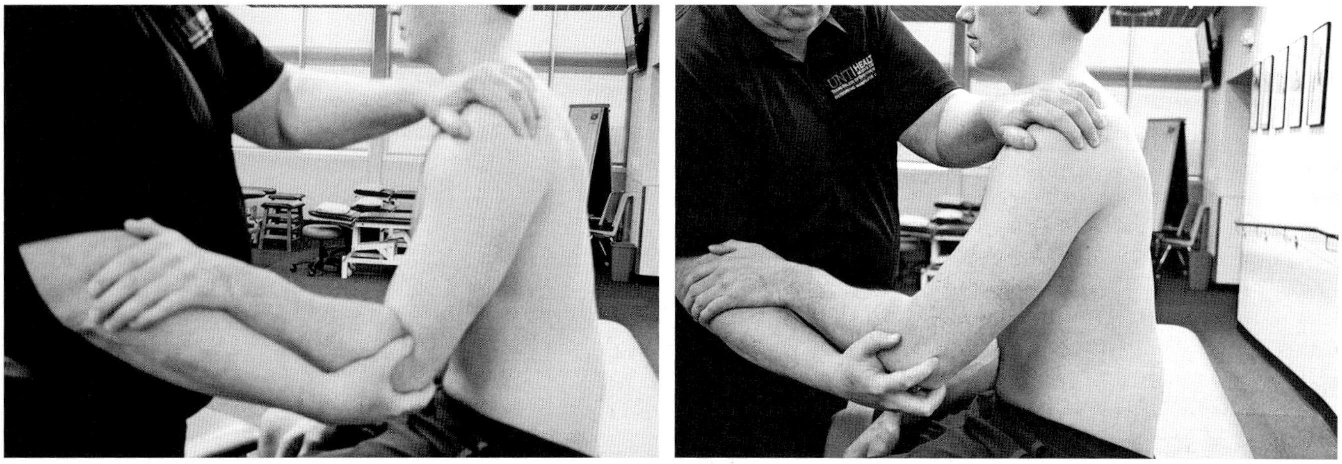

STEPS 1 – 4

1. Place an observing hand (your left hand) on top of the patient's left shoulder
2. With your right hand, take the patient's left arm by the elbow and turn their left humerus into internal and external rotation, and then back to neutral
3. Place your left thumb as near to the head of their left humerus as possible. The humerus is going to function as a fulcrum
4. Keep your left hand on the patient's left shoulder
5. Ask the patient to inhale and let their left elbow come upwards. When they exhale, let their left hand and left elbow drop as far down as it can. When the arm drops it goes into internal rotation. Your hands make a fulcrum to pry the head of the humerus out of the shoulder socket
6. Re-check and see if the internal and external rotation is equal

Wales' Shoulder Technique #2

EXAMPLE: Right shoulder
PHYSICIAN: Seated beside the patient
PATIENT: Seated

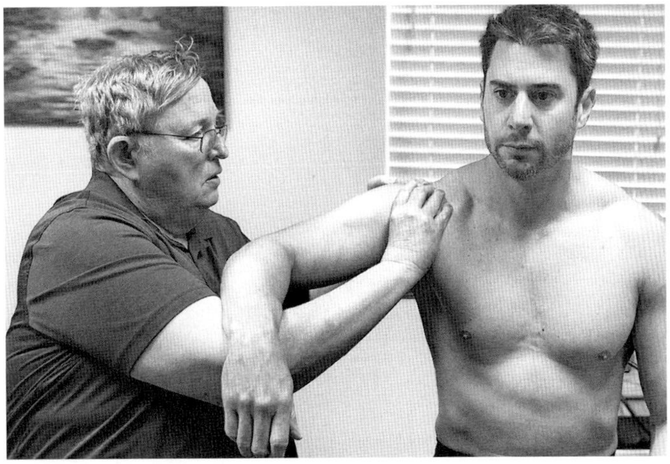

1. Place both your hands on the patient's right shoulder and interlace your fingers
2. Place both your thumbs in their right axilla. This gives you a fulcrum
3. Ask the patient to move their right shoulder backwards
4. Ask the patient to raise their right elbow towards the ceiling
5. Ask the patient to inhale and hold their breath

Wales' Scapula Technique

EXAMPLE: Right scapula
PHYSICIAN: Standing behind the patient
PATIENT: Seated

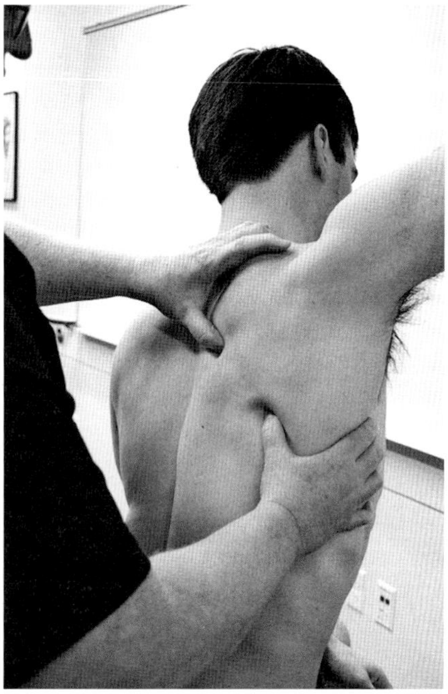

STEPS 1 – 3

STEPS 4 – 5

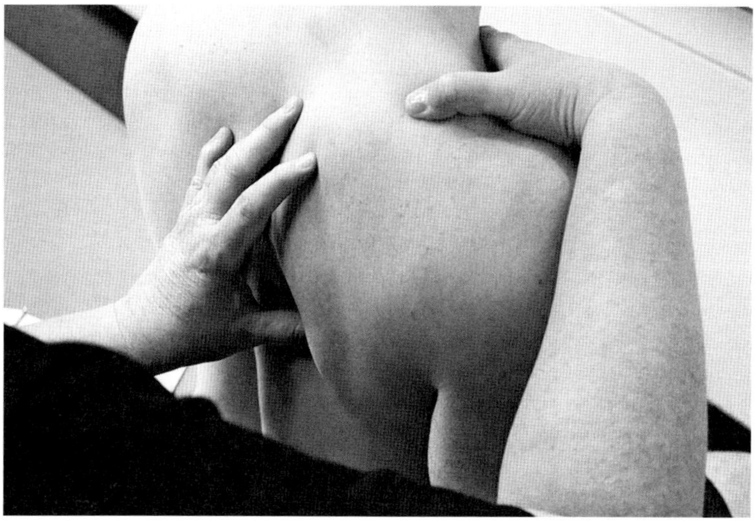

1. Ask the patient to raise their right shoulder
2. Place your left thumb underneath their right scapula posterior to the mid-axillary line
3. Ask the patient to drop their right shoulder over your left thumb. You will meet some resistance in the subscapular musculature
4. Point your left thumb to the middle of the ventral surface of their right scapula so your thumb can function as a fulcrum
5. Take the heel of your right hand and place it on the apex of their right scapula

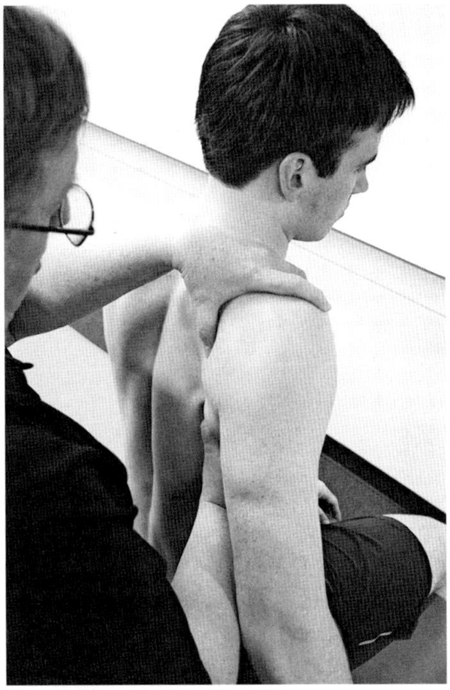

STEPS 6 – 7

6. Turn their right scapula over your left thumb so that the supraspinatus muscle moves back, this reseats the right shoulder girdle
7. The patient is breathing inwards, and you push the apex of their right scapula upward as the upper border moves backwards

Wales: This was a favorite of Dr. Sutherland's, putting a glove on his finger and not shoving. The mid-axillary line is sensitive. This technique is decidedly helpful in patients with stiff necks and aspects of torticollis.

FOREARM, WRIST AND HAND – OSTEOPATHIC CONCEPTS

Lippincott: The bones of the forearm move in relation to each other on a double swivel. The proximal head of the radius rotates in the annular ligament, and the distal head around the end of the ulna. Little motion is possible between the humerus and ulna except flexion and extension. The capsular ligament of the elbow is composed of interlaced and confluent fibers that operate as a unit. Unbalanced tension may be caused by a strain of the elbow joint or result from rotation dysfunctions of the humerus. Strains which disturb the position of the olecranon process prevent complete extension of the arm. Those which affect the coronoid process prevent complete flexion. The semilunar notch between these two processes, which receives the trochlea of the humerus, opens anteriorly at about a right angle to the shaft of the ulna. However, this is frequently at an angle of more nearly 135 degrees.

Sutherland's Ulna Technique

EXAMPLE: Right ulna
PHYSICIAN: Seated in front of the patient
PATIENT: Seated

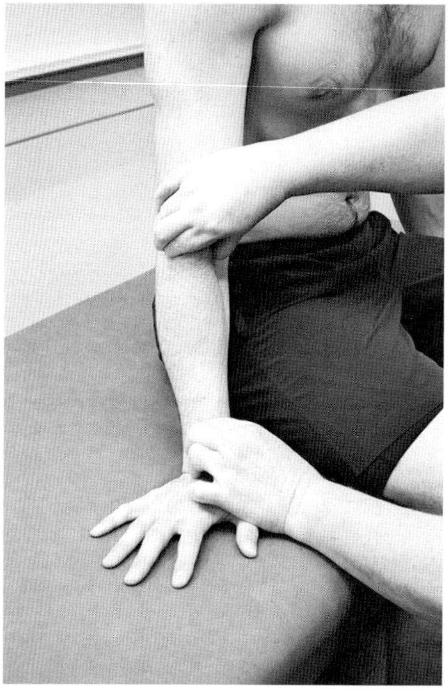

STEPS 1 – 6

1. Ask the patient to place their right hand palm down on the table. Their left fingers are spread open
2. Grasp the styloid process of their right ulna between your left thumb and fingers
3. With your right hand grasp their left olecranon process
4. Ask the patient to invert and evert their right humerus until you have tension in the ligaments
5. Ask the patient to raise their right shoulder to draw their right humerus out of the semi-lunar notch of their right ulna
6. Ask the patient to take in a deep breath and hold their breath

Sutherland's Radius Technique

EXAMPLE: Right radius
PHYSICIAN: Seated in front of the patient
PATIENT: Seated with their palm down on the table. Their fingers are spread open

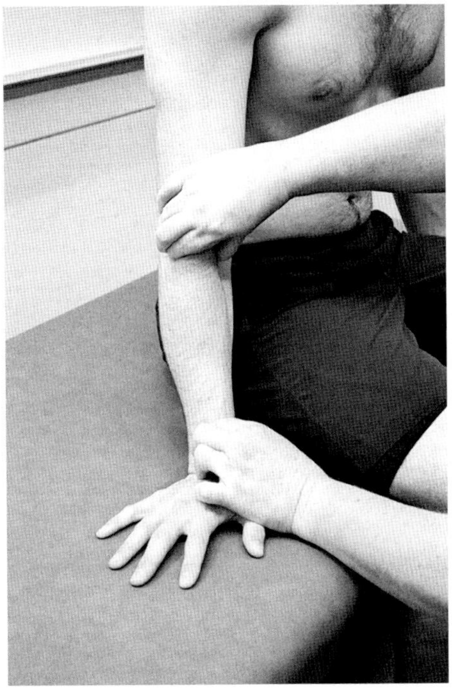

STEPS 1 – 4

1. Grasp the distal end of the patient's right radius between your left thumb and fingers
2. With your right hand grasp the patient's right radial head
3. Ask the patient to circumduct their right elbow ("try to make a circle with your elbow") until you have tension in the ligaments
4. Ask the patient to take in a deep breath and hold their breath

Wales' Radius Technique

EXAMPLE: Right radius
PHYSICIAN: Seated facing the patient
PATIENT: Seated

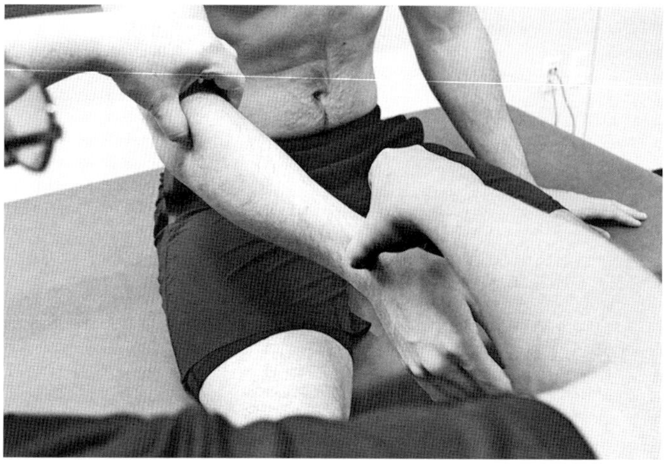

STEPS 1 – 3

1. Hold the distal end of the patient's right radius with right hand and with your left hand hold the proximal end of their right radius
2. Pull up on their right radius at the proximal end so that the weight of the patient's arm puts traction into the interosseous membrane
3. Their right arm should be free from the table so that gravity is helping with the traction of the interosseous membrane

Wales' Elbow Technique

EXAMPLE: Right elbow
PHYSICIAN: Standing in front of the patient
PATIENT: Seated

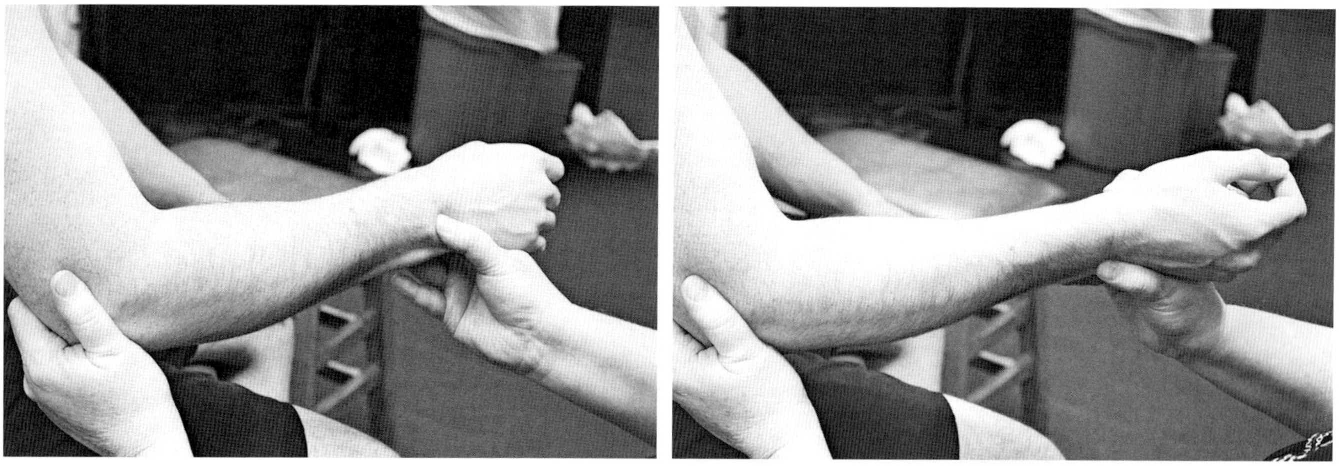

STEPS 1 – 2

1. With your left hand you have contact with the olecranon process of the patient's ulna
2. With their right forearm at a right angle to their right arm, you grip their right ulna with your right hand and turn their right forearm into pronation and supination

Sutherland's Interosseous Membrane Technique

EXAMPLE: Right radius
PHYSICIAN: Seated in front of the patient
PATIENT: Seated

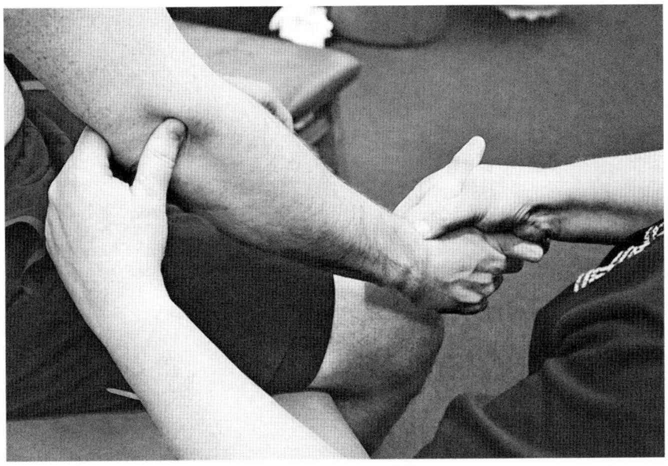

STEPS 1 – 3

1. Hold the distal end of the patient's right radius with your right hand
2. Hold the olecranon process of their right ulna with your left hand
3. Find a point of balance between their radius and ulna by pushing and pulling on them. You want a balanced membranous tension in the radial ulna interosseous membrane

WRIST AND HAND – OSTEOPATHIC CONCEPTS

Lippincott: In dealing with dysfunctions of the wrist and hand it is well to remember the inter-communicating articular cavity of the joints. Additionally, consider the dorsal convexity of the arch formed by the wedge shaped proximal heads of the metacarpal bones, narrowed on their volar aspect.

Sutherland's Hand and Wrist Technique

EXAMPLE: Right hand and wrist
PHYSICIAN: Seated in front of the patient
PATIENT: Seated with their palm down

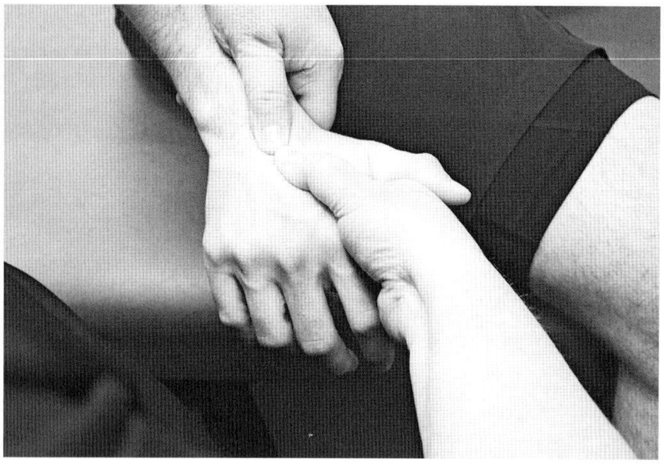

STEPS 1 – 4

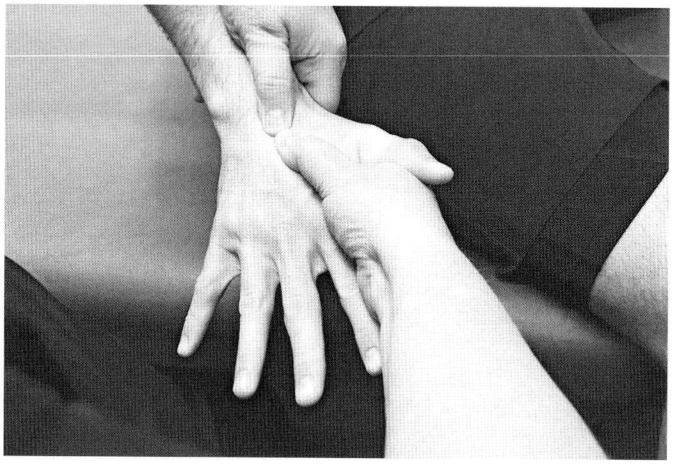

STEPS 5 – 6

1. Take the patient's right hand. Between your right thumb and fingers hold the heads of their right metacarpals at their proximal ends
2. When their right metacarpals are lifted dorsally and separated, they are also rolled on their long axes
3. Your left hand (thumb) stabilizes the carpal bones on the back of the patient's right wrist
4. Your left hand that is holding their carpal bones rotates each carpal bone back and forth until a restriction is found. The ligamentous tension is brought into balance and held
5. The patient then spreads their fingers more widely to disengage the dysfunctional articulations
6. Dysfunctions of the carpal bones as well as the metacarpal bones may be reduced by this technique

Wales' Wrist Technique

EXAMPLE: Right wrist
PHYSICIAN: Seated facing the patient
PATIENT: Seated

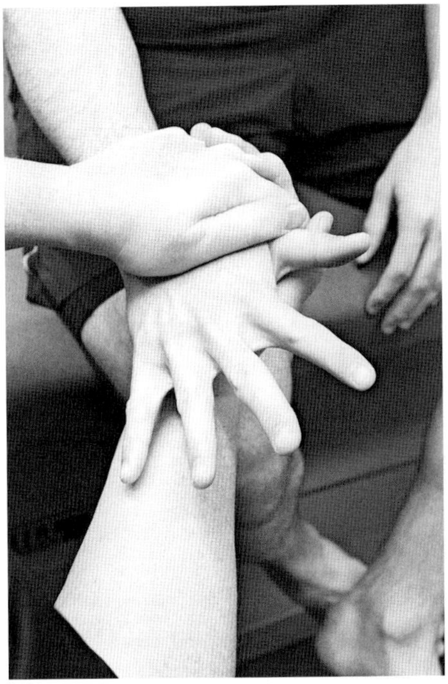

STEP 1

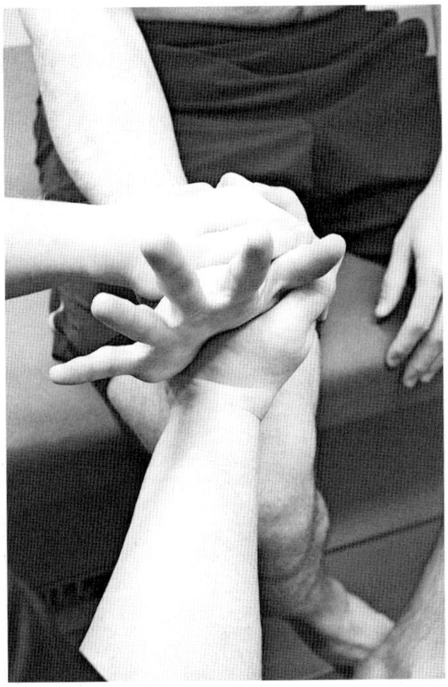

STEP 2

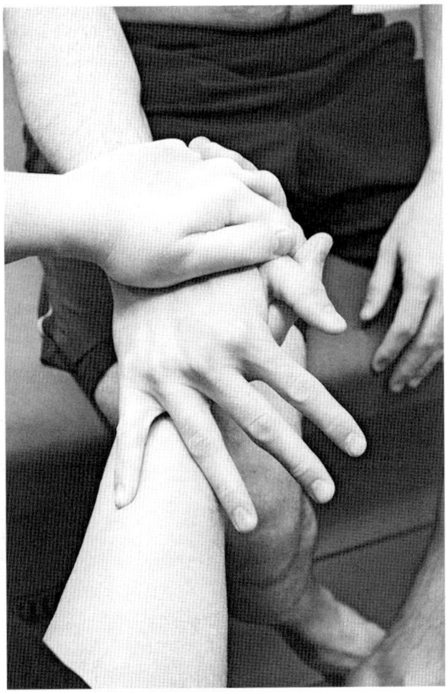

STEP 4

1. Place the patient's right wrist between both your palms and interlaced fingers. Your interlaced fingers and palms are not at the same height. Your right hand on the palmar side of their left wrist is lower than your left hand on the back of their right wrist
2. Ask the patient to open their right hand and move their hand forward at the wrist while you maintain pressure on their carpal bones
3. Return their right hand to a neutral position
4. Ask the patient to move their right hand backwards while you maintain pressure on their right carpal bones

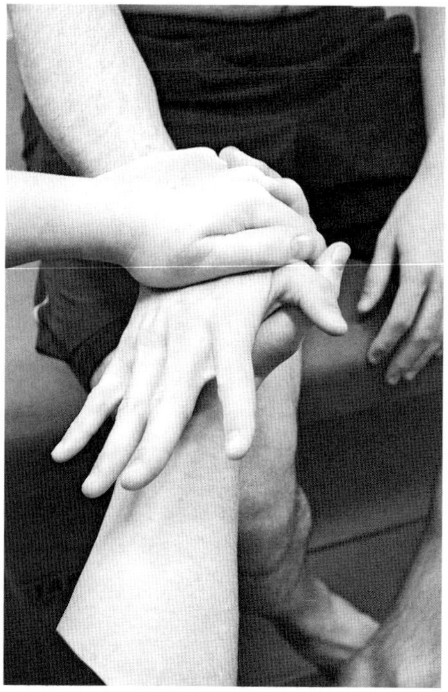

STEP 6

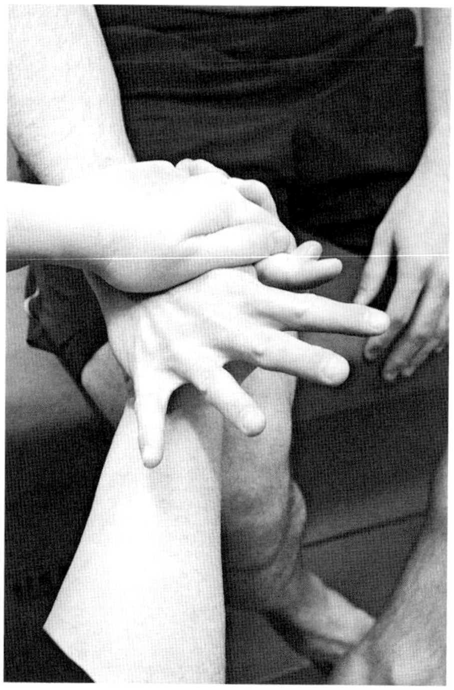

STEP 8

5. Return their right hand to a neutral position
6. Ask the patient to move their right hand toward their head while you maintain pressure on their carpal bones
7. Return their right hand to a neutral position
8. Ask the patient to move their right hand towards their feet while you maintain pressure on their carpal bones
9. Return their hand to a neutral position
10. Ask the patient to move their right hand in a forward circle several times while you maintain pressure on their carpal bones
11. Return their hand to a neutral position
12. Ask the patient to move their right hand in a backwards circle while you maintain pressure on their carpal bones
13. Return their hand to a neutral position

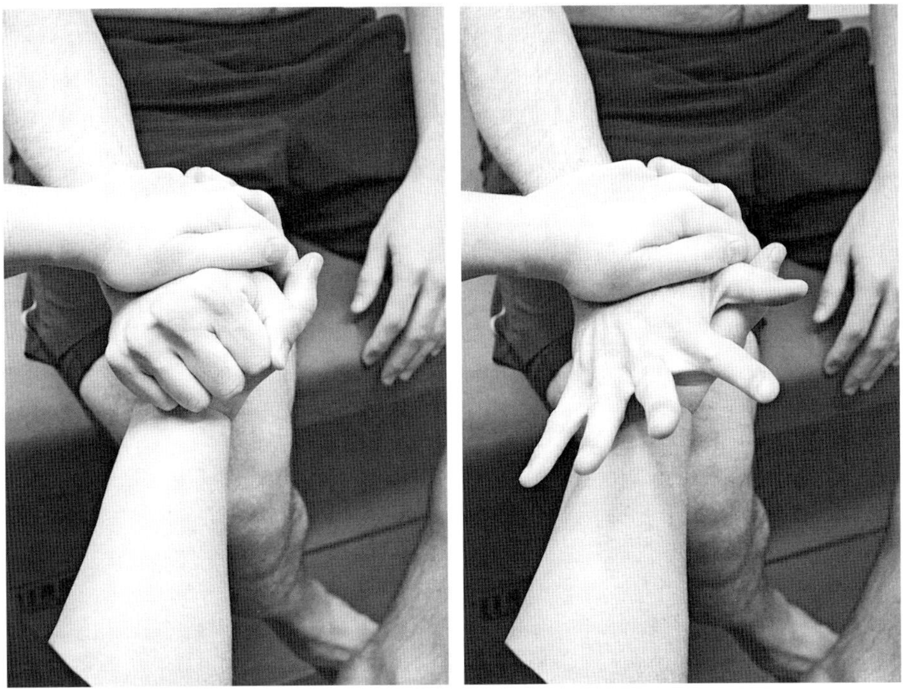

STEP 14

14. Ask the patient to make a tight fist and then to open it fully while you maintain pressure on their carpal bones.

Wales: Dr. Sutherland's first take is that the dysfunction is in the comparative concavity of the wrist. All the little joints (in the wrist) are going to be treated within their limits. You have control over this. You are not running the risk of fixing one thing and putting something else in an undesirable position, because all eight of these bones are ligamentous articular mechanisms. Just a little treatment here and a little there and it's all corrected. This contact protects at the same time as it normalizes. There is the phrase in the profession, I haven't heard it in ages – 'When you do this, and when you get this set up, you just "roll the bones home".'

10

Techniques for the Viscera

Dr. Still developed Osteopathy in the late 19th century. He had been trained as a medical doctor, but found that he could treat most diseases by palpating and treating dysfunctional areas with his hands. He called this new science Osteopathy, meaning "to begin with the bones."

Finding where the bones are not properly aligned or moving correctly can guide the physician to the area of the body that needs to be treated, as they reflect where the forces of life are not "moving with the bones." Many people seeking relief of their affliction flocked to Kirksville for treatment. Due to the large demand, Dr. Still had an infirmary built. It was dedicated on January 10, 1895. He and his students treated all of the known medical diseases of the day.

Notice that he began, but did not end there. In his writing, he constantly talked about joints, fascia, blood supply, nerves, internal organs, and lymphatic flow. He wrote three books on his ideas: *The Philosophy and Mechanical Principles of Osteopathy* in 1892, *Philosophy of Osteopathy* in 1899, and *Osteopathy, Research and Practice* in 1910. His first book was published the same year as the first class started, perhaps serving as a textbook. It primarily outlines his thinking process, and no specific treatment techniques were discussed. Dr. Still described few techniques in his writing. The most specific information is found in his last book, *Osteopathy, Research and Practice.*

Dr. Still palpated for organs that were "out of place", specifically ptosis of the liver, kidneys, bladder and uterus. He mostly treated the organs by lifting them superiorly. In general, Dr. Still's approach for visceral problems was to treat the spine, then lift the organs. Osteopathic manipulation of the viscera began with Dr. Still. He described treating many different digestive, respiratory and urogenital complaints. For Dr. Still, almost all medical conditions had an osteopathic treatment, in some cases curative, in some supportive. Dr. Still left few descriptions of techniques of any kind, but some of his early students did. Here is a sampling of what they and a few others have said about treating the viscera.

DR. WILLIAM GARNER SUTHERLAND

One of Dr. Still's students, William G. Sutherland, credited Dr. Still with the original idea of the cranial concept. Dr. Still often told his students that D.O. stands for "Dig On", encouraging them to expand their view of Osteopathy. While Dr. Sutherland is best known for his work in the cranial area, he never implied that it should be the only area diagnosed or treated. There are multiple references in his writings to treating the viscera. Indeed, in a course he taught in 1947, he never touched the head:

> When you want to observe the abdominal viscera, with the patient supine gently place one hand over or just below the area of interest. This hand is passive; it does nothing. Then place your other hand over it. You use the upper hand for gentle lifts and observation. That gentle application will tell you a great deal about where you are so that you can feel what the tissues can reveal. The lower hand can be permitted to sink into the tissues below, but the upper hand does the lifting in cooperation with the exhalation excursion of the diaphragm.[1]

DR. CHARLES HAZZARD

Dr. Hazzard was quite prolific, writing one of the earliest textbooks on Osteopathy. Along with approaches to most medical diseases, he proposed palpation of the abdomen for temperature changes to find areas of lesions, palpation and treatment for displacement of organs, and direct internal manipulation for female and male complaints. Inspection, palpation, percussion and auscultation are the physical methods employed. The following entry is drawn from his discussion of palpation of the abdomen:

> **Position:** The patient lies supine; the thighs are flexed and the feet rest upon the table; the head and chest are slightly elevated by the inclined head of the table. In this position the abdominal muscles are relaxed. The sides of the body are disposed alike to avoid unequal tension upon the tissues.
>
> **Inspection** reveals enlargement due to gas or fluid, tumor, muscular contraction, etc.; color; distended or retracted walls; restricted or increased motion; pulsation or engorgement of blood vessels, etc.
>
> **Palpation** reveals change in temperature; tumors superficial or deep, fluid or solid; tenseness or flabbiness of the abdominal walls; enlargements and displacements of organs. Pulsations also are to be noted. A marked pulsation of the abdominal aorta is common in nervous people, but generally indicates liver, stomach, or intestinal congestions. Deep palpation of the abdomen in thin persons readily reaches the bodies of the lumbar vertebrae rising quite prominently under the touch. They should not be mistaken for tumor. The examiner should grasp the abdominal walls in the fingers and raise them up away from the abdominal viscera, thus enabling him to tell whether tender places or growths lie in or beneath these walls
>
> **Percussion** reveals the limits of organs, presence of tumors, fluids or gases.
>
> **Auscultation** reveals gases, fetal sounds, and the gurgling with lubrication of the bowel.
>
> Abdominal treatment is generally in conjunction with treatment upon the specific lesion occurring in the spine, or thorax, e.g. typhoid, in which rough abdominal treatment might cause serious injury. It is directed to a specific end and restores mechanical relations of parts, frees nerve and blood-mechanisms, and removes muscular contracture.[2]

---

1. William G. Sutherland, *Teachings in the Science of Osteopathy*, ed. Anne Wales (Portland, OR: Sutherland Cranial Teaching Foundation, 1990), 212.

2. Charles Hazzard, *The Practice and Allied Therapeutics of Osteopathy*, 2nd ed. (Kirksville, MO: Journal Printing Co. 1901).

DR. CARL MCCONNELL

A point often overlooked is that the total ventral side of the body functions under direct diaphragmatic activity as a unit. A pelvic imbalanced state of tension, for example, may be fundamentally dependent on diaphragmatic atony. One of Dr. Still's most enlightening statements, embryologically, physiologically, biologically, and technically, in my opinion, is as follows: "It is only the perfection of the organism and the connected oneness that is the keynote to osteopathic practice." Every part has a duty to perform not only for its own maintenance, but also for the health and harmony of the interrelated whole.

This is part of the law of supply and demand, which is absolute through all of nature. It is important to know the exact place that each organ and tissue occupies in its normal position. It is only by knowing the normal we are able to detect the abnormal. Each organ seems to be a creator of its own fluid substances. We must know the nerve and blood supply and the drainage.[3]

DR. H.V. HOOVER

A brief general discussion of the treatment of viscera is a logical prelude to a discussion of a specific viscus such as the gall bladder. The type of treatment administered in any visceral disease depends on a number of factors.

If acute inflammation is present, what is done therapeutically must achieve quick results without further endangering life. If the disease is chronic, what is done must not cause acute irritation or produce a more fibrotic or diseased organ.

Also, treatment of a disease which is not primary in the organ but of a functional nature caused by un-physiologic autonomic control or mechanical interference differs from the treatment of an inflammation. Prophylactic or preventative treatment differs from the others.

Organs are subject to mechanical interferences which must be removed before function can be normal.[4]

DR. KEN LOSSING

Soft tissue treatment in osteopathy has been frowned upon since the early days when Dr. A. T. Still referred to some types of it as 'engine wiping'. It has been associated in the minds of many of us with rubbing or massage, yet intelligent and scientific adjustment of non-osseous structures is as truly osteopathic as correction of bony dysfunctions. Dr. Still regarded the body as a complex unit composed of interrelated parts working in harmony, each endowed with the inherent desire, intelligence and ability to plan as a Master Mechanic.

When circumstances prevent any part of the body, whether bony or soft tissue, from doing so, the effects are far reaching. Perfect health ensues when each part is in perfect adjustment and free to do its work. Dr. Still had the greatest respect for the humours and the fasciae, the nerves, vessels, viscera and all the other elements that compose the body. They had a remarkable faculty of being able to locate

---

3. Carl McConnell, *The Practice of Osteopathy*, 3rd ed. (Kirksville, MO: Journal Printing Co., 1906).

4. H.V. Hoover, D.O., "A Consideration of an Osteopathic Lesion of the Whole Liver and Its Effect on Hepatic Function," in *Yearbook of the American Academy of Osteopathy* (Chicago: 1948), 135.

maladjusted tissue, of associating cause with effect, and tracing effects back to cause. That quality is reflected in Dr. Sutherland's technique.

The fasciae envelop, separate, protect and support the various structures. Not the least important of their functions is to encourage and direct the movement of tissue fluids and to promote the flow of lymph through its channels. The various layers of fascia interconnect and present continuity from head to foot. Dr. Still recognized 'drags' on the fasciae through his hands on the patient's shoulders caused by hypotonicity, the weight of viscera, strains, and posture. Treatment to restore the normal tension, hence function of the fascial system is extremely effective.

Dr. Still's ideas are clear: all tissues need adequate fluid, and nutritional and neurological exchange, to be healthy. These components come through the blood vessels, lymphatics, and the autonomic nervous system, which all are covered by the peritoneum and pleura, in the form of visceral ligaments. When the attachments are tight, fluid exchange is compromised (tissue perfusion), the nervous system is irritated, and less than optimum function is the result. By treating the attachments, function can be improved. These principles apply to the viscera as well as all other tissues.

DR. ELMER BARBER

Dr. Barber was in one of Dr. Still's first classes. At that time the Osteopathic course was two years, so he would have had only four years of practice when he published his book, *Osteopathy Complete.* It is unclear whether his ideas at that time derived from class notes with Dr. Still, or from his own practice. The book is a textbook of medical conditions, and for each condition he lists an osteopathic approach, including spinal manipulation, visceral manipulation, and lymphatic approaches where appropriate.

> **Infection of the Eyes:** a morbid state, characterized in its simplest form by heat, redness, and pain in the eyes.
>
> *Symptoms:* Often comes on with a sensation of sand in the eyes. In some instances this complaint proceeds no farther, but at other times it is followed by heat, redness, and prickling, with darting pains.
>
> *Cause:* The cause is attributed by the medical profession to a stoppage of function in the microscopic elements of the involved tissues or to changes in the blood-vessels and blood, and exudation of liquor sauguinis, with permeation of white blood corpuscles, without rupture of the vessels, into the contiguous parts, or to altered nutrition of the tissues.[5]

Barber stated that the treatment of the eye began with "General Treatment of the Neck."

5. Elmer Barber, *Osteopathy Complete* (Kansas City: Hudson-Kimberly Publishing Co., 1898), 397.

Barber's General Treatment of the Neck

PHYSICIAN: Standing
PATIENT: Supine

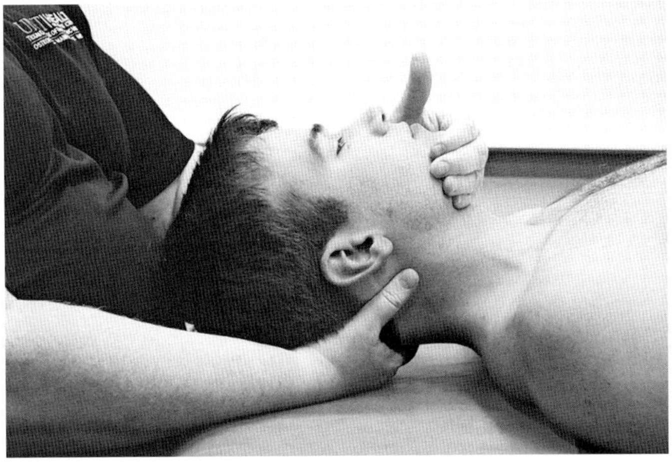

STEPS 1 – 2

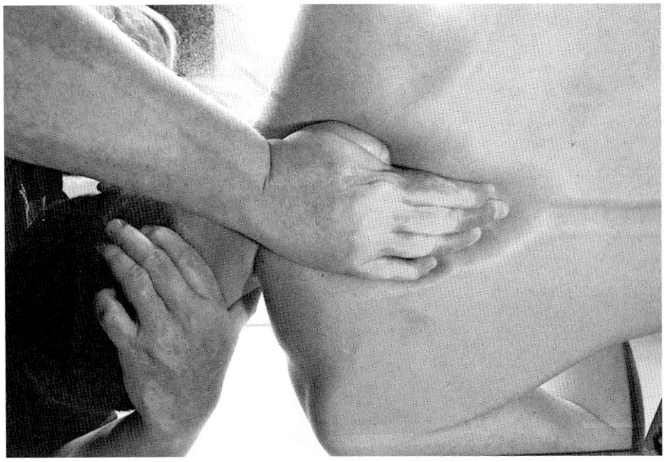

STEP 3

1. Place the patient on the back, with one hand under the chin and the other under the back of the head, pull gently, rotating the head in all directions, slowly but strongly, endeavoring to stretch all muscles of the neck
2. Pull slowly on the head until the body moves
3. Then place the left hand on the top of patient's head, the right hand and arm beneath the head and neck, two fingers upon each side of the fourth thoracic vertebra, the ends of the fingers pressing hard, moving the muscles upward, at the same time press rather hard with the left hand, rotating the head from side to side, the fingers of the right hand working gradually upward, until the occipital is reached

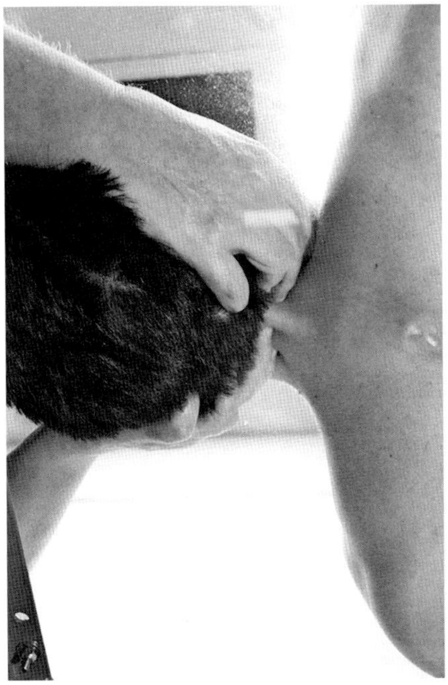

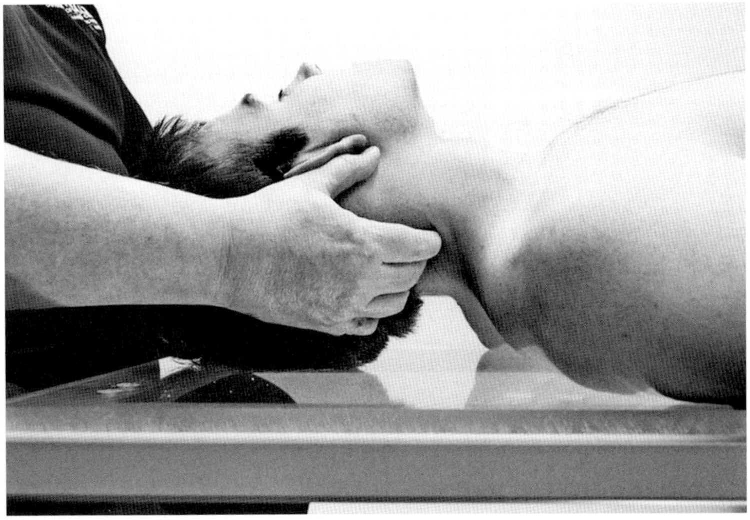

STEP 4

4. Standing at patient's head, place the hands upon the sides of the neck, the fingers just back of the transverse processes of the upper cervicals and give gentle extension, rotating the head to the right, with the left hand moving the muscles forward and over the transverse processes upon the left side, rotate the head in the opposite direction, with the right hand moving the muscles forward and over the transverse processes upon the right side, move the hands downward to the next lower cervicals; rotate the head as before, and repeat until the last cervical is reached

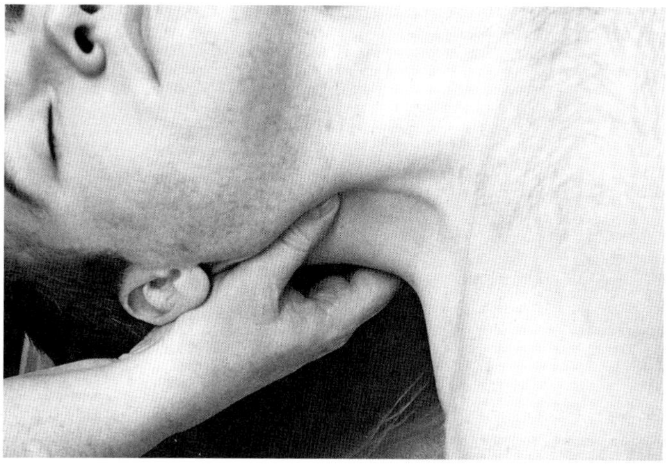

STEP 5

5. Manipulate the muscles thoroughly and deep, in the front of the neck, place the hand under the chin, drawing the head backward, thus giving these muscles extension and work as deeply as possible under the inferior maxillary

Barber's Treatment of the Eye Proper

PHYSICIAN: Beside the patient either standing or seated
PATIENT: Either seated or supine

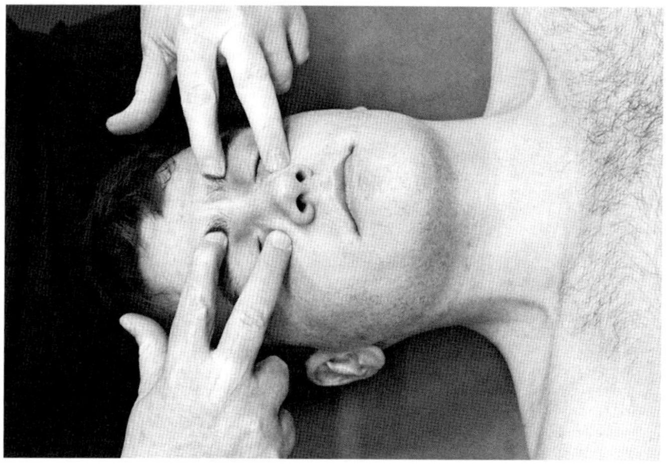

STEP 2

1. With the index finger work gently but deeply under the edge of the bones surrounding the eye, beginning deeply in the corner of the eye, and being particular to press against the bone and not the eyeball. Raise the finger entirely off the flesh as it is moved forward,

in this manner the eye can be treated very thoroughly and deeply without giving pain, while if the physician endeavors to slide his finger over the flesh without removing it from the eye, the operation is painful, and the results not so pronounced. It is always well to manipulate all the muscles in the immediate vicinity of the eye, thus freeing the circulation

2. Place two fingers lightly over the eye and vibrate. Being careful not to move the lid, this should be kept steady on the eyeball so that the vibration may pass through. The vibration should be felt very deeply

Barber: This treatment will require about ten or fifteen minutes, and should be given each day until recovery. We have cured many cases of inflammation of the eyes in a few days when the patient was in such a condition that it was necessary for him to be led to our office. Many cases, however, are more stubborn, requiring from six to eight weeks, and, in chronic cases, often three months' treatment is required to affect a cure. A great many cases of inflammation of the eyes, and other diseases of the head, are due to a slip or partial dislocation of the atlas, which can be readily discovered by making a careful examination, and must be reduced before a cure can be expected.

Barber's Treatment of the Lacrimal Duct

PHYSICIAN: Beside the patient either standing or seated
PATIENT: Either seated or supine

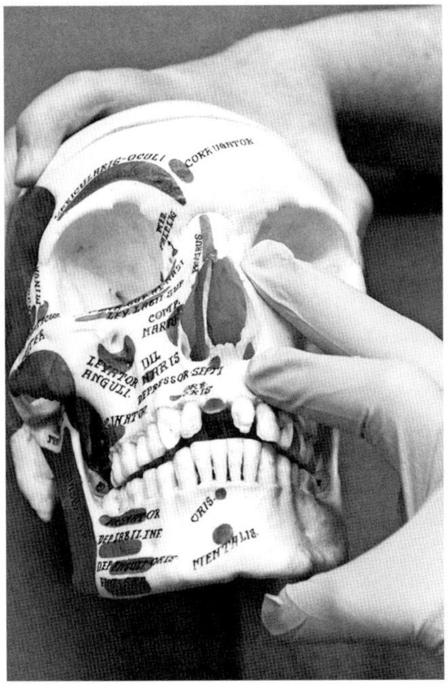

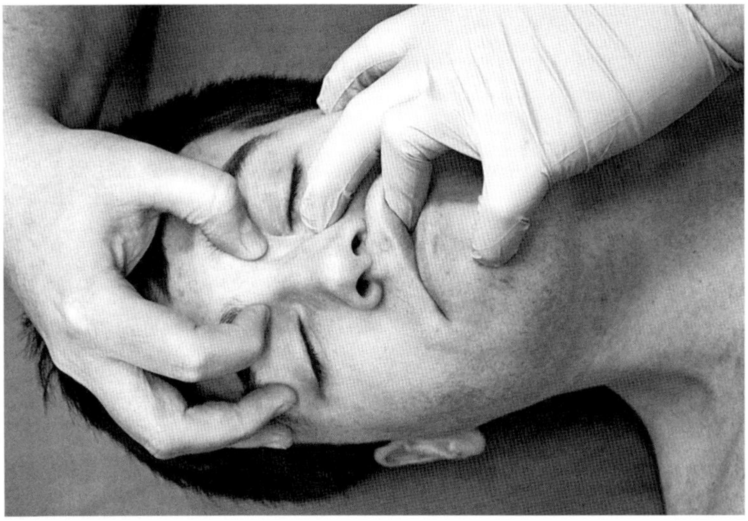

STEPS 1 – 3

1. Place your right index finger next to the eye by the nose next to the lacrimal bone
2. Place your left 4th finger under the lip on the gum line near the nose and pull down
3. Insert a gloved finger into the nose and pull down on the lacrimal gland

Intranasal Technique

Crow: The intranasal technique is useful in patients with recurrent sinusitis. Deason described the technique back in 1929 and 1944, and is simply a way of making sure that the turbinates and nasal bones are moving freely.

PHYSICIAN: Beside the patient either standing or seated
PATIENT: Either seated or supine

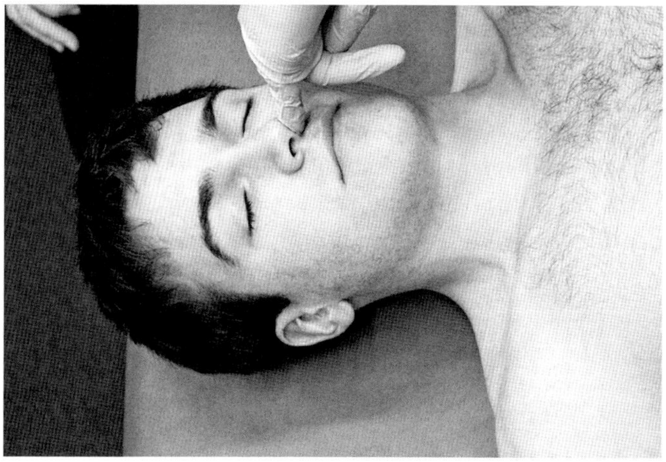

STEPS 1 – 5

1. Place a water based lubricant (i.e. KY jelly) on the little finger of your gloved hand
2. Insert your little finger in their nostril at a 90 degree angle to the treatment table
3. Slowly advance your finger to the turbinate (inferior and middle conchae)
4. When you touch the turbinate slowly externally rotate your little finger
5. Repeat on the opposite side

Most patients will feel drainage going down the back of the throat immediately.

Muncie's Technique (for Eustachian Tube Dysfunction – 1921)

INDICATIONS: Tinnitus, serous otitis media, Meniere's disease
EXAMPLE: Left eustachian tube dysfunction
PHYSICIAN: Seated beside the patient
PATIENT: Supine

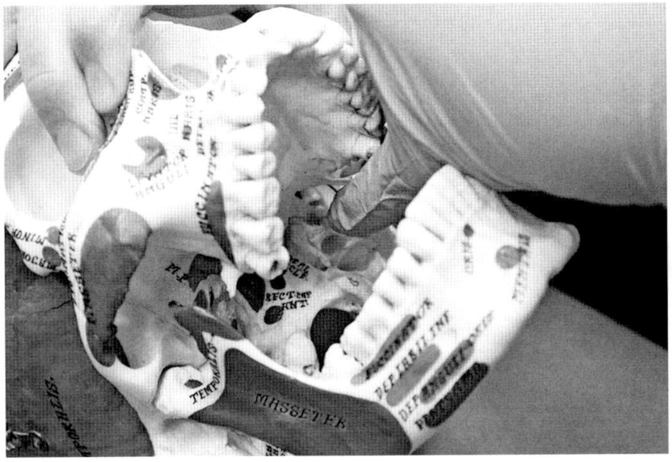

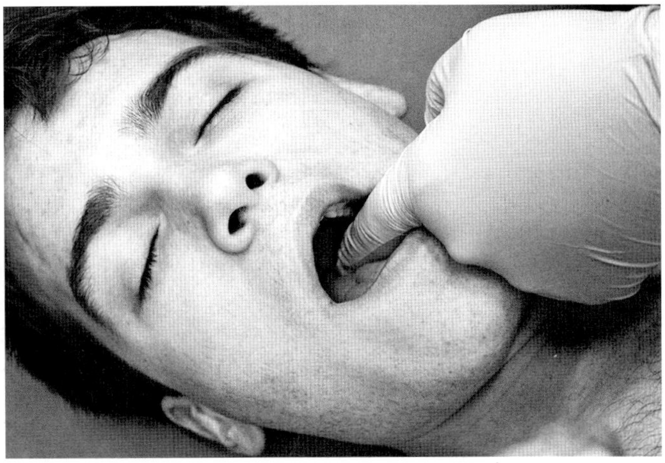

STEPS 1 – 5

1. Place your gloved left index finger in the patient's mouth—going at first along the end of their left upper teeth
2. Go under the molars and place your finger against the inferior part of the posterior pillar of their palatine tonsil. This should be near the opening of the Eustachian tube
3. Move your fingertip cephalad and posterior to the opening of the Eustachian tube
4. Apply a pumping motion with your finger pad to break down any adhesions. This should be done very quickly as the patient is probably going to gag
5. The patient should feel pressure in their ear if you are in the right place. (Note that often times there is blood and a mucus plug on your fingertip when the adhesion is broken)

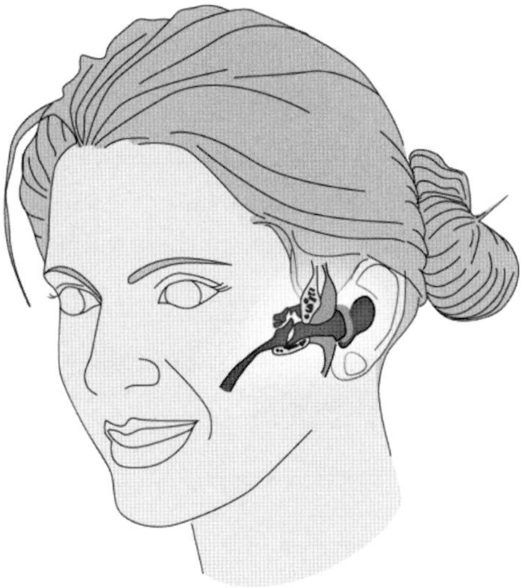

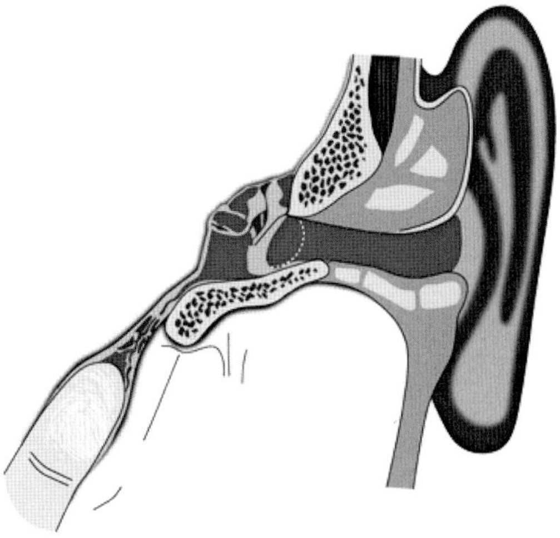

Crow: The Muncie technique was first described in the osteopathic literature in a pamphlet in 1921 and again in a book in the 1960s. In many cases Dr. Muncie was accused of quackery. In his last publication, Dr. Muncie reported his results for improvement in catarrhal deafness, Eustachian tube dysfunction and Meniere's disease, which showed greater than 90% improvement in all cases. Notwithstanding Muncie's exaggerated claims, the technique is still useful.

I have personally used this technique with success on patients with recurrent serous otitis media, tinnitus and Meniere's disease. In the patients with serous otitis media, I have been able to measure improvement of the tympanic membrane movement using the Welch Allyn Portable Tympanometric Instrument. The patients with Meniere's and tinnitus have stated that they had fewer symptoms with the use of this technique.

Miller's Technique (for Root of the Tongue – 2005)

INDICATIONS: TMJ, C1 and C2 restrictions, swallowing difficulties post stroke
PHYSICIAN: Seated beside the table
PATIENT: Supine

Inhibitory pressure is applied to the patient's mylohyoid, geniohyoid, and digastric muscles. Application of steady pressure to the soft tissues reduces reflex activity and produces relaxation of the tissues. The precise 'lesion' point in the range of motion of the connective tissues is where the tension exerted upon these tissues is equalized in all directions.

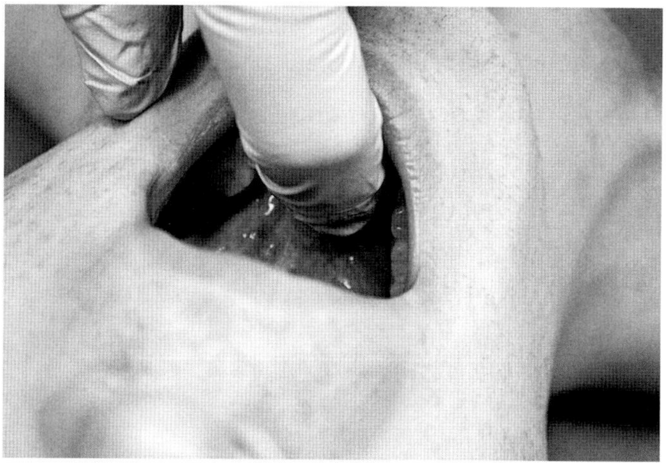

STEPS 1 – 4

1. Your gloved finger is inserted under the patient's tongue at the base of their tongue
2. Your other hand is placed posteriorly behind the cervicals at the level of their C1 and C2
3. Pressure is applied in the midline at one of the four quadrants at the root of their tongue. When you feel the tension let go or 'melt' then go to the next point
4. Going through all four points in sequence is very effective

Crow: The first time I saw the root of the tongue technique was at a course given by the Sutherland Cranial Teaching Foundation. Edgar Miller, D.O. had developed this technique to deal with TMJ problems.

I have found that it was effective for releasing severely restricted C1's and C2's, when other techniques had failed. The suspected physiological basis for this is stimulation of the hypoglossal nuclei on each side. This is a motor region within the medulla of the brainstem. Stimulation of the muscles of the root of the tongue nucleus causes a biochemical cascade to the C1 and C2 nuclei, thus causing a reflex relaxation. In other words, it is going through 'the back door' to release the C1 and C2.

I had a patient who had his head stepped on by a horse. Six months after the injury, he was still unable to eat due to swallowing problems and had a peg tube in his stomach. After several treatments the patient was able to eat and the peg tube removed.

I have treated stroke patients who have had swallowing difficulties with some success using the root of the tongue technique.

Chronic Cough Hyoid Technique

PHYSICIAN: Standing in front of the patient
PATIENT: Seated

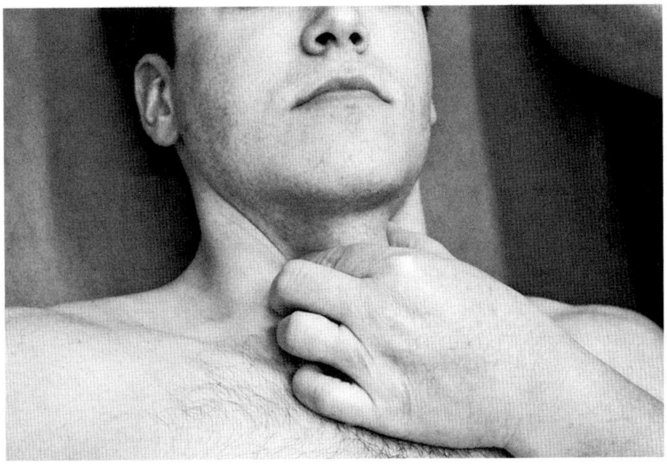

STEPS 1 – 4

1. Place your thumb on one side of the hyoid and the index finger on the other side
2. Balance the tension on the hyoid by pulling the hyoid down on one side and then the other
3. When the balance point is reached hold the position
4. After a minute have the patient swallow. Swallowing resets the strap muscles and frees the inferior laryngeal nerve

Vardy: This is an excellent and highly effective technique.

"Look Well to the Hyoid."[6]

I once overheard a remark of the 'Old Doctor's' that fits very aptly here. I was leaving the Infirmary Building at Kirksville and was passing by the 'Old Doctor' talking to a group of three or four students. One of the ladies was coughing and I heard the 'Old Doctor' say—"Loosen up your Hyoid". I of course didn't know whether his remark was concerning the coughing, or was in reply to some question that had been asked him, anyway, that remark made a deep impression on me, and I have often recalled it when studying this subject and when treating patients with throat involvements. Exceeding gentleness and care must be used in manipulating this thin, delicate fragile bone which is so important to man's happiness, comfort and serviceability to do his job.

Crow: I had a patient who came to me because of a chronic cough that no one could cure. He had been endoscoped because someone thought the cough was due to gastroesophageal reflux. He had seen a cardiologist because his primary physician thought his blood pressure medication was causing the cough.

He went to the respiratory specialist to rule out asthma, which he didn't have. I took his history, and he stated that the cough started after having an upper respiratory infection three years before. The cough never stopped. I treated the hyoid, which was restricted on one side. That was the only treatment given. One visit cured the cough. I'm not stating that this will cure all causes of chronic cough, but after other causes have been ruled out, check the hyoid. The hyoid is suspended by ligaments in the neck. The inferior laryngeal nerve passes around the cornu of the hyoid. If there is restriction on the hyoid, then there is irritation of the inferior laryngeal nerve which will cause a cough.

6. Address presented by G. W. Riley, Ph.D., D.O., and reproduced in the Digest of Papers and Discussion presented at the Manipulative Therapeutic Section of the American Osteopathic Association at Cincinnati, Ohio. Published in volume 1 of the July, 1938 *Yearbook of the American Academy of Osteopathy*.

Sutherland's Anterior Cervical Fascia Technique

PHYSICIAN: Seated
PATIENT: Seated

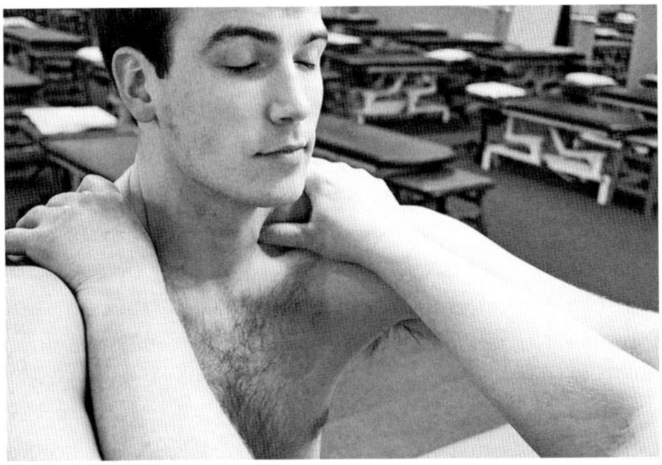

STEPS 1 – 4

1. The patient sits facing you. Their body is flexed with their head hanging down
2. Place your thumbs posteriorly to their clavicles, under their trapezius and your thenar eminences are over their clavicles, just lateral to the attachment of their sternocleidomastoid muscles
3. Ask the patient to rest their hands on your shoulders and slowly drop their weight forward. This advances your thumbs down into their mediastinum, just anterior and to either side of the trachea
4. Lift your thumbs upward as the patient raises their head

Lippincott: The anterior cervical fascia is attached to the base of the skull, the mandible, hyoid, scapula, clavicle and sternum. Through the pretracheal it is connected with the fibrous pericardium, and thence from below with the diaphragm. It surrounds the pharynx, larynx and thyroid gland. It forms the carotid sheath, and by way of the prevertebral fascia is connected with the surrounds of the trachea and esophagus. Therefore, the cervical fascia is concerned quite directly with the lymphatic drainage of the head, neck, thorax and upper extremities. Not only voluntary movements, but respiratory activity, is a factor in this vital function of the fascia by moving it forward in exhalation and backward in approximation to the spine during inhalation. Restoration of free movement of the deep cervical fascia renders unnecessary much of the soft tissue treatment of the neck and helps in overcoming intra-thoracic congestions.

The Respiratory System

Asthma Technique from the 1938 Yearbook

MANIPULATIVE TREATMENT OF ASTHMA

From notes compiled by T.L. Northrup, D.O., at a symposium entitled "Manipulative Treatment of Asthma" presented by Perrin T. Wilson, D.O., T.L. Ray, D.O., and Harry W. Gamble, D.O., at the Manipulative Therapeutic Section of the American Osteopathic Association in Cincinnati, Ohio, July, 1938. Reproduced in the 1938 AAO Yearbook.

Northrup: As I understand Dr. Ray's treatment for an acute attack, he suggests placing your hands on each side of the patient's chest cage in the axillary line on their lower ribs. This provides simultaneous pressure to aid in expelling the air and at the time complete expiration by the patient. After years of practice, I feel that the pelvis and lower spine is a foundation which must be corrected before reduction of lesions higher up can be made and maintained. One of our London writers reports over 100 cases of asthma that he has treated and which revealed bony lesions of the pelvis or 5th lumbar. The Old Doctor said that he found it unnecessary to treat the average asthma case oftener than once a week.

The treatment employed is the pumping treatment, as described for an acute attack. Accompany this with very deep soft tissue work of a boring character with the thumbs between the transverse processes and around between the angles of the ribs. Complete with efforts directed toward loosening of the entire chest.

The mobility of the ribs and vertebrae may well be accomplished by having the patient sitting on a chair or stool. Working on the right side we place the patient's right hand on the back of his head. The operator's right hand is placed on the patient's forehead with his right elbow locking the patient's right elbow. Rotation of the spine is obtained clockwise rotating the head and elbow at the same time the operator's left thumb loosens the tissues around the angle of the rib.

You can see how the pectoralis minor and major raise the front end of the ribs through mechanical leverage, at the same time your thumb performs beautiful rib work. I have his elbow locked in mine. For pressure on his first rib get far enough forward. Many of us fail to depress or loosen the first rib by having our pressure too far back. See what a beautiful leverage you have here. Bend them back, as far as you want, and bring them around so that the pectoral muscles pull the front end of the ribs up. Get straight down on the first rib, not quite as straight down on the second rib and not quite as straight down on the third rib and so forth, pressing down the angles of all the ribs. We alternate to the left and do the same thing. My thumb is near the spine, just inside the angle of the rib. If the patient has a bursitis it may be necessary to modify the technique. You can feel the ribs move. To mobilize the vertebra, hold the one below the one you want to move and prevent it from rotating and pull the one above around on top of the vertebra you are holding.

Crow: The second technique is described below.

PHYSICIAN: Standing behind the patient on their right side
PATIENT: Seated on a stool or chair

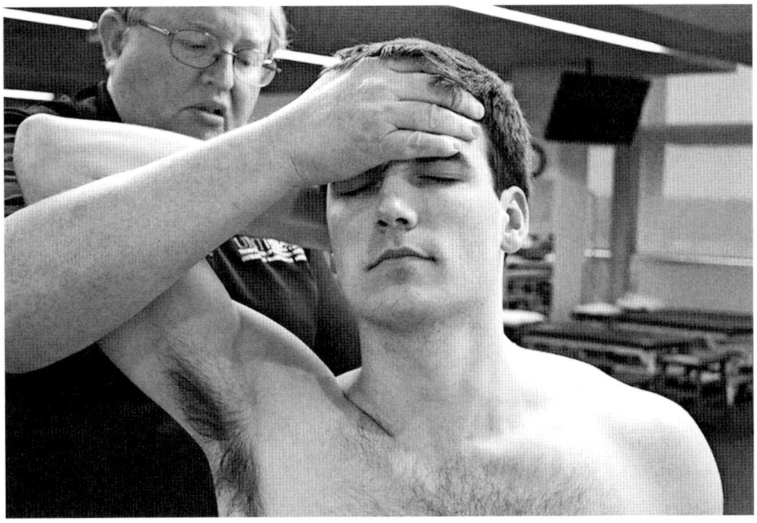

STEPS 1 – 2

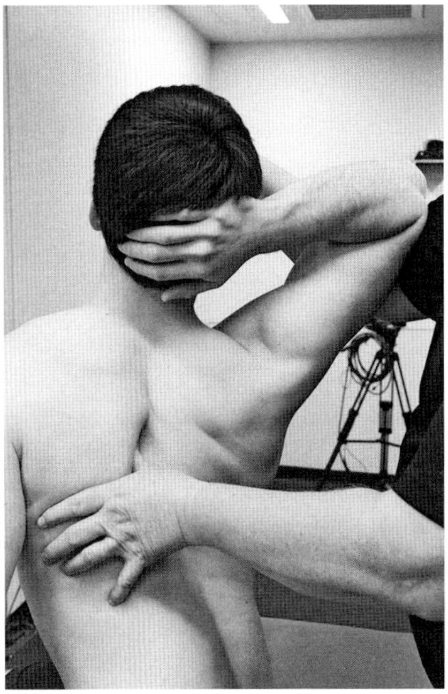

STEPS 3 – 7

1. Place the patient's right hand on the back of their head
2. Place your right hand on the patient's forehead with your right elbow locking the patient's right elbow
3. Place your left thumb around the angle of their rib on their left side
4. Rotate their spine clockwise by rotating their head and elbow at the same time
5. The pectoralis minor and major raise the front end of the ribs through mechanical leverage
6. Move your left thumb higher to the patient's 1st rib
7. Increase the extension as well as rotation of the patient's spine so that their pectoral muscles pull the front end of their ribs upwards

Wales on Asthma

Wales: All the things I may do with this sort of osteopathic treatment are things in the fascial mechanism of balancing and decompression. Mostly it's taking things away when you find resistance. The rest is anatomy. Stimulating the sphenoid palatine ganglia and the superior cervical ganglia are two things which are beneficial to asthmatics. They balance out or undo a predicament where the patients are in a functional crisis with congestion. The autonomic nerve supply is located there and it's part of the picture. So if you can stimulate the sphenoid palatine ganglia and relax the cervico vertebral junction, and ease whatever reflex tensions you find there, this is a good place to start.

But the asthma situation has had its major effects upon the thorax. The point to treating infants as well as adults is their low threshold of tolerance. What I do with my rib technique is to release the lateral chain ganglia in front of the heads of the ribs so that their whole facilitated reactive segments are cooled off. Dr. Perrin Wilson had a particular technique. He positioned the patient prone and up on their elbows on the treatment table. Then he came along from the back and put his thumb under the 4th rib on the left and pushed and held it there. He said that he could stop an asthmatic attack with this treatment.

I have been very successful in the past in treating infants, children and adolescents who were suffering from asthmatic attacks. They didn't have any more attacks. With adults, when I went on a house call, I could stop an attack in the middle of the night so they could get some sleep. Most of my adult patients who were susceptible to asthmatic attacks had some more attacks. I can't think of any patient as an adult who never had another attack. All I think I've been able to do with allergies and their allergic responses and reactions is to have them raise the threshold of their sensitivity. They were then less apt to get an allergic reaction to whatever they usually responded to. This resulted in fewer and fewer attacks. I can't think of anybody that didn't have any more attacks at all, but I didn't change their particular allergy or sensitivity. All I ever felt I had changed was their degree of susceptibility or however you want to express it. But anybody who has asthma or emphysema has labored so much in their breathing that they have really strained and sprained their skeletal mechanism. This includes the cranio base and the focal mechanism including their general postural mechanics and even the whole shape of their thorax suffers.

Crow's Treatment of Acute Asthma using a Tender Point

PHYSICIAN: Standing
PATIENT: Seated

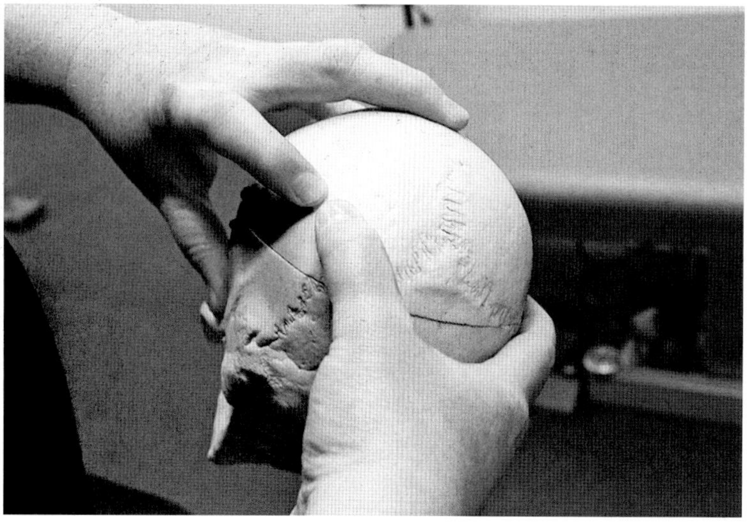

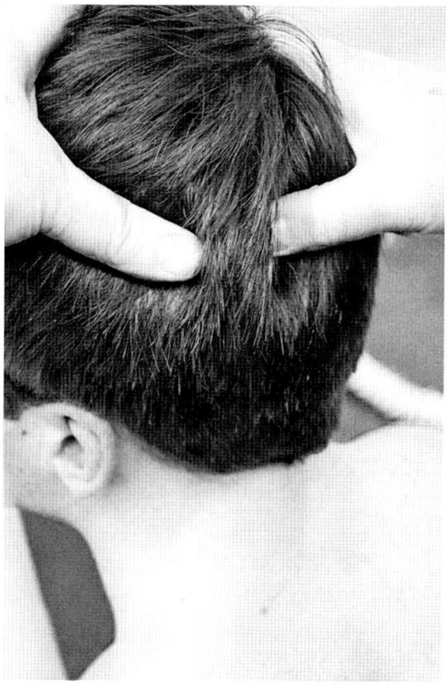

STEPS 1 – 3

1. Place your right thumb on a tender point near the left parietal eminence on the patient's left side
2. Take your left hand and fold the patient's scalp around the tender point

3. Hold until the patient's breathing eases. This is usually within 60 seconds

This technique was first published as a research article 'The Use of a Tender Point on the Skull to Improve Peak Flow Values in Acute Asthma Patients' (Crow, C.T, Kasper, D.A.; Retrospective Study) *Journal Of The American Academy Of Osteopathy,* spring 2006.

Barber's Lung Technique #1 (Two-Person Technique)

PHYSICIAN: Standing with an assistant
PATIENT: Supine

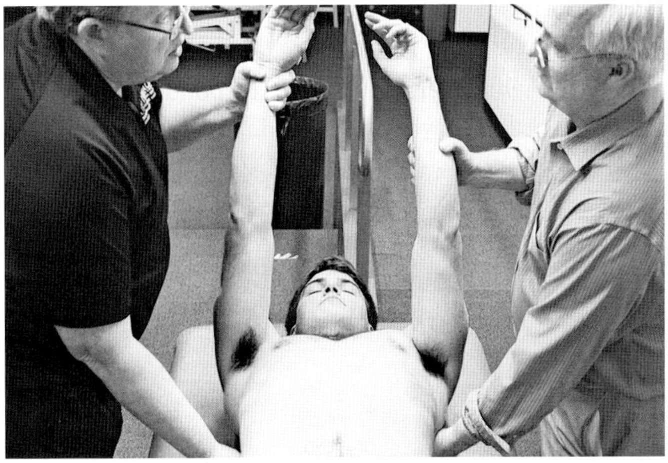

STEPS 1 – 2

1. Have the patient on their back with a pillow under their head. Physician and assistant stand at the head of the table on each side of the patient
2. Both physician and assistant take their upper hand and place it under the patient's shoulders on the angle of the second rib, half way between the scapula (shoulder blade) and spine and one inch above the scapula

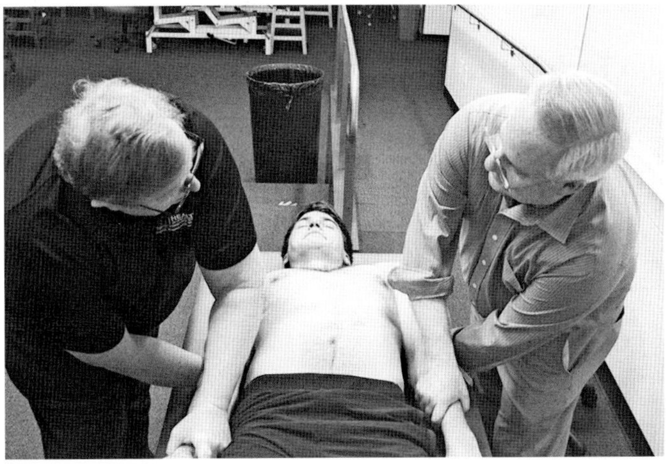

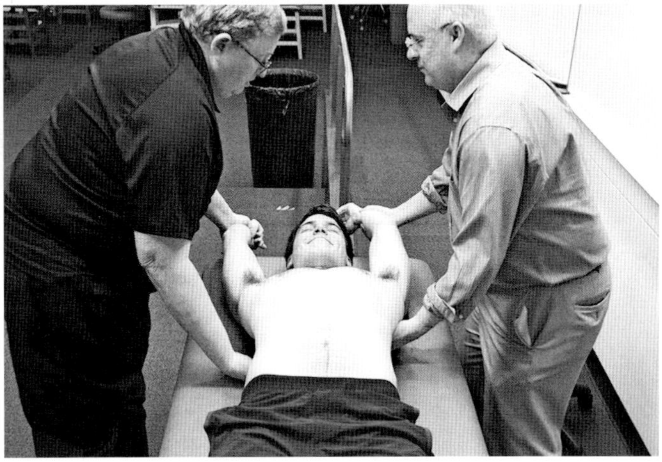

STEPS 3 – 4

3. With the free hand, the physician and assistant take the patient's wrists, and slowly draw their arms upwards high above their head. Pull steadily and strongly for a moment, and at the same time with the fingers of the upper hand press steadily on the angle of the ribs

4. The physician and assistant lower the patient's arms slowly, the patient's elbows passing below and to the sides of the table
5. The physician and assistant move their fingers down the patient's spine one inch, to the angle of the next rib, and draw up the patient's arms as before. Repeat until the physician and assistant have raised the four or five upper ribs. It will also be also observed that this operation stretches the intercostal muscles

Barber's Lung Technique #2

PHYSICIAN: Standing
PATIENT: Seated upon a stool

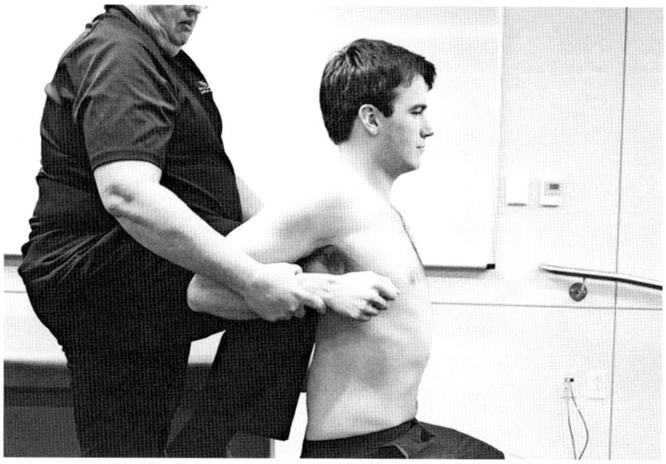

1. The physician places their knee between the shoulders, grasps the patient's wrists and raises the arms slowly but strongly high above the head, pressing hard with the knee and lowering the arms with a backward motion
2. Each time as the patient's arms are drawn upward the patient should inhale, filling the lungs to their utmost capacity, exhaling as the arms reach their normal position

Barber's Lung Technique #3 (Two-Person Technique)

PHYSICIAN: Standing with assistant
PATIENT: Supine

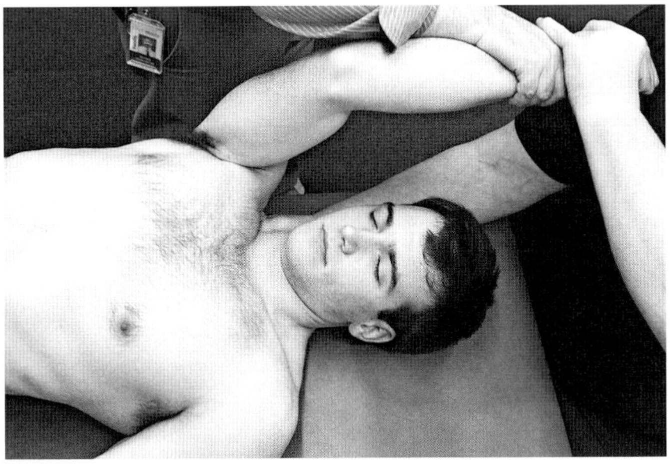

STEPS 1 – 2

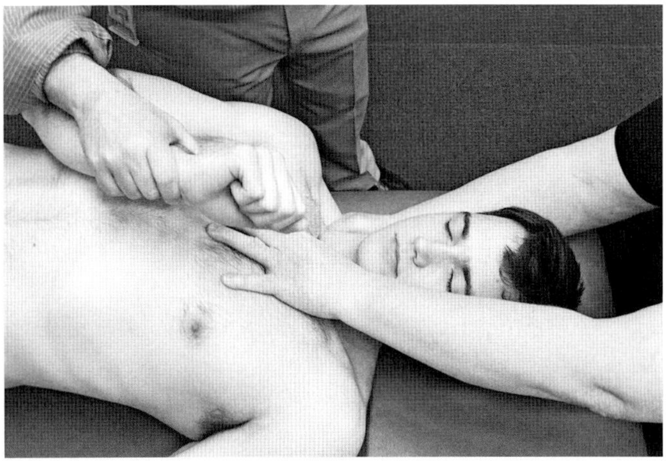

STEP 3

1. With the fingers of one hand the physician presses upon the angle of the first rib, which is depressed. With the other hand press outward and downward upon the cartilages of the ribs that are pushed forward towards the sacrum
2. Have an assistant draw the patient's arm upon the side where the depression has been discovered, high and strong, above the patient's head. Ask the patient to take a deep breath, filling the lungs to their utmost capacity
3. Have the assistant lower the patient's arm with a backward motion. At the same instant the physician presses hard with their fingers upon the angle of the rib, and with the other hand upon the cartilage which is moved towards the sternum

Barber's Lung Technique #4

PHYSICIAN: Standing
PATIENT: Supine

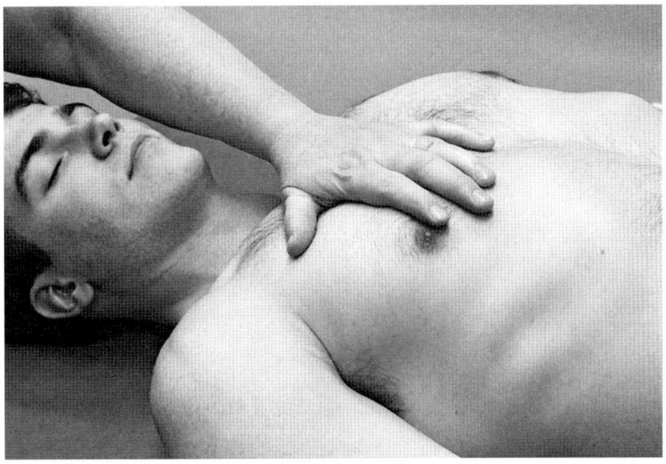

Place the hand lightly upon the thorax, and vibrate gently for two minutes over that portion of the lungs or bronchi which seems to be affected.

The Diaphragm

Lippincott: Because of its relationships the diaphragm deserves consideration other than as a muscle of respiration. The pericardium is firmly attached to it above, the peritoneum below, and the great vessels and esophagus pass through it. Being rather closely associated with the organs of respiration, circulation and digestion, it is important that the full excursion of the diaphragm be unimpeded. This is prevented by a 'drag' on the abdominal fascia and may be restored by a technique known as the diaphragmatic lift. The object of the treatment is to draw the diaphragm cranially, elevating the floor of the thorax, drawing upward on the abdominal contents and promoting venous and lymphatic drainage from the lower half of the body. Visceroptosis and even internal hemorrhoids respond to it.

McConnell on Diaphragm Doming

Have the patient stand sideways to a mirror, pucker the lips as in whistling, and blow out, exhale, while slowly elevating and retreating the abdomen. Do this several times a day, also while walking.

Sutherland's Diaphragm Release

PHYSICIAN: Standing
PATIENT: Supine

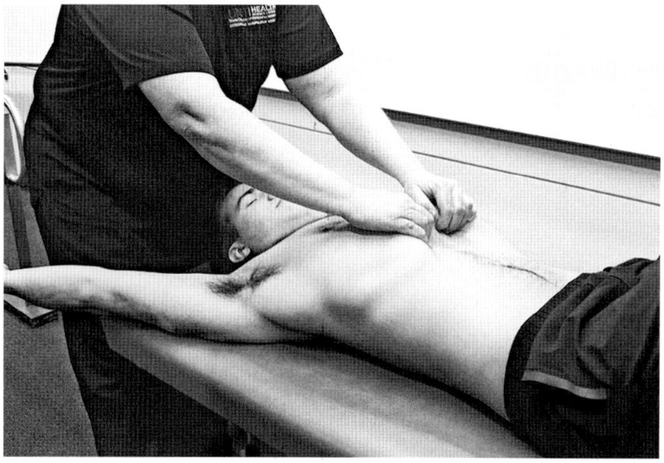

STEPS 1 – 6

1. The physician introduces their fingertips under the costochondral junctions
2. If that area is particularly sensitive ask the patient to hook their own fingers under their ribs and lift on their hands
3. As the patient exhales the physician lifts the lower rim of the thorax in a cranial and slightly lateral direction
4. The advancement that is made is held during inspiration and is increased on exhalation
5. The patient is instructed not to hold the breath in, but to exhale immediately after inhalation

6. After several respiratory cycles there is no further upward progress and the patient is told to breathe out, close the throat and attempt to expand the chest

Wales: Because of its relationships the diaphragm deserves consideration other than as a muscle of respiration. The pericardium is firmly attached to it above, the peritoneum below, and the great vessels and esophagus pass through it. Being rather closely associated with the organs of respiration, circulation and digestion, it is important that the full excursion of the diaphragm be unimpeded. This is prevented by a 'drag' on the abdominal fascia and may be restored by a technique known as the diaphragmatic lift. The object of the treatment is to draw the diaphragm cranially, elevating the floor of the thorax, drawing upward on the abdominal contents and promoting venous and lymphatic drainage from the lower half of the body.

Wales on Fascial Drag and the Diaphragm

Wales: I've been having a little correspondence with Tom Schooley and he said since we were in Will's class you should always tell it. But I'm in favor of everyone who's heard it and understands it making the point if not with that story then in some other way. Because I am convinced that when there is fascial drag, sacral sag whether or not lymph's involved, but if the diaphragm is working at a lower level, the crura of the diaphragm locks down on the aorta. And it does affect the mechanics of the heart. And just how many of heart attacks are brought on by that factor, because I don't know.

I had some patients who have had all valves of their hearts removed in some hospital in Boston. And had some patients that have had bypass surgery for coronary insufficiency or problems with the musculature of the heart. The management is different than what it was in the distant past, but with all the different stress and strains upon the cardiac organ itself, its musculature and its coordination with lungs, and liver and kidneys. I have some insight into something which is not uncommon, and so I take to release the lumbocostal arches and get the diaphragm up, and get the liver turned around so it doesn't drag as well as other things, and I will say what it's worth, except what it's worth to my thinking. I think I have done what is within my power to benefit the patient whether they knew it was or not. I am absolutely focused on releasing the tension across the thoracolumbar junction from the back wall of the abdomen and the lumbocostal arches as well as everything that hangs from the undersurface of the diaphragm and so anything you can do that will provide a lift to the ventral mechanism of the body is good. What you do with what is thoracic to the plane of gravity has a very specific influence on postural mechanics.

Wales on the Diaphragm

Wales: The diaphragm works on the vertebral column so that the crurae of the diaphragm are attached to the anterior longitudinal spinal ligament. The anterior longitudinal spinal ligament is attached to the sacrum at the bottom and the basilar occiput at the top. Being nonextensible ligamentous tissue the diaphragm is shifting to and fro and up and down. If I hold the vertebral bodies in the state of ligamentous balance, breathing moves the vertebral column. And, pretty soon the ligamentous of the heads of the ribs and the discs, everything the anterior longitudinal spinal ligament is attached to starts to move. And this is one of the criteria of the body that makes me say to myself that the anterior longitudinal ligament is the main street or hub of the trunk. It will move everything, and everything moves as everything else is attached to it.

I concentrate my attention on a ligamentous articular mechanism and intervertebral joint and its neighbor and then in a region that operates as a whole. On the thoracic spine in relationships with its original curvature. It's a region in this sense. And the thoracic lumbar junction is a region, because the lumbar lordosis has another curvature.

Sutherland's Arcuate Ligaments

Lippincott: In a technique utilized for relaxation of the external arcuate ligaments, the tension affecting the important structures passing through the arches of the diaphragm is relieved.

PHYSICIAN: Standing
PATIENT: Seated

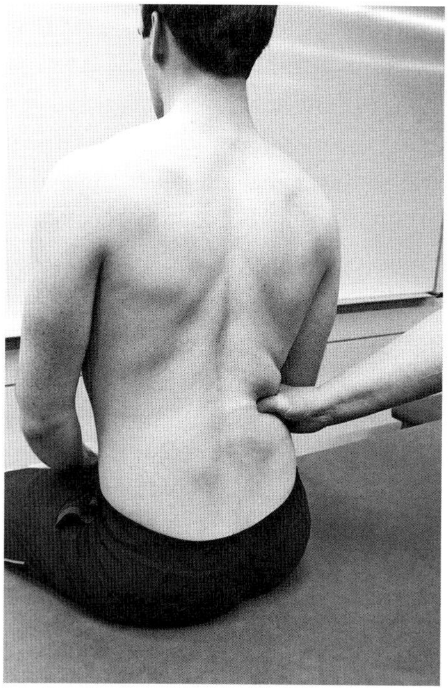

STEPS 1 – 4

1. Place your thumb under the twelfth rib just lateral to the erector spinae mass. The right thumb is used for the right side of the patient and vice versa
2. Have the patient bend their trunk over your thumb which gently and gradually advances upward and posteriorly as the patient exhales
3. Hold your position as the patient inhales
4. When your thumb arrives against or under the ligament, draw it laterally with a rolling motion relaxing the external and usually the internal arcuate ligament

The Cardiovascular System

ARRHYTHMIA TRIGGER POINT[7]

They [Drs. Travell and Rinzler] also saw evidence that the [ethyl chloride] spray could suppress cardiac arrhythmias. On several later occasions, I saw the conversion of atrial fibrillation to normal rhythm when vapocoolant spray was applied over the arrhythmia myofascial trigger point (MTrP) on the lower-right anterior chest wall. The same effect could be achieved by trigger point pressure release applied to that MTrP, as described in *The Trigger Point Manual*. For several reasons, it appears likely that many such unexpected influences, to and from MTrPs, depend on modulation of the autonomic nervous system, in addition to modulation of the sensory nervous system (referred pain).

As fully described in chapters 42 and 43 of *The Trigger Point Manual*, the pain patterns of the pectoralis major and pectoralis minor muscles mimic the pain referral patterns of cardiac ischemia. The early studies by Dr. Janet Travell and colleagues provided convincing experimental evidence that the referred pain of cardiac ischemia and the referred pain of active myofascial MTrPs can be eliminated, or decreased remarkably, by application of vapocoolant spray to the skin over the painful area. Clinical studies showed that the two sources of pain are easily mistaken for each other and that persistence of pain for some time after the ischemia of a myocardial infarction should have resolved is likely to be caused by MTrPs. Symptoms of angina in the absence of demonstrable cardiac disease should be considered as likely due to MTrPs.

Treating the Arrhythmia Point

PHYSICIAN: Standing
PATIENT: Seated or supine

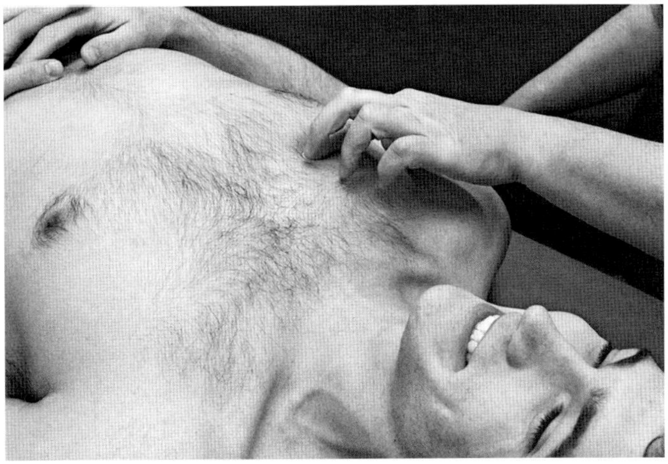

STEPS 1 – 2

1. Palpate the lower right anterior chest wall with your right hand
2. Stimulate the trigger point in a circular fashion with your left hand until the arrhythmia stops and the pain diminishes

---

7. David G. Simons, "Cardiology and Myofascial Trigger Points: Janet G. Travell's Contribution," *Texas Heart Institute Journal* 30, no. 1 (2003): 3–7.

Unwinding the Pericardium

PHYSICIAN: Standing
PATIENT: Supine

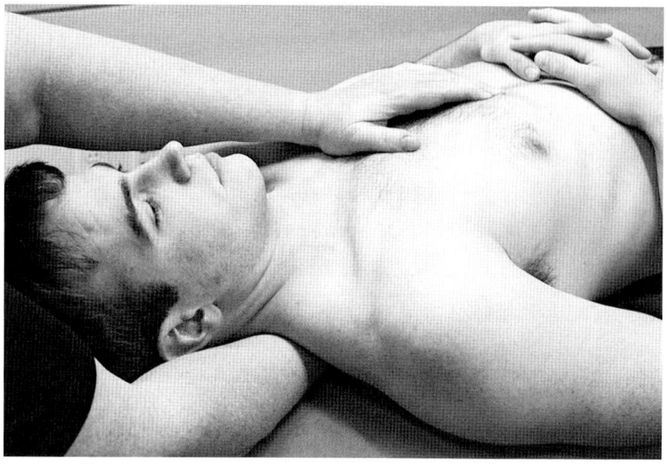

STEPS 1 – 2

1. Place your left hand on the patient's sternum
2. Place your right hand underneath the patient on the thorax opposite your other hand
3. Compress and rotate into the direction of ease usually to the left

The Gastrointestinal System

Fox's Treatment of Gerd

PHYSICIAN: Standing
PATIENT: Supine

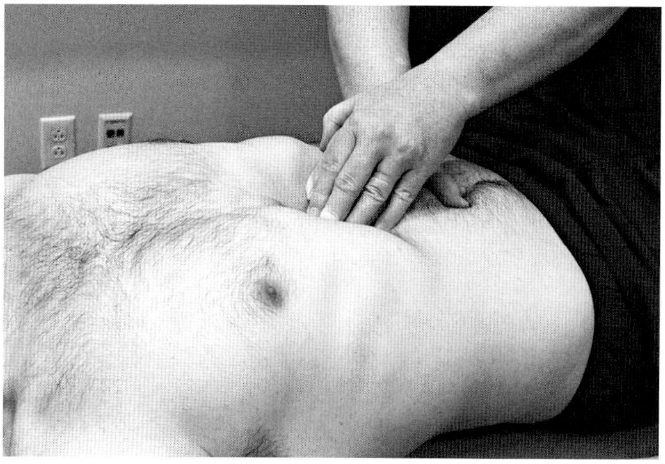

STEPS 1 – 3

1. Place your right hand under the xyphoid process at the central tendon of the crurae
2. Place your left hand on top of your right hand
3. Pull the patient's stomach down

4. Free the crural attachments at L1-L3

Sutherland's Approach to Stomach

PHYSICIAN: Seated
PATIENT: Supine

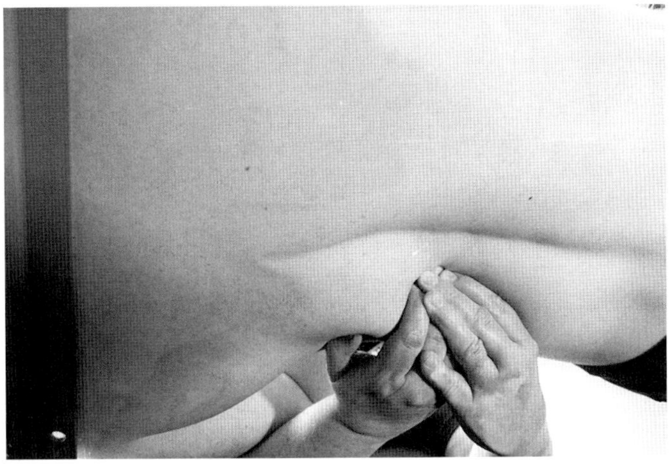

STEPS 1 – 2

1. Use the forefinger of your right hand on the 12th rib (left)
2. Use your left hand behind your right finger to traction inferiorly and laterally until you can feel free and easy movement in the patient's gastroesophageal junction

Still's Stomach Technique

PHYSICIAN: Standing
PATIENT: Right lateral recumbent

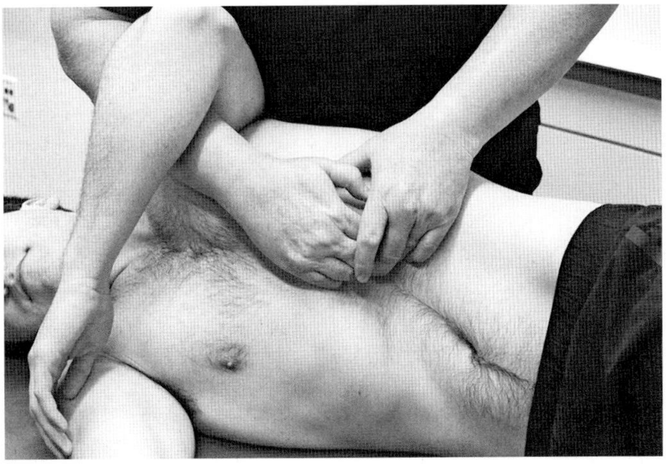

STEPS 1 – 2

1. The physician places one hand over the other and palpates the patient's stomach
2. Using your body weight and arms as long levers, traction the stomach inferiorly and to the left

McConnell's Duodenum Motion with Inhalation Technique

PHYSICIAN: Standing
PATIENT: Kneeling on table in the knee to chest position

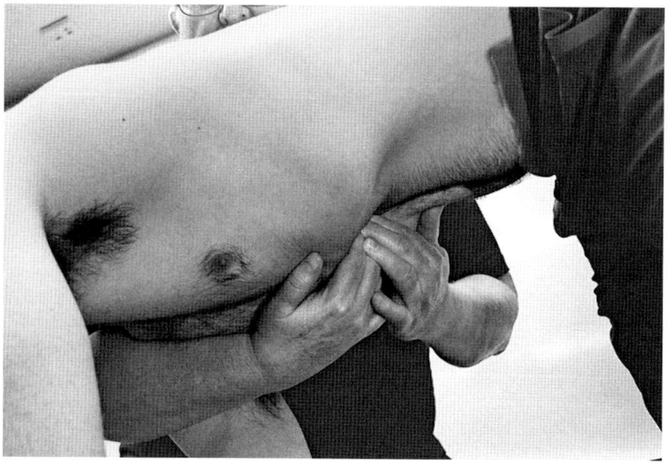

STEPS 1 – 2

1. The physician takes their right hand and places it over the duodenum in the upper right quadrant of the abdomen
2. Place your left hand over your right hand. The physician takes both hands and inhibits and lifts the duodenum toward the ceiling
3. Ask the patient to inhale. This causes the duodenum to descend, and the sides come closer together

Sutherland's Liver Release (Liver Turn) Technique

PHYSICIAN: Seated
PATIENT: Supine

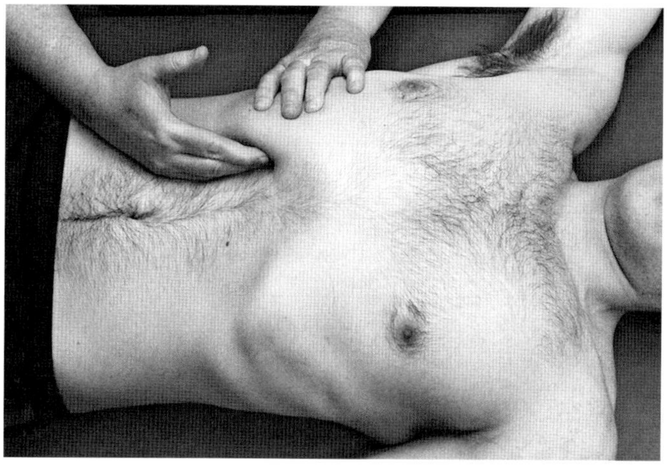

STEPS 1 – 6

1. Ask the patient to bend their knees or place a pillow under the knees
2. Place the fingers of your left hand under their outer ribs and outside of the capsule of the liver. Then observe how the liver moves with breathing and independently

3. Now place your right (lower) hand under the patient's lower ribs
4. The physician's lower right hand is under the costal arch on the outside of the patient's liver capsule.
5. Ask the patient to inhale and hold their breath in
6. Tell the patient, "When you must exhale do so vigorously or force your air all the way out." When the patient exhales the liver goes cephalically, returning freely on its ligaments

Lippincott: That is a procedure called the liver turn. The fingers under the arc forming a fulcrum. The patient is giving you respiratory cooperation. He's doing all the work. You are just assuming a mechanical advantage.

Crow: Now when anybody has been involved in a seated whip-like systemic situation (whiplash) their liver needs to be stirred up. I first see if the diaphragm is working. If the liver is enlarged in the cardiac liver lung mechanism, you'll feel it. It will be out in the epigastrium.

The liver is an encapsulated organ, and a heavy organ with multiple attachments to the diaphragm. So in a car accident the liver goes further than the hollow viscous (intestines) and often will cause pain in the mid back or painful respirations.

It is a good idea to look at the liver when someone has a chronic systemic problem. You do so automatically with a woman in the first trimester of pregnancy. You also see the lifting of the hepatic flexure of the colon. This is also part of the treatment of the 'fascial drag on the abdomen.'

I had heard several of the older doctors talk about using the liver turn or flip in pregnant women who have hyperemesis gravid arum or just plain morning sickness. I have personally used the technique in pregnant women with mixed results, and other patients with intractable vomiting such as occurs after chemotherapy with mixed results, and vomiting after surgery (as long as it wasn't gallbladder) to help calm down the nausea.

Sutherland's Biliary Drainage Technique

PHYSICIAN: Standing
PATIENT: Seated

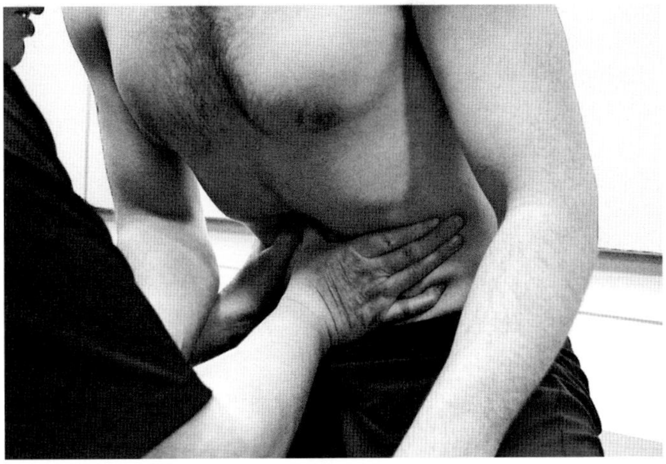

STEPS 1 – 3

1. Place your right thumb firmly in the patients right hypochondrium
2. Ask the patient to lean slightly forward and rotate their body to the left. This causes the thumb to advance further toward the inferior surface of the liver
3. Ask the patient to "suck in your guts." This drains the bile passages and the pancreatic duct

SMALL INTESTINE

The mesentery becomes congested and in cases of small bowel obstruction a mesenteric lift often allows an obstruction to resolve without surgery.

Mesenteric Lift Technique

PHYSICIAN: Standing
PATIENT: Supine

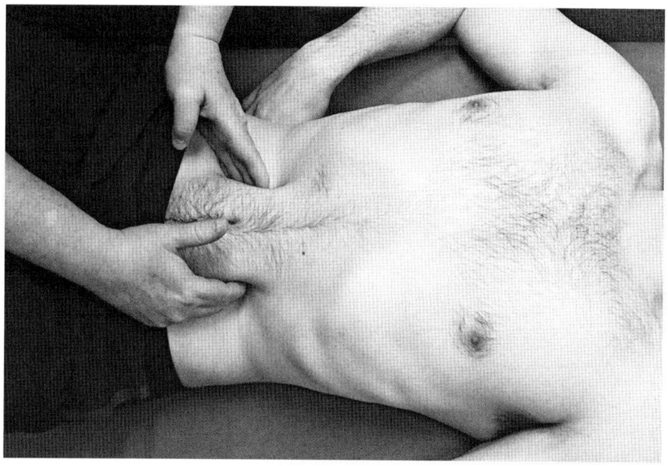

STEPS 1 – 4

1. The physician places their left fingers at the edge of the abdomen and the patient's bowel is gently taken at right angles towards its mesenteric root attachments (which are near the umbilicus) and to the extent allowed by its motion barrier
2. Gentle tension is applied to the attachments with your right fingertips lifting the gut
3. Ask the patient to take shallow breaths to use their respiratory force to drain the bowel and stimulate the lymphatics
4. Repeat 2-3 times

Sigmoid Flexure Technique

PHYSICIAN: Standing
PATIENT: Supine

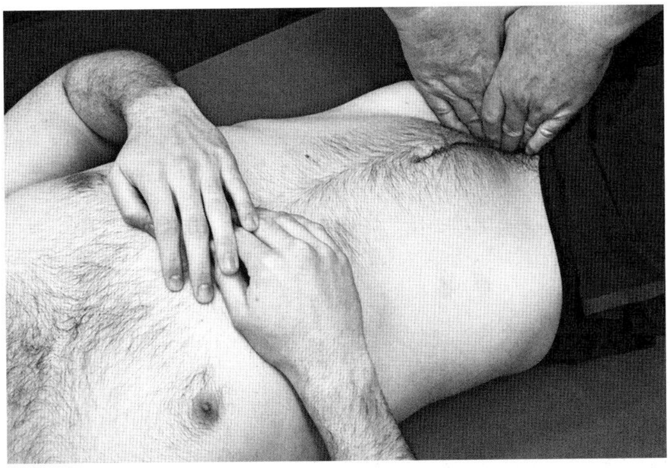

STEP 1

Lift and hold the sigmoid flexure or raise the cecum from the pelvic bowl. The fingers of one hand are introduced close to the ilium and are supported and slowly lifted by the other hand. This requires the use of a keen, tactile sense and the ability to employ the various fingers as needed to restore proper peristalsis, circulation or drainage

The Genitourinary System

Kidney Lift

PHYSICIAN: Standing beside the patient just below their waist
PATIENT: Supine

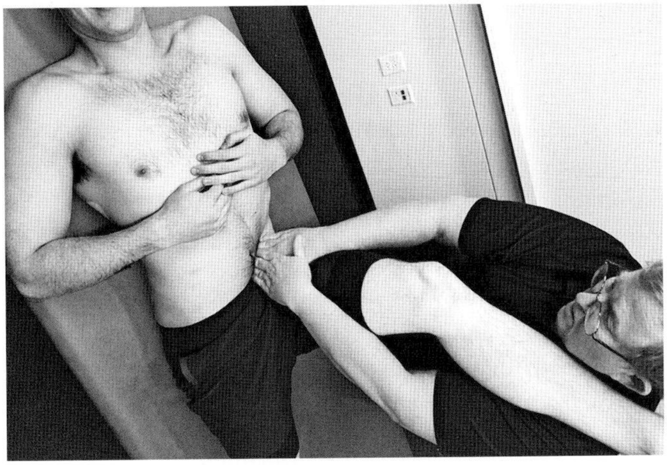

STEPS 1 – 4

1. Place the patient's left leg on your shoulder

2. Place one of your hands on top of the other on the patient's lower abdomen below the kidney trying to touch the psoas muscle
3. Have the patient take a deep breath and exhale fully
4. Slide the kidney up

HAZZARD'S COMMENTS ON THE KIDNEY

Hazzard: Treatment is directed to gain vaso-motor control and is made directly upon the vaso-motor innervation of the kidneys. This consists of spinal stimulation from the 6th thoracic to the 2nd lumbar, for the vaso-motor fibers to the kidneys originating in this spinal area. This includes the whole splanchnic area. As stimulation over the central ends of the splanchnics and of the great sciatic is known to cause renal constriction, it is well to carry this spinal stimulation down over the origin of the sciatic nerve, including the 4th and 5th lumbar and the upper three sacral nerves.

Hazzard's Kidney Technique

PHYSICIAN: Standing
PATIENT: Supine

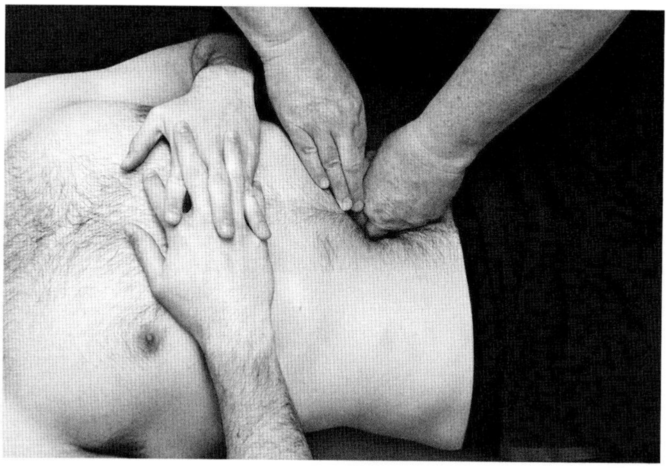

STEPS 1 – 3

1. The physician applies deep pressure with the fingertips of both hands, with a spreading motion, at the umbilicus and about two inches above it. This stimulates the peritoneal nerve centers said to exist at each side of the umbilicus
2. Next the fingers are bent at the metacarpo-phalangeal knuckles, making a fulcrum of the latter upon the table. The cushions of the fingers are pressed deep into the abdominal tissue, the weight of the patient is raised by the fingers thus applied, and the tissues are drawn laterally away from the midline (paraspinal inhibition)
3. Quick repetition of this movement a number of times

Sutherland's Pelvic Lift

PHYSICIAN: Standing in front of the patient
PATIENT: Lying on their right side

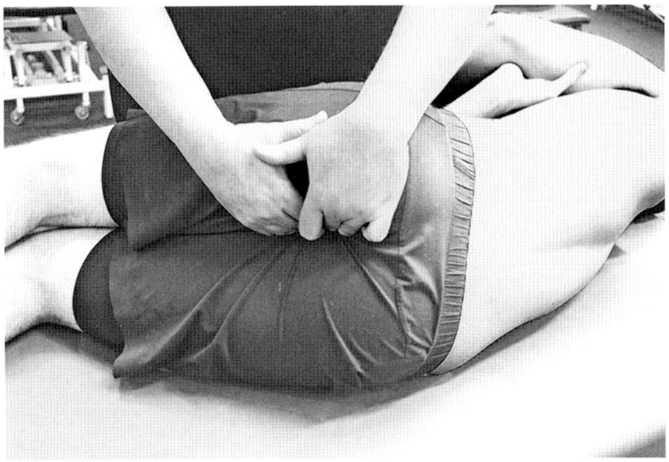

STEPS 1 – 6

1. Ask the patient to bring their thighs to a position in which the floor of their pelvis is most relaxed, either straight or flexed
2. Place the tips of your fingers medial to the left ischial tuberosity and advance them upward in the fascia between the ischial tuberosity and the rectum while the patient exhales
3. During the patient's inhalation your right fingers are held gently, but firmly, not allowing them to recede
4. Support your right hand with your left hand to allow the fingers to hold more steadily
5. After several cycles of deep respiration the resistance will be felt to diminish suddenly and the tissues spring upward in advance of your fingers
6. Your fingers may be directed cranially and medially or anteriorly toward the cecum, uterus, bladder or prostate for specific effect upon those organs

Lippincott: The fascial connections from the neck to the diaphragm have been mentioned. The direct attachment of the diaphragm to the liver and the connections to the stomach, duodenum, psoas and peritoneum complete a chain embracing the viscera all the way down into the pelvis. Fascial 'drag' has an adverse influence on the support and function of the organs and on the circulation and drainage of the lower half of the body.

The aorta lies against the bodies of the vertebrae and is crossed anteriorly by the crura has a constricting effect upon the aorta, throwing an extra load upon the heart and predisposing to cardiac insufficiency. Dr. Still described this phenomenon with the parable of the goat and the boulder:

> The boulder represented the crura, the path the aorta, and the valves of the heart were the tail, the heels and the whole goat. The goat, finding the boulder in its path backed up and gave it a butt and his tail went up. Not to be outdone the goat backed up further and came a-running and gave the boulder another butt. The goat then backed up further and with a supreme effort gave it another butt and the whole d--- works went up.

11
Women's Health

Wales on Pregnancy

You start with a patient who is pregnant and doesn't know it yet. You firstly need to find this out. The frontus pubis tends to get a little heavier and it turns on the levator ani in pregnancy. Weight makes it a little uncomfortable and the patient doesn't sit comfortably. But they don't complain about that. It's just that while they are sitting there talking to you they are squirming. So there is good reason to pay attention to pelvic mechanics. Standing postural techniques are most useful at this time. By the time a patient is at the end of the first trimester the front of the uterus is beginning to rise up in the pelvis, so you are getting other things happening.

The female pelvis is broader and so the hips are further apart with them standing. So their feet are further apart, and then when they want to balance themselves, they externally rotate their legs for security. This pronates both their feet. Any time you're externally rotated you pronate. That's because it's more comfortable. They aren't always doing it symmetrically.

A lot of women I have met through the years who have painful feet have been the ones who had said their feet began to pain after their children were delivered. I think that is a pretty good comment.

Wales on Postnatal Depression

I've noticed that in post natal depression that the feeling of 'drag' down the neural tube seems to also come up the brain stem and into that third ventricle pituitary area. You obviously want to tend to the patient here. But giving them a lift up there, it seems as if these areas hate any kind of drag. It's very sensitive to any drag in that area. The next time you see a sacrum that is dragging, that's where it's bound to drag. Of course, once the mother has delivered her child, her whole neuroendocrine system has to get out of one functional phase and into another. She's got to start the lactation process. She's got to get her own neuroendocrine system back to normal. Will said that sacral 'sag' is the cause of postnatal, post-partum depression or psychosis.

I had a patient who was going to be hospitalized. Her mother had to go and take care of the baby because she wasn't paying any attention to it. Her mother sent her to me. When she walked up my driveway, she walked as a woman has to walk when she's nine months pregnant. She was still in that position, in that posture, and she didn't really know why she was. She was calm and agreeable, and her sacral sag was clearly there. Of course it drags on the occiput and that mucks up the CSF and the whole mechanism and consequently the person is badly influenced.

A post-partum woman has had relaxing from her endocrine system all during her pregnancy, and so these ligaments are still lax. That's why you get the sacral sag. But this is real sacral sag. It's not just the extension position. You set the situation so the patient's postural co-operation can lift their sacrum into position and the spinal dura will help.

When I did discover it, it accounted for the patient's chief complaint. So what you do in the practice of osteopathy is first to balance the mechanism, whether it's the foot or the knee or the shoulder or the spheno-basilar junction. You use your diagnosis to find the position of easy balance, and hold it in that position while the respiratory cooperation operates to release it. If it doesn't release it, you're going to have to think of other treatment plans, but that is a place to start. The patient is always breathing. If you can establish conditions of easy balance at the place where the strain pattern is focused, the release of that strain is most apt to occur. If it does it you'll know it.

I think Dr. Sutherland said it the best possible way. "Sacral sags and fascial drags make chronic rags."

So if the sacrum has sags in relation to the pelvic bone between the ilia, if it's gone into a position between the ilia in a strained way, it's going to drag on the occiput. Under conditions of trauma in the patient's history I have not been able to lift the sacrum with the occiput. I have also had some difficulty in trying to release the occiput from the sacrum. But lots of times you can release the cranial base by rebalancing the low back pelvic hip ligamentous articular mechanism.

The first thing I do is to check the patient's sacrum. I also think of the low back pelvic hip region as a regional mechanism. Now I don't know how many different ways you use for re-adjusting or re-aligning the sacrum between the ilia, but there is one way that is especially appropriate for this.

The sacrum can turn between the ilia on a transverse axis, so that the base goes forward and the apex comes back, and vice versa. We call this the flexion position, because of the spinal dura mater and its relationship to the occiput. So you have the occiput and sacrum doing something together. It's named for what happens at the spheno-basilar junction, and not for what happens locally there. When the extension position occurs the base comes forward and the apex goes back. When the ligaments have become lax and the patient stands or sits vertical it's not only this. There's 'sag'. Dr. Sutherland calls it 'sacral sag'.

This sag pulls on the spinal dura mater which is non-extensionable. It's an extension of the inner layer of dura mater from the cranium. Therefore, when it does this, it pulls the occiput down into the facets of the atlas and buckles the neck. The remark which Dr. Sutherland made about this particular predicament was that it is the cause of post-partum depression and psychosis. Fortunately, it doesn't happen all the time. But in your practice you may have a patient with this problem. I have and I've been asked to see this or that patient by some friend of the family because the family doctor said if she doesn't come out of this she's going to the psychiatric hospital. When you can release the sacrum they don't have to go to the psychiatric hospital. So this is the tool. The sacrum is suspended beneath two ilia by sacroiliac ligaments. There's not a lot of motion there, but Dr. Still said there was some. The early profession worked accordingly, and of course the anatomy books said the sacroiliac joints were fused in the adult and didn't move. The fluctuation of the cerebral spinal fluid confounded this situation.

What I had to do was simply use osteopathic procedures to get the patient's postural mechanics together, and to get the ligaments at the hip joints and the low back pelvic bowl together. I did treat these. That gave them a lift. Dr. Sutherland was quite emphatic about it. "This postpartum psychosis is just because the venous drainage out of the head isn't efficient. There is depression and the cerebellum is smack down on the roof of the 4th ventricle. Their neck is locked up and their ligaments are lax. Their sacral sag is there holding the occiput down."

As pregnant women get further along in the process, the pelvic bone either rolls forward and the abdomen comes forward, or it's rolling in the other direction and it's just not showing. Then you don't know if the patient is pregnant or not until practically the last moment. So there are these postural mechanics to be considered. These are related to the feet, the hips, the pelvic bone and the thoracolumbar junction, where the line of gravity crosses the sagittal plane.

I have acquired a habit of watching all of my patients, but particularly my pregnant patients when they didn't think I was looking at them. I could see how they stood, how they sat, how they moved and walked when they were simply directing their bodies as their automatic reflexes dictated. Then I could see what I could do to help them to a more comfortable arrangement in their postural mechanics if I saw a stress there.

Crow: The treatments used are Anne Wales' Anterior Sacral Release and the Differential Technique. Freeing up the pelvic floor and the respiratory diaphragm are also important.

Wales on Dysmenorrhea

When I got to the sacrum we covered the differential, but this is also the anterior sacral ilial approach. When I was interning I was often asked by some nurse who was on duty, but who was suffering from dysmenorrhea, if I could make her comfortable enough so she could stay on duty. So I would say 'sure'. I would have the nurse lie prone on the table and I would just put my hand on the dorsum of the sacrum and lean a little bit, and she would get free of her dysmenorrhea. I did not at that time know that I was establishing a state of balance ligamentous tension. I had no concept of the link between the sacrum and the occiput, but I've never forgotten how many times in the past I've been asked to do that. Therefore, I have used this technique in my practice. It is not a thrust technique. But I have had the experience that when I was leaning on the sacrum like this, the ligaments allowed the sacrum to just drop and I got my wrist bones all tangled up.

I've often wondered what I may have done that I didn't realize. That is not as exact a technique as the others, but it is worth a lot to have a variety of ways in which you can deal with the low back pelvic hip mechanism and the sacrum in particular.

Now there are no muscles relating the sacrum to the ilia. You can look at the 'low back pelvic hip' as a ligamentous articular mechanism as a whole. When you look at the muscular system, you see that the opponents of this region are the abdominal and the gluteal musculatures. The line of gravity is in the sagittal plane. It's the coronal plane that's at right angles to it, and it is also in the transverse plane. The thoracolumbar junction is where two of these planes intercept.

You have the respiratory diaphragm with the crura attached to the anterior longitudinal spinal ligament, and the clime and domes of the two halves of the diaphragm are attached to the inside of the rib cage. You have the central tendon of the diaphragm with the pericardium sitting on it. The mediastinal fascia is going up in the midline to the upper thorax and the base of the neck.

12
Pediatrics

Lippincott's Basion Technique

Since we cannot contact the basion directly, this is a procedure to affect the basion-condylar part (B-CP) junction by applying tension on the lining of the posterior cranium. This procedure is applicable to infants and young children. The B-CP junction has a cartilaginous union. This junction is subject to compression and possible twisting or buckling.

PHYSICIAN: Seated behind the patient
PATIENT: Supine

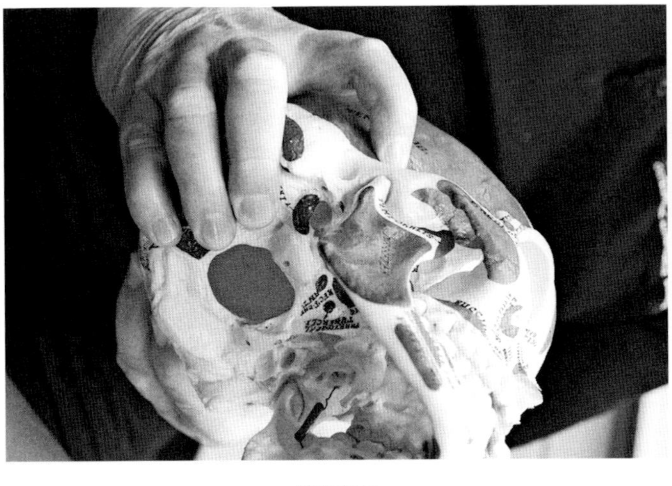

STEP 1

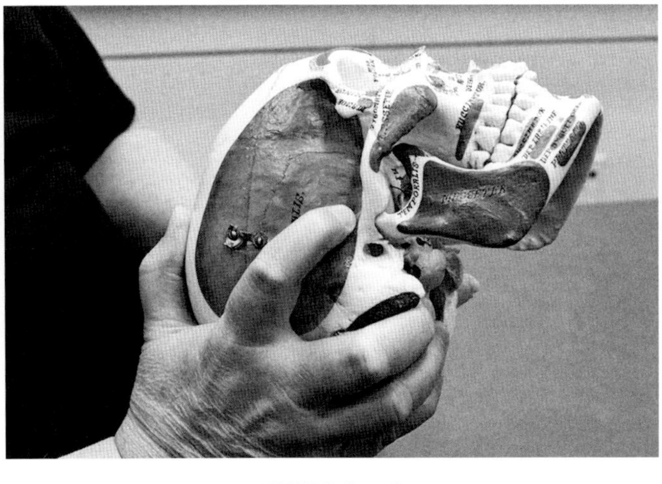

STEPS 2 – 3

1. To release the right condylar part of the patient's skull, the fingers of your right hand are placed beneath their cranium with your right index finger on the inferior surface of their right temporal. Your middle finger is on their occiput, as near the posterior end of their right condylar part as possible. Your 4th finger is under their external occipital protuberance
2. The placement of your left hand (thumb) is on the posterior aspect of their left parietal
3. The fingers of your left hand contact the left side of their head lightly. The intention is to

draw the patient's right condylar part posteriorly, while carrying the eminence anteriorly (toward their left frontal)

4. The tension on the dura moves down the posterior and inferior aspect of the left side of their occiput and across the basion. This is accomplished by the direction of the dural fibers. They sweep down and around across the basion and into the foramen magnum
5. The physician applies this tension steadily and for a prolonged period to get the release. This takes some time and patience. This procedure may be applied to both left and right B-CP junctions
6. After the release of one or both sides, it is imperative that their parietal is returned to its physiological position and function. You have intentionally carried it anterior. You must, with finger pads, carry it posterior
7. Check their parietals and frontals as well as the base to assist their cranium to balance

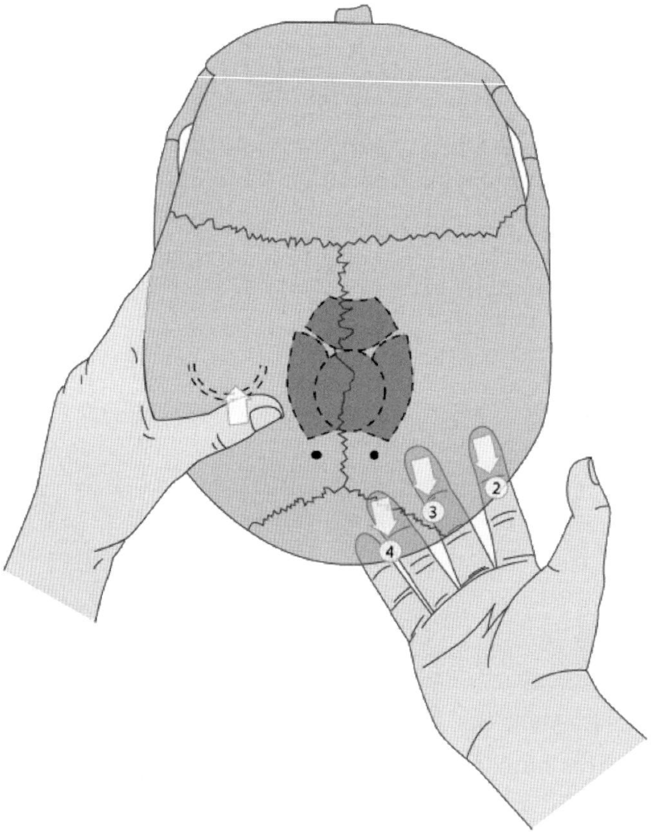

Wales on Treating Children

When it comes to children, if they have been brought by their parents they have their own ideas. Somewhere between the age of two and a half and four, girls as well as boys object to having you put your hands on them. They object to being laid down on the table. They object vigorously, but you can use this as postural co-operation. Once I was treating a lad about the age of eight. He was a handicapped child. His parents brought him and he sat down on the table. So I suddenly had a bright idea. I thought—well, I'll hang on and let him do the work. So I got hold of his innominates, and I got a position that I thought was somewhere near a ligamentous balance. Then I leaned on the table and I held on. He just kept on moving around and working, and he was very successful in decompressing and releasing his pelvic mechanism. He got so much better that he got out of special education and into the mainstream and even the right grade in his school. So I actually thought that he did it. All I had to do was hang on.

With children, you can take hold of the innominates and carry them laterally if you have a parent there to see they don't roll off the table. If they kick and yell, all you have to do is hold the innominates and they'll get their sacrum twisted. Then you hold the ribs laterally and they bellow nicely. They get their diaphragm up and so on. You can thus work with the children who are not disposed to work with you.

When it comes to teenagers I don't know all the answers. I've treated many teenagers beneficially and they have committed to treatment with a condescending attitude. The thing is that many people in their teenage era don't like to be told to go to the doctor by a parent. 'There's nothing wrong with me. I don't know why I'm here' and yet they are here. But you have been given the chief complaint over the telephone by the parent so fortunately you don't have to question them. This is a big help because they don't like to be questioned. I don't know whether it is better if the doctor is a man or when the doctor is a woman. I certainly have been aware of the fact, and not just from boys, that I was a very peculiar doctor anyway. This business of going to an osteopath who would put his or her hands on you was for the birds. You can't put your hands on anybody unless they let you do it.

Wales on Treating the Newborn

You put a clean towel over you and you just put the patient over your shoulder. That way they are prone. You can then treat their backs with your fingertips. You can make the diagnosis and find out how the sacrum is, and whether it is staying up. Gravity is operating to stretch them out, and this little mass that was all bunched up has already done a lot of stretching out. Then you put them on their backs.

I have a little towel or something like that so I can move them around without jarring them. You get your fingertips under their ilia. Your thumb is up under the crest of their ilia and you just take them laterally. The spinal dura mater will release the sacrum.Then I go up and do the same with their ribs and their lower back.

What you have in this human framework, whether it's the mother or the infant, is still the same path. It's just at different stages of development. The first thing you want to be sure of is that the sacrum is free. You have to start with the way your patient is when they come in. Understand that you have a mental picture of how the patient was at the earliest moment you saw them, because there isn't any chance of changing a patient to become an ideal, an absolute symmetrical abstract ideal.

As a physician who practices osteopathy you have to work with things the way they are, and the way they will work in the patient's machinery as they bring themselves to you. You can't impose an abstract pattern on the patient's body. It's going to do its own thing. However, you should understand the ideal or normal, and have it as the pattern in your mind as you right their body.

Wales on Treating Children's Sacrum

For the sacrum in infants and small children, instead of the anterior sacral ilia approach or anything that requires patient cooperation, you've now got the patient small enough to take one innominate in each hand. So you get your thumbs on their anterior superior spine, and you get your fingers around underneath on their tuberosity. So you've got one innominate in each hand, and you take them laterally at the same time. It's not easy to do, but with infants and small children it is possible. Their breathing is sufficient, but usually they will only cooperate by yelling. That really gets their sacral lifted while you have their innominates held back.

13

Dr. Fulford's 'Putting It All Together'

Crow: Dr. Robert Fulford was made somewhat famous by Dr. Andrew Wyle MD, because he was able to help kids with recurrent otitis media. He is also known for his use of the Foredom Percussor to help free fascia. He worked with kids and adults in a treatment sequence that he personally liked to use. That is not to say that he never deviated from it, but this was his way of treating a patient. I had the privilege of working with him at several conferences. However, I am not one of his followers or students who worked with him in his office. Some of his close students could no doubt expand on his treatment sequence.

Dr. Fulford almost always started off treating the lower extremity first. He stated that he usually treated the left leg because in utero it was tucked up and under the right leg. If the leg is turned on the left side you will see problems in the left hip, scapula on the right, distortion of the lumbar spine, and distortion in the left ribs. The skull will be distorted in the parietal bones at the ossification center on the right side, with the right parietal being higher than the left. Also, the left hip and left scapula both will be restricted because they work together fascially. So restriction in one will cause a restriction in the other.

Dr. Fulford stated that congestion builds up in the left tarsal bones in infants. Unless you correct the left foot and tibia in the infant, you cannot correct the deformation in the infant/child's skull.

Fulford's Technique for the Lower Extremity

▶ DIAGNOSIS

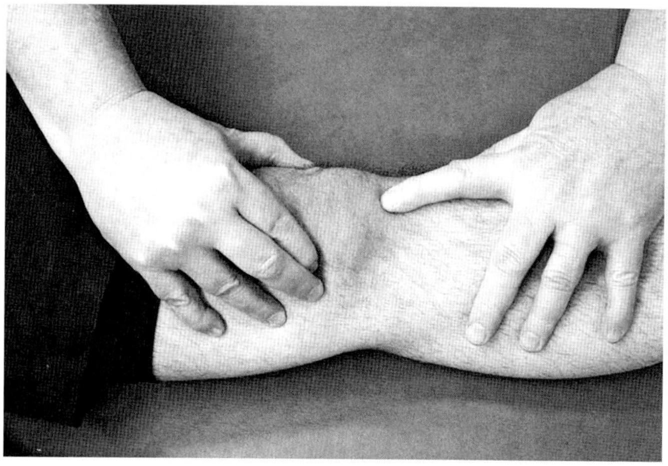

STEPS 1 – 3

1. Take the patient's patella between your thumb and first finger
2. Locate the center of their patella
3. With your other hand place a finger midline on the ridge of their tibia and see if it comes into the midline of the patella

▶ TREATMENT

EXAMPLE: Left leg
PHYSICIAN: Standing facing the patient on the table
PATIENT: Supine

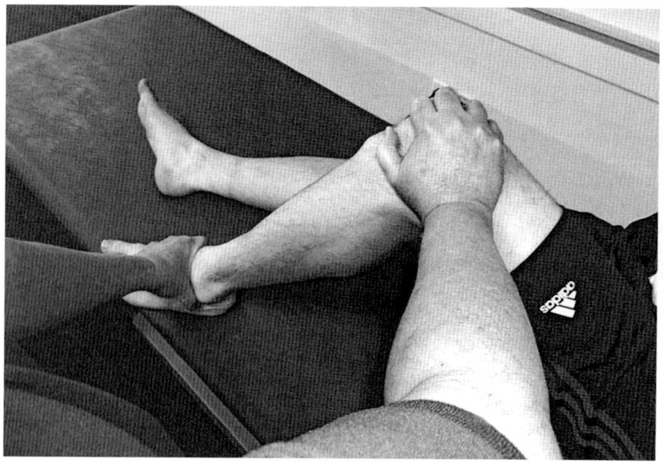

STEPS 1 – 2

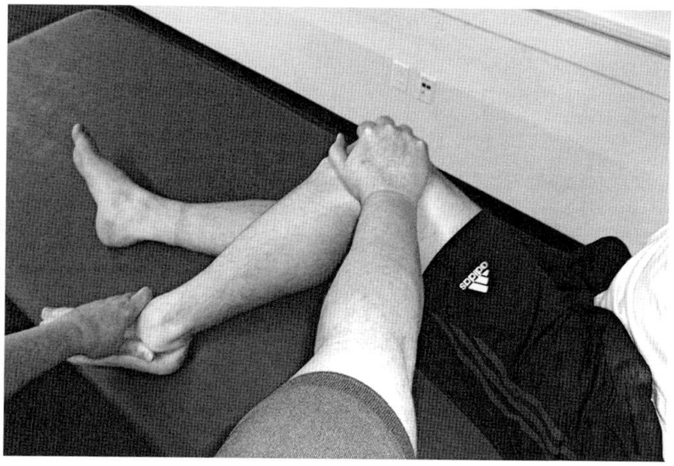

STEPS 3 – 4

1. Place the patient's left foot on the table and place your right hand on their left knee
2. Hold their left foot with your left hand
3. Rotate their left knee inward to the barrier with your right hand
4. As the fascia frees follow the barrier as it loosens until their left hip is free

Crow: Dr. Fulford stated that this treatment left you with a twist in the pelvis. However, he did not immediately treat the sacrum and pelvis until later in the treatment sequence.

SHOCK OR TRAUMA RELEASE

Crow: Any person who has had any kind of trauma or shock will have a shock point or trauma point in the chest region of the body. Dr. Fulford stated that the recess was on the left side of the sternum at about the level of T6 and about the size of your little finger. He believed that this shock or trauma point can come about from either an accident, surgery or emotional trauma. He stated that he learned about this from the German psychiatrist Wilhelm Reich. "As you examine the patient you have to place your left hand on the left side of the chest wall on the anterior aspect of the body. This is the sensory side of the body. On the level of the 6th rib on the left side there is a trauma point. It is a little divot."

He related a story at multiple conferences about a young man, 24, who had hit his head when diving into the river. He had use of his hands, but no use of his legs. When you touched his legs, they would quiver. He had been through the standard medical work-up. The patient had been told that he had a "disturbance in the cervical part of his spinal cord." Dr. Fulford stated that the only thing he did on the first visit was to take the shock out of the patient's body. When the patient took his first deep breath, he stated "That's what I've been telling them all the time. It felt like something was pressing on my chest. It felt like an elephant's foot standing there." On the next visit, Dr. Fulford was able to take the patient's leg in any direction he wanted. He stated that the patient made about an 80% recovery.

Treatment of the Trauma or Shock Point

PHYSICIAN: Stand on the left side of a male and stand on the right side of the female
PATIENT: Supine

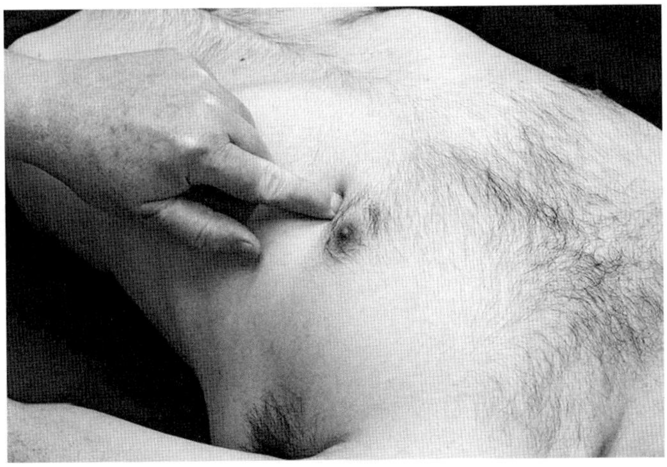

STEPS 1 – 4

1. Using the pads of your fingers place your little finger on the tip of the xiphoid process of their sternum and your other little finger in their umbilicus
2. As the patient breathes out take the slack out of the linea alba and hold while the patient breathes in

3. You then apply a little more pressure on the xiphoid process end
4. As it frees you might be down to the level of the abdominal aorta in a thin patient. If you have not completely released the tissue, then draw your hands down to the side of their aorta

To take the shock out of the babies and infants up to age one, place your hand above the vertex of their head. The other hand is on their xiphoid process.

Fulford's Technique for the OA and Atlas / Axis Release

PHYSICIAN: Standing on the right side of the patient
PATIENT: Supine

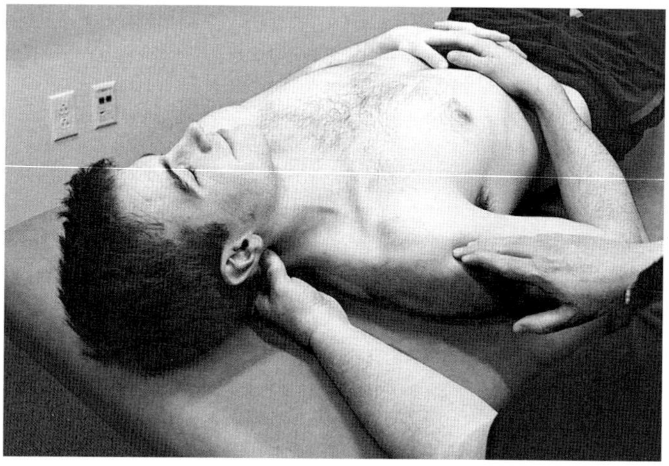

STEPS 1 – 3

1. Place the fingers of your right hand over their right deltoid recess (bursa) or use a Foredom Percussor
2. Place your left hand on top their head or at their OA junction
3. Pump the patient's deltoid bursa on the right rapidly until their OA releases

Fulford's Technique for the Sphenoid and Frontal Bone

PHYSICIAN: Standing on the left side of the patient
PATIENT: Supine

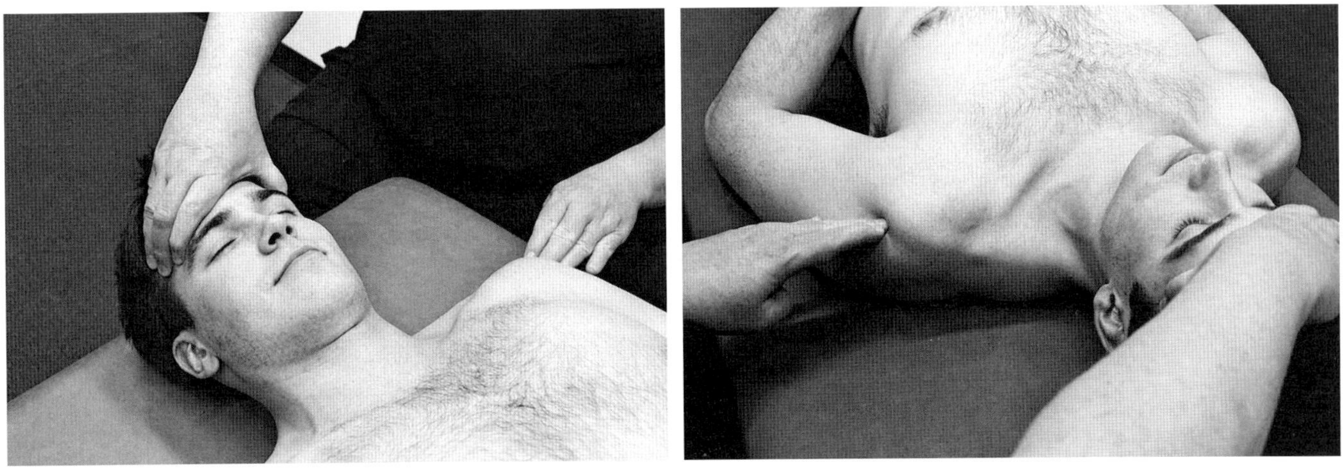

STEPS 1 – 3

1. Place the fingers of your left hand over their left deltoid recess (bursa) or use a Foredom Percussor
2. Place your right hand over the frontals and wings of the patient's sphenoid
3. Pump their deltoid bursa on the left rapidly until their sphenoid and frontals release

Fulford's Technique for the Pelvis – Part 1

PHYSICIAN: Standing beside the patient
PATIENT: Prone

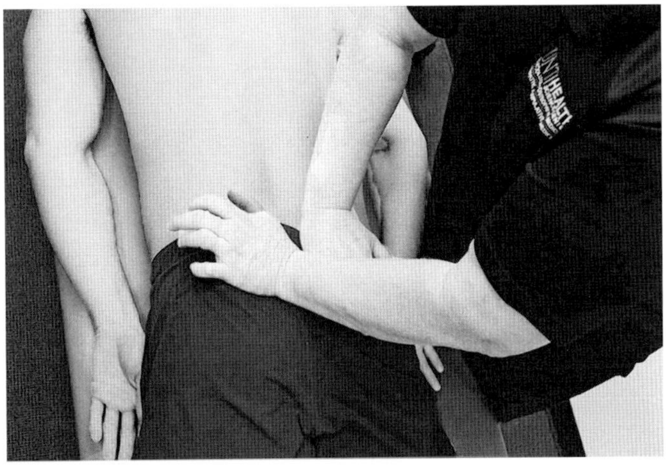

STEPS 1 – 4

1. Place your palms on the patient's SI joints bilaterally
2. Press down on each side
3. On the tight side apply more pressure and lock it

4. With your opposite hand pump the patient's SI joint until the tight side releases. Alternatively use the Foredom Percussor on the loose SI joint

Fulford's Technique for the Pelvis – Part 2

PHYSICIAN: Standing beside the patient
PATIENT: Prone

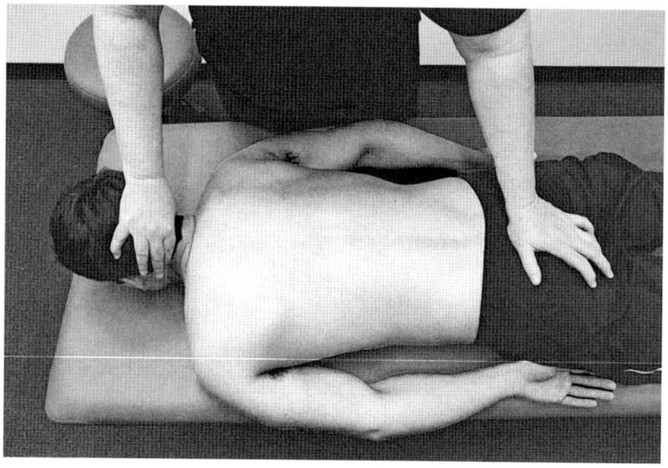

STEPS 1 – 3

1. Place your right hand on the base of the patient's occiput
2. Place your left hand on their sacrum
3. Stabilize their head and gently pump their sacrum. This straightens out the meninges along their spinal cord

Fulford's Technique for the Scapula and Pelvis

▶ DIAGNOSIS:

PHYSICIAN: Standing behind the patient
PATIENT: Seated

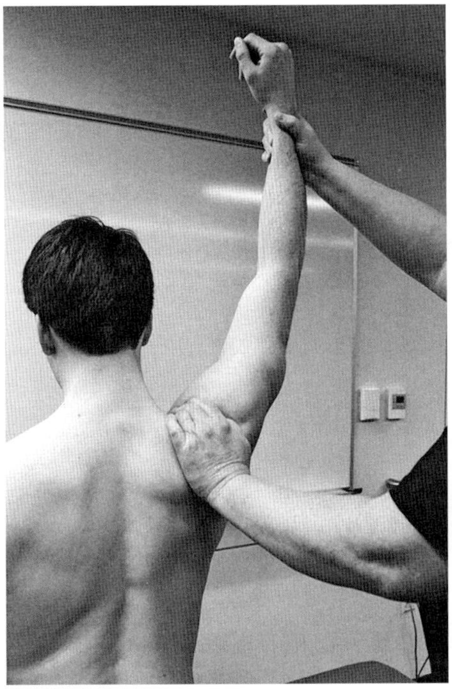

STEPS 1 – 3

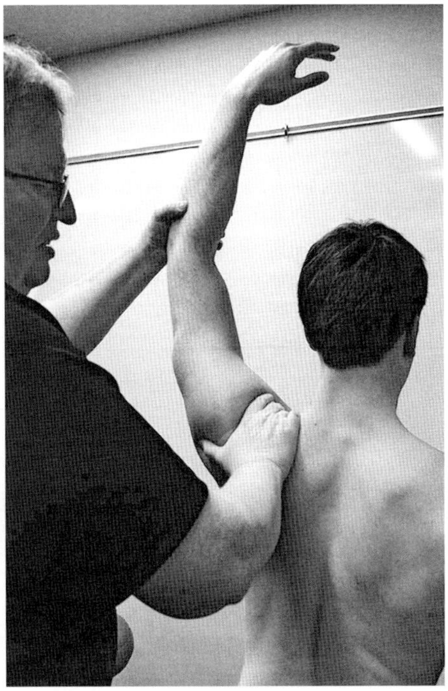

STEPS 4 – 6

1. Ask the patient to raise both their arms at a 90 degree angle to their body
2. Place your left hand on their right shoulder and with your right hand raise their right arm straight up and over their head. Note if there is a sudden stop or slowing
3. Bring their right arm back down to 90 degrees
4. Place your right hand on their left shoulder and with your left hand raise their left arm straight up over their head. Note if there is a sudden stop or slowing
5. Bring their left arm back down to 90 degrees
6. If there is a restriction on either side there will be a sternal restriction noted

▶ TREATMENT:

PHYSICIAN: Standing
PATIENT: Supine

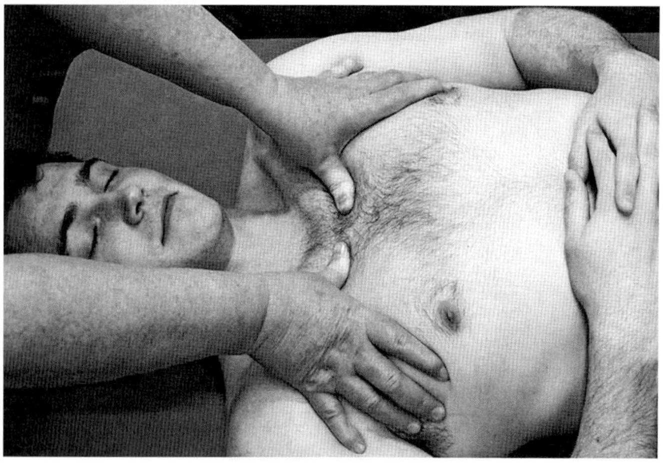

STEP 1

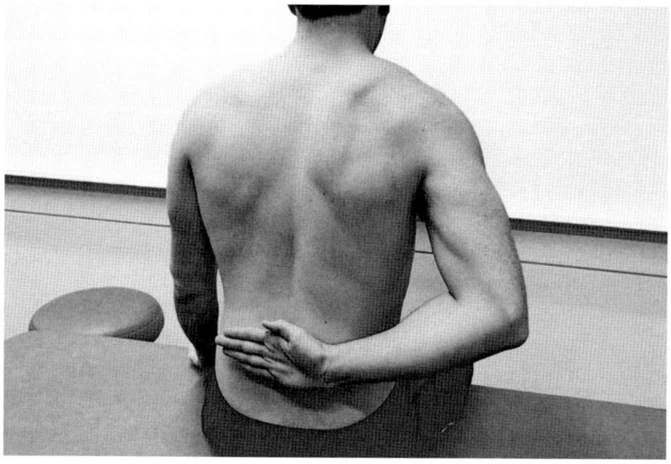

STEP 3

1. Place your thumbs on each side of their sternal angle (manubrium and body of the sternum) and rock back and forth
2. Ask the patient to sit up
3. Place the diagnosed dysfunctional arm behind the patient's back with the palm out. This locks down their clavicle on that side

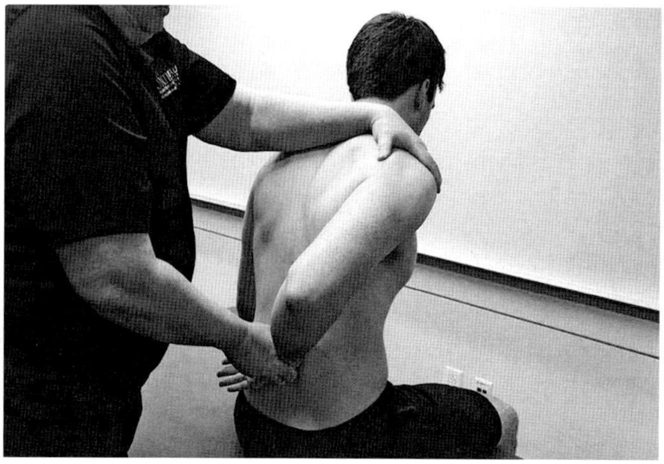

STEPS 4 – 5

4. Place your hand on the dysfunctional shoulder
5. Take the patient's hand from around their back and swing it up and around and back down

Fulford's Falx and Tentorium Release

PHYSICIAN: Standing
PATIENT: Seated

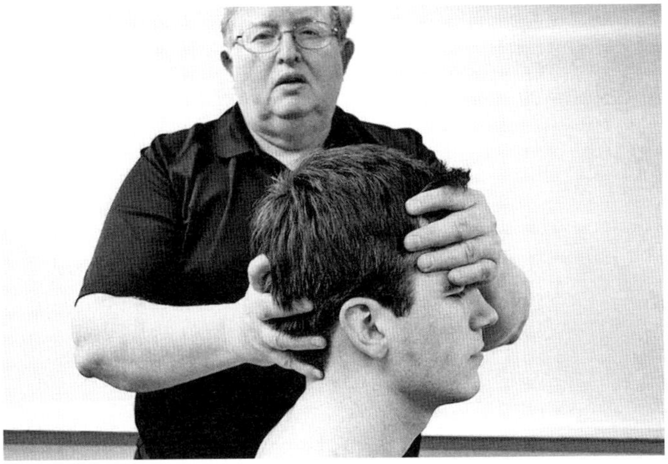

STEP 1

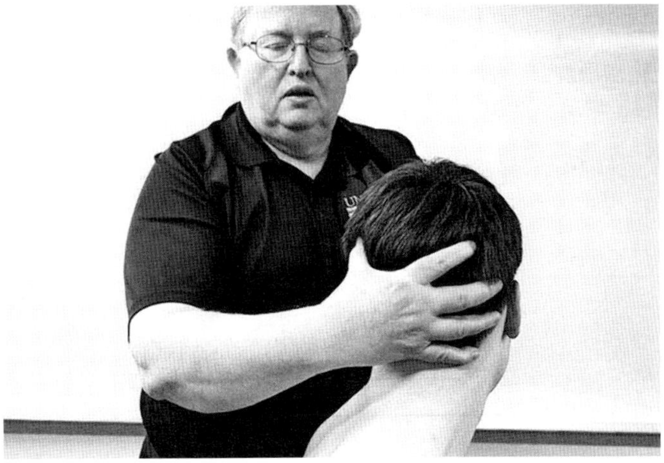

STEP 2

1. Place your left hand on the midline on the frontal bone and your right hand on the midline of the occiput
2. The physician rotates the head to the left until it reaches its barrier. This stretches the membranes until they balance themselves out

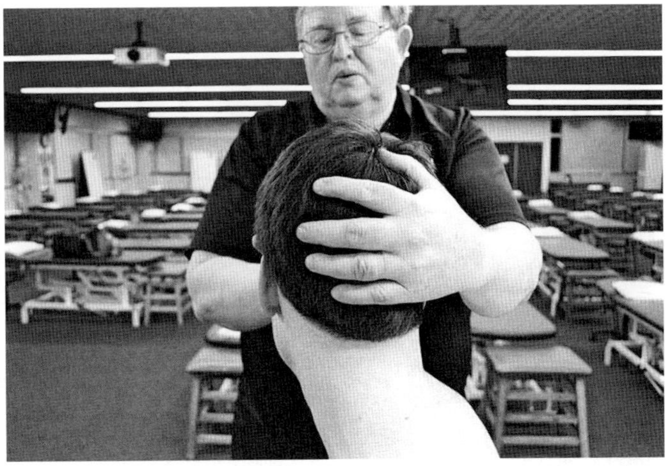

STEP 3

3. Reverse your hands so the right hand is on the frontal and the left hand posterior. Turn the head to the right shoulder
4. This should release the cranium

General Index

A

abdominal palpation, Hazzard's, 198
acromio-clavicular ligament, 175
acute asthma, tender point treatment, 212–213
adaptation, 3
alignment
  versus lesion reduction, 14
  versus pathology relief, 12
ankle mortise, 168
  as fulcrum, 168
  origin of stability, 158
  as universal joint, 163
ankle sprains technique, Crow's, 167
ankylosis, 13
anterior cervical fascia technique, 209
anterior cervical technique, William West's, 47–48
anterior innominate rotation
  Sutherland's diagnosis, 139
  Sutherland's treatment, 140–141
anterior longitudinal spinal ligament, crura attachments, 217
anterior sacral release technique, Wales', 233
anterior sacroiliac technique, Wales', 134–135
anterior spinous ligament, 118
anterior superior iliac spine, 147
approximation lesions, 117
arcuate ligaments, 113
arrhythmia trigger point technique, 219
arterial blood, as master tissue, 20
arterial integrity, role in health, 16
arterial obstruction, 20
arthritis, upper extremity, 175
articular dysfunction, causes of, 8
articular pillars, 53, 62
articular processes, 57, 58
asthma
  low threshold of tolerance in, 211
  manipulative treatment of, 210
  treatment of acute, 212–213
  Wales on, 211–212
asthma technique, 1938 Yearbook, 210–211
atlas, 41
  articular pits, 59
  articular processes, 50
  divergence, 42
  stabilization techniques, 42–43
atlas dislocation, eye problems and, 203
atlas techniques
  Hazzard #1, 49
  Hazzard #2, 50–51
  Hazzard #3, 51–52
atlas/axis release technique, Fulford's, 242
atonized muscle, 17
atony, of ligaments, 18
atrial fibrillation, conversion with vapocoolant spray, 219
atrophic fibrotic musculature, 11
atrophy, 9
auscultation, abdominal, 198, 199
auto-regulation, 2
autopsy proof, 22
axon degeneration, 20

B

backing sacrum into the garage, 135

balance point, 31, 59, 60, 159
  cervical flexion dysfunction, 57
balanced ligamentous tension, 132, 135, 233
balanced ligamentous tension (BLT) techniques, 45
balanced position, 31
Barber, Elmer, 197
  on duration of eye treatment, 203
  eye infection treatment, 200
  eye treatment, 202–203
  general neck treatment, 201–202
  lacrimal duct treatment, 203
  lung technique #1, 213–214
  lung technique #2, 214
  lung technique #3, 214–215
  lung technique #4, 215
  Osteopathy Complete, 198
  on visceral manipulation, 198
base spread technique, Anne Wales, 42–43
basion technique, Lippincott's, 235–236
biliary drainage technique, Sutherland's, 223–224
biological law, 5
Blackman, Elliott, occiput technique, 40–41
bladder, ptosis, 197
body, as vital mechanism, 19
body distortions, 16
bone, as support tissue, 9
bony contact theory, 52
bony lesions, leading to ligamentous lesions, 18
bootjack technique, Wales', 165–166
brachial neuralgia, 175
brachial neuritis, 175
bunion technique, 166
bunions, 164
Burns, Louisa, 8

C

C1/C2 restriction, 207
  Miller technique for, 206–207
C3 dysfunction
  West's anterior cervical technique, 47
  West's lateral cervical technique, 45–46
C3 posterior right lesion, 53
C3 right anterior lesion, 55
C3 rotation left, 60
C3 side-bent left, 60
C4 on C5, 63
calcaneus, 162
callouses, 164
capsular ligaments, 10, 113
  balancing tension in, 56
cardiovascular system techniques, 219–220
  arrhythmia trigger point, 219
  pericardium unwinding, 220
carpal tunnel syndrome, 175
cell, as inherent structural/functional unit, 3
central motor neuron, 21
cerebral palsy, roots of, 43
cerebro-spinal fluid, 129
cervical curve, anterior convexity, 56
cervical extension dysfunction techniques, 57–58
cervical flexion dysfunction techniques, 57
cervical lesions
  anterior lesions, 52
  flexion lesion, 52
  lateral lesions, 52
  multidirectional potentials, 52
cervical ligamentous articular strains, 56
cervical region techniques, 45
  Anne Wales cervical vertebrae technique, 60–61
  Crow's lower cervicals technique, 63
  Crow's OA and upper cervical techniques, 62
  Ernest Eckford Tucker cervicals, 52
  Hazzard's atlas technique #1, 49
  Hazzard's atlas technique #2, 50–51
  Hazzard's atlas technique #3, 51–52
  Hazzard's cervical technique, 48
  Sutherland's cervical extension dysfunction techniques, 57–58
  Sutherland's cervical flexion dysfunction techniques, 57
  Sutherland's cervical rotation side-bending dysfunction techniques, 58–59
  Sutherland's cervicals, 56
  Sutherland's condylo-atlantal dysfunctions, 59–60
  Tucker anterior cervicals, 55–56
  Tucker posterior cervicals, 53–54
  William West anterior cervical technique, 47–48
  William West lateral cervical technique, 45–46
  William West scalene technique, 46–47
cervical rotation side-bending dysfunction techniques, 58–59
cervical vertebrae technique, Anne Wales', 60–61
chemotherapy, liver turn technique after, 223
children, Wales on treating, 236–237
Chopart's joint, 163
chronic cough, hyoid relationship to, 208
chronic cough hyoid technique, 207
chronic disease, visceral treatment in, 199
cicatricial tissues, 10
cisterna chyli, 112
clavicle
  as strut, 175
  warp lesions, 176

clavice technique
- Sutherland's, 177
- Tucker's, 176–177
- Wales' #2, 179
- Wales' depressed clavicle technique, 178

clinical proof, 22
coccygeal ligaments, 146
coccyx technique, Wales', 146
Cochrane, Dr., foot exercise, 177
Colley's fracture, 175
common cold, 91
compensation, 19
composite lesions, 18, 21
- examples, 18–19

condylo-atlantal dysfunctions, 59–60
configuration, 6
coracoid processes, caution, 72
cork screw movement, 102, 103
corkscrew lumbar technique, 124–125
corns, 163, 164
coronoid process, 187
correction
- directing force of, 28
- principles, 28–30

corrective technique
- focusing on lower dorsals, 68
- principles, 33–34
- for side-bending, 69
- upper dorsals, 68

costo-central articulation, 89
cracking, cautions in cervical techniques, 54
Cranial Academy, 45
cranial bones, 129
cranial bowl, link to pelvic bowl, 32
cranial concepts, Dr. Still and, 198
cranial manipulation, limits of, 45
cranial nerve, 12th, 43
cranial vertebral junction, 61
cranio-cervical junction, as tension spring, 61
Crow, Dr.
- acute asthma treatment, 212–213
- alternate pubic symphysis technique, 143
- ankle sprains technique, 167
- on Dr. Fulford's techniques, 239
- lower cervical technique, 63
- on Miller technique, 207
- on Muncie technique, 206
- OA and upper cervical technique, 62
- on Sutherland's pubic symphysis technique, 142
- on Wales pelvic fascial release technique, 133

crura, 112, 229
- locking on aorta, 217

crurae, 113
cuboid bone, 169
cuneiform bone, 169, 170
- dropping, 165

D

deafness, Muncie technique for catarrhal, 205
Deason, Wilborn J., 1
degenerative process, 21
density, 6
depressed clavicle technique, Wales', 178
depression, postnatal, 231–232
deviation, 16
diagnosis
- bicipital tendon, 183
- differential for bicipital tendon, 183
- femur and hip dysfunctions, 147–148
- first and second ribs, 85–86
- as first step in osteopathy, 23
- floating rib dysfunctions, 114
- hip dysfunction, 149, 152
- lower extremity, 240
- osteopathic lesions, 8–10
- palpation in, 7
- rib lesions, 102
- sacral respiratory dysfunction, 130
- scapula and pelvis technique, 245–246
- tibiofemoral, 156
- treatable, 12–14

diaphragm, 32
- anatomy and physiology, 216
- attachment to liver, 229
- crura of, 113
- fascial drag and, 217
- movements, 127
- *versus* primary respiratory mechanism, 129
- role in ventral body function, 199
- Sutherland's release technique, 216–217
- Wales on, 217–218
- Wales on fascial drag and, 217

diaphragm release technique, Sutherland's, 216–217
diaphragmatic atony, 199
diaphragmatic breathing, 79
diaphragmatic lift technique, 216
differential diagnosis, bicipital tendon, 183
differential gears analogy, 132
differential technique, 233
- sacrum and pelvis, 131–133

differentiation
 of cells, 3
 and proneness to failure, 3
"dig on," 198
digastric muscle, 206
direct action technique, 33
direction of ease, 31
disease
 causes of, 8
 micro-organic theory of, 4
 predisposing factors, 7
disease causes, osteopathic interpretation, 14
disease processes, osteopathic interpretation, 14
disease-fear, 27
disengagement method, 33
displacement, complete, 16
distraction techniques, 60
dorsal region movements, 66–69
drag, postnatal depression and, 231
dropped navicular/cuneiform technique, Wales', 170
duodenum motion with inhalation technique, 222
Dupuytren's contracture, 175
dural membranes, 129
Dutch yoke analogy, 175
dysfunctions
 first and second ribs, 86
 floating ribs, 113
 Sutherland on rib, 89
dysmenorrhea, Wales on, 233–234

E

edema, 9, 10
eighth rib elevated on right, 104
elastic ligaments, 10
elasticity, 6
elbow technique, Wales', 190–191
emphysema, 212
engine wiping, 200
environmental influences, as etiological factor, 16
erector spinae muscles, 69
 release technique, 79–80
etiology
 inherited and environmental influences, 16
 osteopathic concept, 5–8, 14
eustachian tube dysfunction, Muncie technique for, 205–206
exhalation, association with extension/internal rotation, 59
experimental proof, 22
extension, 13, 14
 association with exhalation, 59
 respiratory, 129
 sacral dysfunction, 130
external hip rotation technique #1, Sutherland's, 151
external hip rotation technique #2, Sutherland's, 153
external humerus rotation technique, Sutherland's, 182
external rotation, association with inhalation, 59
eye infection treatments, 200–201
eye techniques, Barber's, 200–203

F

falx, 61
falx and tentorium release, Fulford's, 247
fascia, 200
 roles, 200
 strain in, 31
fascia drags, 200
fascial drag
 on abdomen, 223
 diaphragm and, 217
fascial envelopes, 32
feet
 Anne Wales on, 163–164
 prehensile in children, 164
femur, Tucker on treating, 147–148
femur and hip technique, Tucker's, 148–149
fibroblastic infiltration, 10
fibrosis, 10
fibrotic musculature, 10–11
fibula and interosseous membrane release technique, 168
fibula technique, Wales', 158–159
first and second rib technique, Wales', 91–92
first rib, left, 82–83, 85
first rib supine technique, 85
first rib technique
 Sutherland's, 89–90
 Tucker's, 86
 Tucker's #2, 88
 West's #1, 82–83
 West's #2, 84
 West's supine, 85
fixation, 13
 of joints, 11
flexion, 13
 association with inhalation, 49
 respiratory, 129
 sacral dysfunction, 130
flexion lesions, in thoracic region, 65
floating ribs 11/12 technique
 Sutherland's, 111
 Tucker's, 113–114, 114–115
 Wales', 111–113

floating ribs dysfunctions, 113
flu, 91
fluid, tissue needs, 200
foot, as ligamentous articular mechanism, 163
foot exercise, Dr. Cochrane's, 172
foot pain, origins in leg, 163
foot pronation, 165
foot technique, Sutherland's, 171
foramen magnum, 41, 42, 43
  deformation, 43
forearm, osteopathic concepts, 187
fourth metatarsal phalangeal junction, 165
fourth right rib, 100
fourth to tenth rib technique, Sutherland's, 106
Fox, John, 45
  GERD treatment technique, 220
freedom of motion, palpating for, 75
fulcrum leverage, 30, 31, 54
  ankle mortise, 168
  in thoracic spine, 65
Fulford, Robert
  falx and tentorium release, 247
  lower extremity technique, 240
  lower extremity treatment rationale, 239
  OA and atlas/axis release technique, 242
  pelvis technique #1, 243–244
  pelvis technique #2, 244
  scapula and pelvis technique, 245–246
  shock or trauma release treatments, 241–242
  sphenoid and frontal bone technique, 243
  treatment sequences, 239
function
  differentiated/specialized, 1
  structure as determinant of, 1–5, 6
functional relationship, 3

G

Gamble, Harry W., 210
gastrointestinal system techniques, 22–225
  John Fox's GERD treatment, 220
  McConnell's duodenum motion with inhalation technique, 22
  mesenteric lift technique, 224
  sigmoid flexure technique, 225
  Still's stomach technique, 221
  Sutherland's biliary drainage technique, 223–224
  Sutherland's liver release technique, 222–223
  Sutherland's stomach approach, 221
geniohyoid, 206
genitourinary system techniques, 215–219
  Hazzard kidney technique, 226
  kidney lift technique, 225–226
  Sutherland's pelvic lift, 229
  Sutherland's psoas technique #1, 227–228
  Sutherland's psoas technique #2, 228
  ureter and psoas muscle relationship, 227
gentle technique, 30
GERD treatment technique, 220
goat and boulder parable, 229
greater trochanter, 147, 155
  arc abnormalities, 147
grippe, 91

H

habit lesions, 28
hand, osteopathic concepts, 187, 191
hand and wrist technique, Sutherland's, 192
hand positioning, in visceral manipulation, 198
Hazzard, Charles
  abdominal palpation contributions, 198
  atlas technique #1, 49
  atlas technique #2, 50–51
  atlas technique #3, 51–52
  cervical technique, 48
  kidney comments, 226
  kidney technique, 226
  Practice and Applied Therapeutics of Applied Osteopathy (1905), 199
  rib technique, 96–97
  rib technique for ribs 3 to 10 seated, 98–100
  rib technique for ribs 3 to 10 side lying, 100
  on visceral manipulation, 198–199
head techniques, 35, 200
  Anne Wales base spread, 42–43
  Anne Wales occiput technique, 39–40
  Brooks Walker and Elliott Blackman occiput technique, 40–41
  chronic cough hyoid technique, 207
  eustachian tube dysfunction, 205–206
  eye infection, 200–203
  intranasal technique, 204
  Miller technique, 206–207
  Muncie technique, 205–206
  OA release (1938 yearbook), 38–39
  Sutherland's anterior cervical fascia technique, 209
  Tucker technique for posterior OA, 35–36
health
  and functional relationship, 3
  role of artery and nervous system in, 16

heart lung complex, pericardium and, 127
heel lift therapy, contraindications, 172
hepatic flexure, 223
hepatic flexure of colon, 127
hip dislocation, 147
hip dysfunction
  Sutherland's diagnosis, 149
  Sutherland's diagnosis #2, 152
  Sutherland's method #1, 149
homeostasis, 2
Hoover, Dr., on visceral manipulation, 199
humerus, internal rotation technique, 182
humours, 200
hyaline cartilage, 9
hyoid bone, Riley's address on, 208
hyoid technique, for chronic cough, 207
hyperemesis gravidarum, 223
hyperplasia, 9
hypertonic musculature, 10
hypertrophy, 9

I

iliolumbar technique, West's, 145
immunity, 7
  dependence on structural intactness, 6
  Dr. Still's theory, 4
  natural chemical, 8
infants, occiput compression in, 42
inferior vena cava, 127
inhalation, association with flexion/external rotation, 59
inheritance, as etiological factor, 16
inion, 42
inner longitudinal arch, 164
interosseous membrane, 158, 167
  Sutherland's technique, 191
innominates, 135
  left anterior, 140
  left posterior, 137
  in pediatric treatment, 236, 237
  relation to sacrum and spine, 18–19
  right posterior, 136
  Sutherland's technique for posterior rotation, 137–138
  Sutherland's techniques, 135
inspection, abdominal, 198
inspiration, 100
  deep, 116
  rib 3 stuck in, 96
inter-segmental articular lesions, 8
inter-segmental motion, 11
intercostal aponeurosis, 101
intercostal muscles, 101
internal hip rotation technique #1, Sutherland's, 150
internal hip rotation technique #2, Sutherland's, 154–155
internal humerus rotation technique, Sutherland's, 181
internal medical therapeutics, 3
internal pudic nerve, 141
internal rotation, association with exhalation, 59
interspinous ligaments, 118
interstitial fluids, 112
intervertebral articulation, 13
intervertebral discs, 119
  in thoracic spine, 65
intranasal technique, 204

J

joint fixations, 11
joint functions, 8–9

K

keystone, 164, 170
kidney
  Hazzard's comments, 226
  kidney lift technique, 225–226
kidney lift technique, 225–226
kidney technique, Hazzard's, 226
kidneys, ptosis, 197

L

lateral cervical technique, William West's, 45–46
lateral malleolus, 158
learn the normal, 4
leg-ankle-foot, as whole region, 168
lesion. *See also* osteopathic lesion
  acromial clavicular, 179
  alteration of nervous tissue and vascular channels by, 15
  composite, 18
  direct effects on blood vessel or nerve, 21
  discerning among types, 19
  exaggerating, 49, 50
  as functional and organic disorder, 15
  habit, 28
  inter-segmental articular, 8
  ligamentous, 17–18
  ligamentum teres, 147
  muscular, 17
  osseous, 18
  osteopathic, 15–19
  posterior cervical, 52
  primary, 28

- visceral, 18
- warp, 28

lesion en bloc, 18
lesser trochanter, 172
leukocytosis, 10
ligament
- elastic, 9
- fibrous, 9
- relaxation, 17
- role in osteopathic lesion maintenance, 33
- strain in, 31
- as support tissue, 9
- thickening and adhesion, 17

ligament laxity, postpartum, 231, 232
ligamentous articular strain (LAS) techniques, 45
ligamentous lesions, 17–18, 21
- bony lesions leading to, 18

ligamentous structures, 9
- elastic/capsular, 10
- tension supporting, 9–10
- three types, 9–10
- weight supporting, 9

ligaments
- reseating in pelvis, 132
- stretching, 118

ligamentum flavum, 118
ligamentum teres lesions, 147
limited movement, quality of, 13, 14
limiting factor, release from, 14
Lippincott, Rebecca
- on anterior cervical fascia, 209
- basion technique, 59, 60, 235–236
- on diaphragm anatomy and physiology, 216
- forearm, wrist and hand anatomy/physiology, 187
- on forearm, wrist, hand physiology, 187
- on liver turn, 223
- on liver turn technique, 223
- on pubic symphysis anatomy, 141
- on sacral and pelvic anatomy, 129–130
- on Sutherland's arcuate ligaments, 218
- on Sutherland's humerus diagnosis, 180
- on Sutherland's thoracic technique principles, 74
- on Sutherland's tibiofemoral diagnosis, 156
- wrist and hand physiology, 191

lipping, 9
liquor sanguinis, 200
liver ptosis, 197
liver turn technique, Sutherland's, 222–223
long lever, in erector spinae release, 80
longitudinal spinal ligaments, release technique, 79–80
Lossing, Ken, 200
- on non-osseous anatomy/physiology, 200

low back pelvic hip region, 233
- as regional mechanism, 232

lower extremities techniques, 147
- Anne Wales on feet, 163–164
- Anne Wales on short leg syndrome, 172
- Anne Wales' bootjack technique, 165–166
- Anne Wales' bunion technique, 166
- Anne Wales' dropped navicular/cuneiform (keystone) technique, 170
- Anne Wales' fibula and interosseous membrane release technique, 168
- Anne Wales' fibula technique, 158
- Anne Wales' Morton's neuroma technique, 164–165
- Anne Wales' outer longitudinal arch/cuboid release technique, 169
- Anne Wales' psoas/soleus contraction, 173
- Anne Wales' subtalar joint technique, 160
- Anne Wales' talus, calcaneus, tarsal arch technique, 162
- Anne Wales' tarsal arch technique, 161
- Anne Wales' tibia technique, 159
- Cochrane's foot exercise, 172
- Crow's ankle sprains technique, 167
- diagnosis, 147–148
- Ernest Tucker femur and hip technique, 148–149
- Sutherland's external hip rotation #1, 151
- Sutherland's external hip rotation #2, 159
- Sutherland's foot technique per Anne Wales, 171
- Sutherland's hip joint diagnosis #2, 152
- Sutherland's hip techniques, 143
- Sutherland's internal hip rotation #2, 154
- Sutherland's internal hip rotation technique #1, 150
- Sutherland's lateral condyle technique, 157
- Sutherland's medial condyle technique, 156
- Sutherland's tibiofemoral diagnosis, 156
- Sutherland's tibiofemoral technique, 156, 157
- Tucker on femur and hip treatments, 147–148
- William West's sartorius technique, 155

lower extremity technique, Fulford's, 240–241
lumbar region techniques, 117
- corkscrew technique, 124–125
- side-bending rotation, 118
- Sutherland's lumbar/sacral region technique, 126
- Tucker on lumbar spine, 117–120
- Tucker's lumbar spine technique #1, 121–122
- Tucker's lumbar spine technique #2, 122–123
- Tucker's lumbar spine technique #3, 123–124
- Tucker's lumbar spine technique #4, 124–125
- Wales on thoracic lumbar junction, 127

lumbar/sacral region technique, 126

lumbosacral convexity, 129
lung techniques. *See* respiratory system techniques
lymphatic approaches, 198
lymphatic drainage, role of anterior cervical fascia, 209
lymphatic fluids, moving, 133
lymphatic pump, 112
lymphatic system, 112

M

manipulation, direct action technique, 33
manipulative treatment, 8
manubrium, 69
  bone to bone connection, 175
  movement in, 82
master tissues, 20
McConnell diaphragm doming technique, 216
McConnell, Carl, 5, 197
  on visceral manipulation, 199
McConnell, Dr., duodenum motion with inhalation technique, 222
mechanical instinct, 23
mediastinal fascia, 82, 127
membranes, strain in, 31
Meniere's Disease, 206
  Muncie technique for, 205
mesenteric lift technique, 224
metacarpal bones, reducing dysfunctions, 192
metatarsals, 164
Miller technique, for tongue root, 206–207
Miller, Edgar, 207
minimum force, 26, 27
mobility, 6
  voluntary, 31
morning sickness, 223
Morton's neuroma, 163, 165
Morton's neuroma technique, Wales', 164–165
motion
  in 1st and 2nd ribs, 85
  freedom or restriction, 56
  intersegmental, 11
  palpating for freedom of, 75
  in sacroiliac ligaments, 233
  sterno-clavicular joint, 175
  in thoracic facets, 67
motion limits, 28
  articulations at, 29
  in cervical techniques, 56
  in dorsal region, 65
  in lumbar spine, 117–120
  ribs, 101
  rotation in thoracic spine, 66
  rotation/side-bending, 66
  thoracic extension, 65
  thoracic flexion, 65
movement
  of diaphragm, 127
  dorsal region, 66–69
  as joint function, 9
  limitations to, 9
  planes of, 14
  sacrum, involuntary, 129
  stoppage, 14
Muncie technique, 205–206
Muncie, Dr., 205
  accusations of quackery, 205
muscle
  relaxed, overstretched, atonized, 17
  as support tissue, 9
muscle changes, 16
muscle conditions, 10
  atrophic fibrotic musculature, 11
  fibrotic musculature, 10–11
  hypertonic musculature, 10
muscle tissue
  encroachment on nerve fiber, 17
  encroachment on vascular channel, 17
muscular lesion, 17, 21
  causes, 17
mylohyoid, 206

N

naked nerve endings, 12
neck treatment, Barber's for eye health, 201–202
nerve endings, naked, 12
nerve fiber, muscle tissue encroachment on, 17
nerve intactness, dependence on normal circulation, 21
nervous system
  proneness to failure, 3
  role in health, 16
  as software operating system, 2
nervous tissue
  alteration by lesions, 15
  factors in integrity, 20
  as master tissue, 20
neural axis, motility, 129
neuromuscular mechanisms, 10–11
neuromuscular physiology, 11
neutral position, 31
  direction of ease and, 31
newborn, treatment for, 237

nodding motion, 40
non-osseous structures, manipulation of, 200
normal, as key to detecting abnormal, 199
normal bone, visualizing, 117
Northrup, T.L., 210
noxa, 22
nut and bolt principle, 94
nutritional effects, 16

O

OA and upper cervical technique, Crow's, 62
OA junction technique, Fulford's, 242
OA release technique, 1938 yearbook, 38–39
obturator internus, sitting problems, 172
obturator notch, 147
occipital axis (OA)
  release technique (1938 yearbook), 38–39
  Tucker technique, 35–36
occipital condyles, 42
occipital protuberance, 48
occiput, sacral sag effects on, 232
occiput compression, in infants, 42–43
occiput technique, Anne Wales, 39–40
olecranon process, 187
omentum, 127
opisthion, 39, 42
organ lifting methods, by Dr.Still, 197
osseous lesion, 18, 21
osseous tissues, 17
osteopathic articular dysfunction, 30
osteopathic lesion, 30
  defined, 15–19
  as disease factor, 23
  as etiologic factor, 19
  etiology, 27–29
  Lippincott on, 33
  role in etiology, 16
  role in immunity breakdown, 8
  treatable diagnosis, 8–10
osteopathic philosophy, 23
  Lippincott on, 33
  McConnell's and Teall's, 14–15
  Sutherland's, 33
  Tucker's, 23–27
osteopathic technique
  etiology and principles, 27–29
  exacting nature, 24
  first principles, 26–27
osteopathy
  in cranial field, 45
  etiology in, 5–8
  etymology, 197
  ideals, 25–26
  parasitic imitators, 25
  popular conceptions, 25
  relationship to surgery, 5
  as system/science, 15
  ten-fingered, 24
Osteopathy Complete, 198
Osteopathy, Research and Practice (1910), 197
osteoporosis, contraindications for, 95
otitis media, 206
outer longitudinal arch, weight bearing attributes, 169
outer longitudinal arch/cuboid release technique, Wales', 169
over-rotating, 78
overstretched muscle, 17

P

pain, 11–12
  law of referred, 12
  misleading nature, 12
  nondiagnostic nature, 12
palpation
  possible findings, 198–199
  for thoracic motion, 74–76
  value of, 7
paraspinal inhibition, 226
paresthesias, upper extremitics, 175
parietal tracks, 43
pathology
  osteopathic concept, 14
  in osteopathy, 19–23
  successive developments, 10
patient participation, importance, 34
patient retention, 26–27
Peckham, Russell R., 8–10
pectoralis major, pain patterns, 219
pectoralis minor, pain patterns, 219
pectoralis minor and major, 211
  in asthma, 210
pediatrics techniques, 235
  basion technique, 235–236
  children's sacrum treatment, 238
  newborn techniques, 237
  Wales on, 236–237
pelvic and lower extremity fascial release technique, 133
pelvic bowl, link to cranial bowl, 32
pelvic dysfunction, right, 144, 145
pelvic lift technique, Sutherland's, 229
pelvic mechanics, 231

pelvis. *See* sacrum and pelvis techniques
pelvis technique
  Fulford's, 243–244
  West's, 144
percussion, abdominal, 198, 199
pericardium
  attachments, 216
  and heart lung complex, 127
  unwinding technique, 220
periosseous tissues, 9
Perrin, Dr., 210
philosophy
  osteopathic masters, 1
  Wales', 30–32
Philosophy and Mechanical Principles of Osteopathy, The, 197
physio synthesis motion exercises, 172
physiological economy, 2
physiology
  neuromuscular, 11
  non-osseous structures, 200
  wrist and hand, 191
planes of movement, 14
plantar callous, 165
plantar warts, 165
pop, significance, 29–30
position, 6
  for abdominal palpation, 198
  balanced, 31
  maintenance of, 1
  neutral, 31
  relative, 12
  structural, 7
posterior cervical lesions, 52
posterior innominate rotation
  Sutherland's diagnosis, 136–137
  Sutherland's treatment, 137–138
posterior OA, Tucker technique, 35–36
posterior superior iliac spine, 137. *See also* innominates
postnatal depression, Wales on, 231–233
postpartum depression, venous drainage insufficiency and, 233
postural co-operation, in pediatrics, 236
postural defects, 18
Practice and Applied Therapeutics of Applied Osteopathy (1905), 199
pregnancy, Wales on, 231
primary lesions, 28
primary respiratory mechanism, 129
prognosis, ligament changes and, 18
progression, stage, 14
prophylactic treatment, 199
psoas, chronic contraction, 173
psoas technique #1, Sutherland's, 227–228
psoas technique #2, Sutherland's, 228
ptosis, Still's palpation for, 197
pubic symphysis, Lippincott on anatomy, 141
pubic symphysis technique, 142
  Crow's alternate, 143
pumping treatment, for acute asthma, 210
pyloric spasm, in infants, 113

Q

quadratus lumborum, 113, 134

R

radical technique, 30
radius technique
  Sutherland's, 189
  Wales', 190
rallying call, need for new, 25
Ray, T.L., 210
Reich, Wilhelm, 241
relative position, 12
  of lesioned segments, 13
relaxation, securing by gentleness, 27
relaxed muscle, 17
release, from limiting factors, 14
Research and Practice (1911), 197
resistance, avoiding patient, 27
respiration
  correct technique, 79
  as power within body, 32
  role in thoracic side-bending rotation correction, 78
  sacral as primary, 129
respiratory co-operation, 57, 59
  Wales on, 61
respiratory dysfunction, sacral, 130
respiratory system techniques, 210–218
  acute asthma tender point technique, 212–213
  asthma technique, 1938 Yearbook, 210–211
  Barber's lung technique #2, 214
  Barber's lung technique #3, 214–215
  Barber's lung technique #4, 215
  diaphragm related, 216
respiratory techniques
  Elmer Barber lung technique #1, 213–214
  McConnell diaphragm doming technique, 216
  Sutherland's arcuate ligaments technique, 218
rib 3, stuck in inspiration, 96

rib dysfunctions, from hyper extension of thoracic vertebrae, 109–110
rib lesions, 91
  diagnosis, 102
  head *versus* tubercle, 101
  secondary deviations, 102
rib movements, 101
rib techniques, 81
  Anne Wales 11th/12th ribs technique, 111–113
  Anne Wales first and second rib technique, 91–92
  Anne Wales on ribs, 90–91
  Anne Wales rib technique, 94–95
  Anne Wales sternal release technique, 81–82
  diagnosis, 102
  Ernest Tucker's first and second ribs, 85–86
  Ernest Tucker's first rib technique #1, 86–87
  Ernest Tucker's first rib technique #2, 88
  Ernest Tucker's floating rib technique #1, 114–115
  Ernest Tucker's floating rib technique #2, 115–116
  Ernest Tucker's floating ribs technique, 113–114
  Ernest Tucker's rib technique #1, 103
  Ernest Tucker's rib technique #2, 104
  Ernest Tucker's rib technique #3, 105
  Ernest Tucker's third through 10th ribs technique, 101–102
  Hazzard's rib technique, 96–97
  Hazzard's rib technique for ribs 3 to 10 seated, 98–100
  Hazzard's rib technique for ribs 3 to 10 side lying, 100
  Sutherland's 4th to 10th rib technique, 106
  Sutherland's alternate technique for upper ribs, 94
  Sutherland's first rib technique, 89–90
  Sutherland's floating ribs 11 and 12 technique, 111
  Sutherland's rib dysfunctions and technique, 89
  Sutherland's second and third rib technique, 92–93
  Sutherland's techniques for rib dysfunctions associated with hyper extension of thoracic vertebrae, 109–110
  William West's 6th through 10th seated rib technique, 107
    side lying position, 108
  William West's first rib technique #1, 82–83
  William West's first rib technique #2, 84
  William West's second to sixth rib technique, 97–98
ribs, 17
  venetian blinds analogy, 79
  Wales on, 78–79, 90–91
ribs 3 to 10 seated technique, Hazzard's, 98–100
ribs 3 to 10 side lying technique, 100
right 12th rib, 114–115
Riley, G.W., 208
roll the bones home, 195
rotation, 13, 14
  limits in thoracic spine, 66
  posterior, innominate, 136–138
  strain in thoracic segments, 68
  in thoracic spine, 66, 67
  trunk, 67–68
rotation\side-bending, 118, 119, 120
  flexion tendencies at limits, 122

S

sacral ala, 135
sacral lesions, 52
sacral release, for newborns, 237
sacral sag, 231
  effects on occiput, 232
sacroiliac lesion, 27, 28
sacrum
  backing into the garage, 135
  flexion position, 232
  links to occiput, 233
sacrum and pelvis techniques, 129–146
  Anne Wales anterior sacroiliac technique, 134–135
  Anne Wales coccyx technique, 146
  Anne Wales differential technique, 131–133
  Anne Wales pelvic and ower extremity fascial release technique, 133
  Crow's alternate pubic symphysis technique, 143
  Lippincott on anatomy, 129–130
  pubic symphysis anatomy, 141
  Sutherland's diagnosis of innominate anterior rotation, 139
  Sutherland's diagnosis of innominate posterior rotation, 136–137
  Sutherland's diagnosis of sacral respiratory dysfunctions, 130
  Sutherland's innominates techniques, 135
  Sutherland's pubic symphysis technique, 142
  Sutherland's technique for innominate posterior rotation, 137–138
  Sutherland's treatment of innominate anterior rotation, 140–141
  William West's iliolumbar technique, 145
  William West's pelvis technique, 144
sartorius technique, West's, 155
scalene technique, William West's, 46–47
scalenes, in spasm, 46
scapula and pelvis technique, Fulford's, 245–246
scapula technique, Wales', 186–187
scar tissue, 10
Schooley, Tom, 217

second and third rib technique, Sutherland's, 92–93
second rib, dysfunction, 97
second to sixth rib technique, West's, 97–98
secretory nerve supply, ribs' influence on, 90
semilunar notch, 187
serous otitis media, Muncie technique for, 205
serratus magnus muscle, 105
shock
  absorption through inner longitudinal arch, 164
  avoiding in cervical techniques, 54
shock release treatment, Fulford's, 241–242
short leg syndrome, Wales on, 172–173
short lever, in erector spinae release technique, 80
short ligaments, in subtalar joint, 160
shoulder diagnosis, Wales', 184
shoulder dislocation, 175
shoulder elevation, in thoracic technique, 74
shoulder girdle analogy, 175
shoulder joint technique, Tucker's, 179–180
shoulder pain, 175
shoulder technique
  Wales' #2, 185
  Wales', 184
  Wales' #2, 185
side-bending, 13, 53, 55
  in lower dorsals, 68, 69
  OA release technique, 39
  rib movement in, 101
  in thoracic spine, 66, 67, 68
  upper thoracic technique, 73–74
side-bending rotation, 119, 120
  flexion tendencies at limits, 122
  in lumbar region, 118
sigmoid flexure technique, 225
Simons, David G., 219
sinusitis, intranasal technique for, 204
sixth through tenth seated rib technique, West's, 107
small bowel obstruction, 224
soft tissue work, 31
soft-tissue treatment, 200
soleus muscle
  role in back, sacral, sacroiliac problems, 173
  role in short leg syndrome, 172
sphenobasal synchondrosis, 43
sphenoid and frontal bone technique, Fulford's, 243
sphenoid palatine ganglia, 211
sphincter of Odi, 113
spinal anatomy, study of, 25
spinal curvatures, 18
spinal dura mater, 32
  sacral sag and, 232
spinal manipulation, 198
spinal organ, 32
splenic capsule, 127
spring technique, 29
springing motion, 29
standing position, sacroiliac strains in, 135
sternal release technique, 81–82
sterno-clavicular articulation, 175
sternocleidomastoid muscle, 55
stiff neck, 175
Still, A.T., 4, 15, 27, 30
  on arterial system, 22
  atlas settling technique, 51–52
  early visceral techniques, 197
  goat and boulder parable, 223
  infirmary, 197
  interest in humours and fasciae, 200
  organ lifting methods, 197
  origination of cranial concepts, 198
  Osteopathy, Research and Practice (1910), 197
  palpation methods, 197
  paucity of technique descriptions, 197
  Philosophy and Mechanical Principles of Osteopathy (1892), 197
  *Philosophy of Osteopathy (*1899*),* 197
  Research and Practice (1911), 197
  rib technique, 96
  on sacroiliac ligament motion, 233
  on soft-tissue treatment as engine wiping, 200
  stomach technique, 221
  survival of technical training, 24
  on technique, 24
stomach technique, Still's, 221
stomach treatment technique, Sutherland's, 22
stretching, 30
  prior to cervical techniques, 54
stroke patients, Miller technique for, 206, 207
structural derangement, 16
structural freedom, 22
structural intactness, 8
structural mal-adjustment, 19
structure
  as determinant of body function, 1–5, 6
  differentiation and resistance, 2
  immunity and, 6
  palpation of, 7
subtalar joint technique, Wales', 160
superior cervical ganglia, 211
superior cervical ganglion, 61
support, as joint function, 9
support tissues, 9

supraspinatus muscle, 187
surgery
physical restructuring through, 5
relationship to osteopathy, 5
Sutherland Cranial Teaching Foundation, 207
Sutherland, Dr., 32, 78
4th to 10th rib technique, 106
alternate technique for upper ribs, 94
anterior innominate rotation technique, 140–141
anterior sacroiliac technique from, 135
arcuate ligaments technique, 218
biliary drainage technique, 223–224
cervical extension dysfunction techniques, 57–58
cervical flexion dysfunction techniques, 57
cervical rotation side-bending dysfunction techniques, 58–59
cervicals technique, 56
clavicle technique, 177
condylo-atlantal dysfunctions, 59–60
on cranial vertebral junction, 61
cranial work, 198
diagnosis of anterior innominate rotation, 139
diagnosis of posterior innominate rotation, 136–137
diaphragm release technique, 216–217
external hip rotation technique #1, 151
external hip rotation technique #2, 153
external humerus rotation technique, 182
first rib technique, 89–90
floating ribs 11 and 12 technique, 111
on foot anatomy and physiology, 163
foot technique per Anne Wales, 171
hand and wrist technique, 192
hip diagnosis #1, 149
hip joint diagnosis #2, 152
hip techniques, 149
humerus diagnosis, 180
interosseous membrane technique, 191
innominates techniques, 135
internal hip rotation technique #1, 150
internal hip rotation technique #2, 154–155
internal humerus rotation technique, 181
involuntary sacral movement, 129
on limits of cranial manipulation, 45
liver release technique, 222–223
lumbar/sacral region technique, 126
occiput compression emphasis, 42
psoas technique #1, 225–226
psoas technique #2, 228
pubic symphysis technique, 142
radius technique, 189
rib dysfunction techniques associated with thoracic vertebral hyper extension, 109–110
rib dysfunctions and technique, 89
on ribs as venetian blinds, 79
sacral respiratory dysfunction diagnosis, 130
sacral sags saying, 232
scapula technique, 187
second and third rib technique, 92–93
stomach treatment technique, 221
thoracic diagnosis, 74–76
thoracic extension dysfunctions technique, 76–77
thoracic flexion dysfunctions technique, 76
thoracic side-bending rotation dysfunctions technique, 78
thoracic vertebrae principles of technique, 74
tibiofemoral diagnosis, 156
tibiofemoral/lateral condyle technique, 157
tibiofemoral/medial condyle technique, 156
ulna technique, 188
on visceral manipulation, 198
Wales' differential technique from, 132
on wrist and hand dysfunction, 195
Sutherland's technique for thoracic side-bending rotation dysfunctions, 78
swallowing difficulties, post stroke, 206–207
sympathetic nervous system, ribs' role in, 90, 91
symphysis pubis. *See* pubic symphysis
synovial membrane, 9

T

T3 rotation right and side-bent left, 72, 73
tactile sensitivity, 26
importance of, 34
talo-calcaneal ligament, 163
talus, calcaneus, tarsal arch technique, 162
tarsal arch, restoration of mechanics, 165
tarsal arch technique, 161
Wales', 162
Teachings in the Science of Osteopathy, 198
technical skill, 24
technique
adequate, 23
corrective, 33–34
exacting, 24
gentle, 30
principles of, 27–29
radical, 30
Technique of removing lesions usually found in gallbladder diseases (1948), 199
techniques
cervical region, 45–63
head, 35–43

lower extremities, 147–173
lumbar region, 117–127
ribs, 81–116
sacrum and pelvis, 129–146
thoracics, 65–80
upper extremities, 175–193
visceral, 197–200
teenagers, challenges in treating, 237
temporal bone, 42
ten-fingered osteopathy, 24
tender point, use in acute asthma, 212–213
tennis elbow, 175
tension, point of balanced, 33
tension supporting tissues, 9–10
tentorium, 61
Thinking Body, The, 32
third through tenth ribs technique, Tucker's, 100–102
thoracic
dorsal region movements, 66–69
slight flexion and extension in, 66
thoracic diagnosis, by palpation for motion, 74–76
thoracic extension dysfunctions technique, Sutherland's, 76–77
thoracic flexion dysfunctions, Sutherland's technique, 76
thoracic hyperextension, rib dysfunctions associated with, 109–110
thoracic lumbar junction
as region, 218
Wales on, 127
thoracic side-bending rotation dysfunctions, Sutherland's technique, 78
thoracic techniques, 66
Anne Wales, 78–79
erector spinae muscles release, 79–80
longitudinal spinal ligaments release, 79–80
side-bending technique, 73–74
Sutherland's technique for thoracic extension dysfunctions, 76–77
Sutherland's technique for thoracic flexion dysfunctions, 76
Sutherland's technique for thoracic side-bending rotation dysfunctions, 78
Sutherland's thoracic diagnosis, 74–76
Sutherland's thoracic vertebrae principles of technique, 74
Tucker's prone thoracic technique, 70–71
Tucker's supine thoracic technique, 71–72
Tucker's thoracic technique, 69–70
Tucker's upper thoracic technique #1, 72–73
Tucker's upper thoracic technique #2, 73–74
thoracic vertebrae, rib dysfunctions from hyper extension of, 109–110
thoracics, Tucker on, 65–66
thorax, Wales on, 78–79
thyroid notch, 147
tibia technique, Wales', 159
tibiofemoral diagnosis, Sutherland's, 156
tibiofemoral joint, 157
tibiofemoral techniques
Sutherland's lateral condyle technique, 157
Sutherland's medial condyle technique, 156
tibiofibular syndesmosis, 167
tilted pelvis, 18
tinnitus, 206
Muncie technique for, 205
tissue integrity, factors determining, 22
tissue nutrition, 16
TMJ, Miller technique for, 206–207
Todd, Mabel Elsworth, 32
tone, 6
tongue root technique, 206–207
tonic osteopathic treatment, 91
torticollis, 175, 187
touch
importance to osteopathic technique, 26
locating by sense of, 26
traction, for hip dislocation, 147
training, in tactile sensitivity, 26
transverse atlanto ligaments, 42
transverse processes, thoracic vertebra, 75
trauma, 16
trauma release treatments, Fulford's, 241–242
trauma/shock point, 241
traumatic injury, rib dysfunctions after, 109
Travell, Janet G., 219
Trigger Point Manual, 11, 219
Tucker, Ernest Eckford
on acromial clavicular lesions, 179
anterior cervicals technique, 55–56
bicipital tendon diagnosis, 183
bicipital tendon technique, 183–184
cervical lesion cautions, 54
cervical techniques, 52
clavicle technique, 176–177
on clavicular area sensitivity, 177
diagnosis of first/second ribs, 85–86
diagnosis of rib lesions, 102
differential diagnosis, bicipital tendon, 183
on dorsal region movements, 66–69
dysfunctions of first/second ribs, 86
femur and hip technique, 148–149
first and second ribs technique, 84–85
first rib technique #1, 86–87

first rib technique #2, 88
on floating rib diagnosis, 114
floating rib technique #1, 114–115
floating rib technique #2, 115–116
floating ribs technique, 113–114
on hip treatment, 147–148
on lumbar spine, 117–120
lumbar spine technique #1, 121–122
lumbar spine technique #2, 122–123
lumbar spine technique #3, 123–124
lumbar spine technique #4, 124–125
osteopathic philosophy, 23–27
posterior cervicals technique, 53–54
posterior OA technique, 35–36
prone thoracic technique, 70–71
rib technique #2, 104
rib technique #3, 105
shoulder joint technique, 179–180
supine thoracic technique, 71–72
third through tenth ribs technique, 100–102
thoracic technique, 69–70
on thoracics, 65–66
upper thoracic technique #1, 72–73
upper thoracic technique #2, 73–74
Tucker's prone thoracic technique, 70–71
Tucker's supine thoracic technique, 71–72
Tucker's thoracic technique, 69–70
Tucker's upper thoracic technique #1, 72–73
Tucker's upper thoracic technique #2, 73–74
twelfth cranial nerve, 43
two-person techniques
Barber's lung technique #1, 213–214
Barber's lung technique #3, 214–215

U

ulna, 187
ulna technique, Sutherland's, 188
unilateral dysfunction, sacral, 130
upper cervicals technique, Crow's, 62
upper extremities techniques, 175
anatomy and physiology, 175
Anne Wales' clavicle technique #2, 179
Anne Wales' depressed clavicle technique, 178
Anne Wales' elbow technique, 190–191
Anne Wales' radius technique, 190
Anne Wales' scapula technique, 186–187
Anne Wales' shoulder diagnosis and technique #1, 184
Anne Wales' shoulder technique #2, 185
Anne Wales' wrist technique, 193–195
diagnosis, 176
Ernest Tucker's bicipital tendon technique, 183–184
Ernest Tucker's clavicle technique, 176–177
Ernest Tucker's shoulder joint technique, 179–180
forearm, wrist and hand osteopathic concepts, 187
Sutherland's clavicle technique, 177
Sutherland's external rotation of humerus technique, 182
Sutherland's hand and wrist technique, 192
Sutherland's humerus diagnosis, 180
Sutherland's interosseous membrane technique, 191
Sutherland's internal rotation of humerus technique, 181
Sutherland's radius technique, 189
Sutherland's ulna technique, 188
Tucker on clavicular issues, 175–176
wrist and hand osteopathic concepts, 191
upper ribs alternate technique, Sutherland's, 94
upper thoracics
corrective technique, 68
difficulty or correcting, 72
limited motion in, 68
uterus, ptosis, 197

V

vapocoolant spray, in arrhythmia, 219
vascular channels
alteration by lesions, 15
muscle tissue encroachment on, 17
vasomotor blood supply, ribs' influence on, 90
vertebral segments, role in ctiology, 16
visceral displacement, 18
visceral lesion, 18, 21
visceral ligaments, 200
visceral manipulation, 198
visceral techniques, 197–200
cardiovascular system, 219–220
gastrointestinal system, 220–225
genitourinary system, 225–229
hand positioning in, 198
head related, 200–209
respiratory system, 210–218
voluntary mobility, 31
vomiting, intractable, 223

W

Wales, on postnatal depression, 231–233
Wales, Anne, 61
11th and 12th ribs technique, 111–113
anterior sacroiliac technique, 134–135
on asthma, 211–212
base spread technique, 42–43

bootjack technique, 165–166
bunion technique, 166
cervical vertebrae technique, 60–61
on children's sacrum, 238
clavicle technique #2, 179
coccyx technique, 146
depressed clavicle technique, 178
on diaphragm, 217–218
on diaphragm release, 217
differential technique for sacrum/pelvis, 131–133
dropped navicular/cuneiform (keystone) technique, 170
on dysmenorrhea, 233–234
elbow technique, 190–191
on feet, 163–164
fibula and interosseous membrane release technique, 168
fibula technique, 158–159
first and second rib technique, 91–92
on manubrium movement, 82
Morton's neuroma technique, 164–165
on newborn treatments, 237
occiput technique, 39–40
osteopathic philosophy, 30–32
outer longitudinal arch/cuboid release technique, 169
pelvic and lower extremity fascial release technique, 133
on pregnancy, 231
radius technique, 190
rib technique, 94
on ribs, 90–91
scapula technique, 186–187
on short leg syndrome, 172–173
shoulder diagnosis and technique #1, 184
shoulder technique #2, 185
sternal release technique, 81–82
subtalar joint technique, 160
on Sutherland's foot technique, 171
on Sutherland's innominate rotation techniques, 141
on Sutherland's scapula technique, 187
talus, calcaneus, tarsal arch technique, 162
tarsal arch technique, 161
Teachings in the Science of Osteopathy, 198
on thoracic lumbar junction, 127
on thorax and ribs, 78–79
tibia technique, 159
on treating children, 236–237
on upper extremity anatomy and physiology, 175
wrist technique, 193–195
Walker, Brooks
atlas control technique, 43
occiput technique, 40–41
warp lesions, 28
weight supporting ligaments, 9
Weill, Andrew, 239
West, William
6th through 10th rib technique, side lying position, 108
anterior cervical technique, 47–48
first rib supine technique, 85
first rib technique #1, 82–83
first rib technique #2, 84
iliolumbar technique, 145
lateral cervical technique, 45–46
pelvis technique, 144
sartorius technique, 155
scalene technique, 46–47
second to sixth rib technique, 97–98
whiplash, liver turn for, 223
Willard, Frank, 32, 43
Wilson, Perrin, 212
Wilson, T., 210
women's health, 231–234
dysmenorrhea, 233–234
postnatal depression, 231–233
pregnancy, 231
wrist, osteopathic concepts, 187, 191
wrist technique, Wales', 193–195

Y

Yearbook
1938, 208
asthma technique, 210–211
hyoid address, 208
1948, 199

About the Authors

William Thomas Crow, D.O. has been a professor at the University of North Texas Health Science Center in Fort Worth, Texas and the Philadelphia College of Osteopathic Medicine. He has individually authored or contributed to over 40 osteopathic textbooks and scholarly articles, and is the recipient of two national research awards. He lectures widely in the United States and abroad. Dr. Crow is dually board certified by the American Osteopathic Board of Family Practice and the American Osteopathic Board of Neuromusculoskeletal Medicine, and served as a residency director for almost 20 years.

Terence Cecil Vardy, D.O., N.D., M.App. Sc. (musculoskeletal medicine) has been a visiting lecturer and has conducted practical workshops in a wide range of osteopathic techniques at osteopathic schools in the United States and Australia, and under the auspices of the American Academy of Osteopathy and the American Osteopathic Association. A 1979 graduate of the Windsor College of Applied Osteopathy (Sydney), Dr. Vardy has published articles on balance, osteopathic treatment, replicating human touch, brain fluid dynamics and neurodegeneration, and has conducted medical research on behalf of the U.S. Department of Defense. He is currently a practicing clinician in Australia and is a member of the AAO, AOA, American Orthopedic Association and the American Academy of Sports Medicine. He is completing a doctorate in the Department of Neuroscience at Cambridge University.